R Y P I N S' **Questions & Answers for Basic Sciences Review**

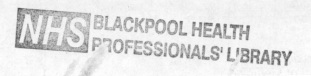

Edited by

E D W A R D   D.   F R O H L I C H ,   M.D.

Alton Ochsner Distinguished Scientist
Vice President for Academic Affairs
Alton Ochsner Medical Foundation

Staff Member, Ochsner Clinic

Professor of Medicine and of Physiology
Louisiana State University School of Medicine

Adjunct Professor of Pharmacology and Clinical Professor of Medicine
Tulane University School of Medicine
New Orleans, Louisiana

With 11 contributors

RYPINS'

Questions & Answers for Basic Sciences Review

Second Edition

J. B. LIPPINCOTT COMPANY Philadelphia

Acquisitions Editor: Richard Winters
Sponsoring Editor: Jody Schott
Production Editor: Virginia Barishek
Cover Designer: Leslie Foster Roesler
Production: Spectrum Publisher Services, Inc.
Compositor: Bi-Comp, Inc.
Printer/Binder: Courier Book Company/Kendallville

Second Edition

Library of Congress Cataloging-in-Publication Data

Rypins' questions & answers for basic sciences review / edited by
   Edward D. Frohlich ; with 11 contributors. — 2nd ed.
      p.   cm.
   Rev. ed. of: Rypins' questions & answers for boards review. c1987.
   Companion suppl. to: Rypins' medical licensure examinations. 16th
ed. c1993.
   ISBN 0-397-51247-3
   1. Medical sciences—Examinations, questions, etc.   2. Medicine—
Examinations, questions, etc.   I. Frohlich, Edward D., 1931–
II. Rypins, Harold, 1892–1939. Rypins' medical licensure
examinations. 16th ed.   III. Rypins' questions & answers for boards
review.   IV. Title: Rypins' questions and answers for basic sciences
review.   V. Title: Questions & answers for basic sciences review.
   [DNLM: 1. Medicine—examination questions.   W 18 R9955]
R834.5.R963   1993 Suppl.
610'.76—dc20
DNLM/DLC
for Library of Congress   92-49898
                                                                    CIP

The editor, authors, and publisher have exerted every
effort to ensure that drug selection and dosage set forth in
this text are in accord with current recommendations and
practice at the time of publication. However, in view of
ongoing research, changes in government regulations, and
the constant flow of information relating to drug therapy
and drug reactions, the reader is urged to check the
package insert for each drug for any change in indications
and dosage and for added warnings and precautions. This
is particularly important when the recommended agent is
a new or infrequently employed drug.

PREFACE

My fellow contributors and I are pleased to offer this special supplement to the 16th edition of RYPINS' BASIC SCIENCES REVIEW. As most readers of RYPINS' are aware, this textbook was first published more than 60 years ago. Because of its long-standing acceptance and the general expectations of the text during these many years, it was with a great deal of hesitancy that I initiated a number of changes in the 13th edition when I assumed editorship. Among these changes was the addition of National Board–type questions and answers to the more rhetorical and essay-type questions included at the end of each chapter in former editions. I was delighted to receive a number of letters encouraging me to invite the contributors to continue with this departure in future editions.

With publication of the 14th edition, I received still more encouragement from our readers to expand the question-and-answer section further. There is, however, a limit to the number of questions and answers that should be included in a textbook, beyond which limit the primary necessity for well-thought-out and well-structured didactic material may become lost. Even in the current 16th edition of RYPINS' we continue to add more National Board–type questions and answers. We now believe we have supplemented the main body of the text to its maximum. It was, therefore, with mixed feelings that we added a relatively inexpensive softcover companion to the parent textbook in the 15th edition. Because clinical considerations are more variable and now involve, in modern testing, much greater complexity in the elaboration and sequencing of questions, we concluded at the time that a companion text would be feasible if we restricted the material primarily to the preclinical science chapters. However, we included questions and answers for the Public Health and Community Medicine and Behavioral Sciences areas in that supplement because these disciplines are more adaptable to the straightforward factual material that has been included in the preclinical (or basic science) areas. The first QUESTIONS AND ANSWERS supplement was so well received that we are encouraged to offer this updated and expanded revision with our 16th edition of RYPINS'.

In framing test questions, there is always the fear of vagueness and ambiguity. The danger of misstatements is ever-present—particularly in a text that prepares the student for a formal examination. To obviate some of these concerns, we have included, wherever the contributor thought it necessary, an explanation for the answer given. Nevertheless, these decisions are arbitrary, and should the reader have any difficulties with the questions presented herein, I would welcome any comments and will review them with our contributors for future editions. Indeed, I am always grateful and flattered to receive letters from our worldwide readers with their comments and suggestions as well as their warm notes of appreciation and encouragement.

Another concern presented itself with respect to the sequencing of questions in each chapter. Again, we elected to present questions in the manner preferred by the individual contributors rather than to impose a uniform style throughout. We thought that doing so might prove more beneficial to the reader than by employing a more standardized format.

Finally, this companion to RYPINS' is offered with the sincere hope that it will provide to the person preparing for licensure examination an opportunity for pretesting and a means to identify areas of possible weakness. Hopefully, this additional learning technique will stimulate the reader to return to the review chapters and other source material as necessary.

Once again, I offer my deep appreciation to each of the contributors, and to Richard Winters and Charles McCormick, our faithful sponsoring editors at Lippincott. And I express my ongoing personal appreciation to Lillian Buffa, Caramia Fairchild, and Debby Smith for their continuing support in the office, and to my family for their understanding for the time spent in mounting this edition that would otherwise have been spent with them.

Edward D. Frohlich, M.D.

C O N T E N T S

Rypins' Questions & Answers for Basic Sciences
Review, Second Edition, edited by Edward D.
Frohlich. J. B. Lippincott Company, Philadelphia
© 1993.

C H A P T E R

1
Medical
Qualifying
Examinations

Edward D. Frohlich, M.D.

Alton Ochsner Distinguished Scientist, Vice President for
Academic Affairs. Alton Ochsner Medical Foundation;
Staff Member, Ochsner Clinic;
Professor of Medicine and of Physiology, Louisiana State
University School of Medicine; Adjunct Professor of
Pharmacology and Clinical Professor of Medicine,
Tulane University School of Medicine

THE OBJECTIVE, OR MULTIPLE-CHOICE, EXAMINATION

Rationale

In recent years more and more examiners have been turning to the objective, or multiple-choice, examination. With each question in this type of test the examinee is faced with a problem, the correct answer to which is included in the question and must be selected and indicated on the answer sheet by a mark made in the appropriate place. The characteristic feature of these tests is that the examinee answers the questions by filling in spaces on answer sheets. Although this is considered a written examination, no actual writing of sentences is required. This kind of test has two important advantages: a great many more questions covering a much wider range of subjects can be asked in a given time than is possible with the essay examination, thereby effectively broadening the scope of the examination; and the answers can be graded more objectively and with greater speed and accuracy than with any other type of examination.

At first the objective, or multiple-choice, examination met with considerable disapproval, on the examinee's part because the technique was new and unfamiliar, and on the examiner's part because the construction of valid, unambiguous, and reliable questions was difficult (far more difficult, in fact, than the preparation of essay questions). But as time passed the objective examination came into its own as a valid, comprehensive, and dependable test of a person's knowledge and, when applied effectively, of that person's competence and ability. Moreover, this type of examination seems to be the most searching, valid, and comprehensive type of test to administer to large groups of examinees.

Many different forms of objective, multiple-choice questions have been devised for medical qualifying examinations to test not only medical knowledge but also subtler qualities of discrimination, judgment, and reasoning. Certain types of questions may test a person's recognition of similarities or dissimilarities of diseases, drugs, and physiologic, or pathological processes. Other questions test judgment about cause and effect. Case histories or patient problems are used to simulate the experience of a physician confronted with a diagnostic problem; a series of questions then tests the examinee's understanding of related aspects of the case, such as associated laboratory findings, treatment, complications, and prognosis. In this type of examination each question has only one correct response among a number of possible choices, most often five.

Scoring

Objective, multiple-choice examinations are usually scored by electronic machines. To the casual observer, this machine scoring may seem highly mysterious. The answer sheets are loaded into the machine, a button is pressed, and the machine reads the sheets, matches the answers against an answer key, and punches the examinees' scores into the automated machine data card. However, the scoring is not completely impersonal and mechanical; a manual check is also made to avoid the possibility of any technical error, and the responsible examiners are the ones who finally determine whether an individual should pass or fail.

A grade of 75 has been established as the passing score for the examinations of the National Board. But it is not necessary to respond correctly to 75% of the questions to obtain this grade; the scoring procedure is such that correct answers to 50% to 60% of the questions usually result in a passing grade of 75. A passing score is determined in part by the distribution curve of the scores of all those taking the examination.

As already mentioned, examinations of the multiple-choice type have certain advantages over the time-honored essay test. Although essay tests may probe more deeply into a limited number of subjects, multiple-choice examinations sample a much greater breadth of knowledge. Because multiple-choice answer sheets can be scored by machine, grading can be accomplished rapidly, accurately, and impartially. With this type of examination it is possible to standardize level of difficulty and thus to make truly comparable different tests used in different places and at different times. Moreover, tests and individual questions within the tests can be subjected to thorough and rapid statistical analysis, thus providing a sound basis for comparative studies and for improvement in the quality of the tests themselves.

EXAMPLES OF QUESTIONS

The following questions are presented as a guide to preparing for the medical qualifying examination. They are samples of the types of multiple-choice questions used in such examinations.

Completion Type

The so-called completion type is the most common. Completion questions usually are placed together at the beginning of the test with directions similar to the following:

Directions. Each of the following questions or incomplete statements is followed by five suggested answers or completions. Select the one that is best in each case and blacken the corresponding space on the answer sheet.

The following is an easy example of a completion type of question:

Question 1

To which one of the following systems of the body does the heart belong?

(a) The digestive system
(b) The central nervous system
(c) The circulatory system
(d) The endocrine system
(e) The musculoskeletal system

The correct answer, of course, is (c). To make this question somewhat more difficult and avoid naming the correct system among the choices, one could omit the circulatory system and instead include the choice, "None of the above." Then the question would appear as:

Question 2

To which of the following systems of the body does the heart belong?

(a) The digestive system
(b) The central nervous system
(c) The endocrine system
(d) The musculoskeletal system
(e) None of the above

The fifth choice, (e), now becomes the correct response. In this manner the candidate is made to think of the various systems of the body and must know the right answer without its being suggested directly as one of the possibilities. Of course, the choice "None of the above" will sometimes be a correct and sometimes be an incorrect response.

Another variant of the completion type of item is in the negative form, where all but one of the choices are applicable, and the candidate is asked to mark the one that does not apply. The following is an example:

Question 3

All of the following are associated with prerenal azotemia except:

(a) Shock
(b) Dehydration
(c) Pernicious vomiting
(d) Gastrointestinal hemorrhage
(e) Multiple myeloma

The correct answer is (e).

Association and Relatedness Questions

Items of a somewhat different nature may be used effectively to determine, for example, the candidate's knowledge of the action and the use of closely related drugs or the distinguishing features of similar diseases.

Below are directions and questions of this type taken from a pharmacology test and from a medicine test. To answer such questions correctly, the candidate must have a well-organized knowledge of a number of related drugs and a considerable understanding of the differential use of these drugs.

Directions. Each group of questions below consists of five lettered headings followed by a list of numbered words or phrases. For each numbered word or phrase, select the one heading that is related most closely to it.

Questions 4–9

(a) Quinidine
(b) Theophylline
(c) Amyl nitrite
(d) Glyceryl trinitrate
(e) Papaverine

4. Relaxes smooth muscle of the arterial system; causes fall in arterial pressure; commonly administered in tablets sublingually *Answer:* (d)
5. An opium alkaloid; has direct vasodilator action; used in instances of coronary occlusion and peripheral vascular disease. *Answer:* (e)
6. Commonly effective in relieving symptoms of bronchial asthma *Answer:* (b)
7. The best for quick treatment of cyanide poisoning *Answer:* (c)
8. Increases the contractile force of the heart and is diuretic *Answer:* (b)
9. May be used in auricular fibrillation *Answer:* (a)

Questions 10–17

(a) Coarctation of the aorta
(b) Patent ductus arteriosus
(c) Tetralogy of Fallot
(d) Aortic vascular ring
(e) Tricuspid atresia

10. Benefitted by systemic pulmonary artery anastomosis *Answer:* (c)
11. Most common type of congenital cyanotic heart disease *Answer:* (c)
12. Corrected surgically by resection and end-to-end anastomosis *Answer:* (a)
13. Possible cause of dysphagia in infants and children *Answer:* (d)
14. Wide pulse pressure *Answer:* (b)
15. Associated frequently with atrial septal defects *Answer:* (e)
16. A continuous murmur *Answer:* (b)

17. Hypertension in the arms and hypotension in the legs *Answer:* (a)

A further elaboration of association and relatedness items is considerably more involved and calls for a discriminatory understanding of a number of similar but distinguishable factors. For example, the following question is designed to reveal considerable information about the candidate's knowledge of the causes of hypoglycemia and the related functional disturbances: four of the five conditions in the numbered list below are commonly associated with one of the three functional disturbances designated by letters. The candidate is instructed to select the one condition that is the exception and the functional disturbance that is common to the remaining four.

Question 18

(a) Clinically significant hypoglycemia
(b) Clinically significant hyperglycemia
(c) Clinically significant glycosuria

(1) Overdose of insulin
(2) Functional tumor of islet cells
(3) Renal glycosuria
(4) Hypopituitarism
(5) von Gierke's disease

The candidate who selects (a) and (3), the correct answer, demonstrates that he or she knows that (1), (2), (4), and (5) may produce clinically significant hypoglycemia; that (3) does not; and that no combination of four of the five conditions is associated with hyperglycemia or glycosuria. This question thus probes the possession of both positive and negative information. Specific directions for handling this form of discriminatory question read as follows:

Directions. There are two responses to be made to each of the following questions. There are three lettered categories; four of the five numbered items are related in some way to one of these categories. (1) On the answer sheet blacken the space under the letter of the category in which these four items belong. (2) Then blacken the space under the number of the item that does not belong in the same category with the other four.

Items of this type may be used to determine knowledge of disease symptomatology, laboratory findings, or therapeutic procedures, as shown by the following:

Questions 19–21

19.

(a) Multiple neurofibromatosis (von Recklinghausen's disease)

(b) Hemangioblastomas of the central nervous system

(c) Multiple sclerosis

(1) Neurofibromas of the skin
(2) Meningeal fibromas
(3) Congenital angiomas of the eye
(4) Lipomas of subcutaneous tissue
(5) Cystic disease of the pancreas

Answer:
1. (a)
2. (5)

20.
(a) Contraindications to saddleblock anesthesia
(b) Contraindications to continuous caudal analgesia
(c) Contraindications to local anesthesia

(1) Deformity of the sacrum
(2) Cutaneous infections
(3) Perforated dura
(4) Decreased perineal resistance
(5) Prodromal labor

Answer:
1. (b)
2. (4)

21.
(a) Eosinophilia of diagnostic significance
(b) Plasmacytosis of diagnostic significance
(c) Lymphocytosis of diagnostic significance

(1) Trichinosis
(2) Multiple myeloma
(3) Löffler's syndrome
(4) Hodgkin's disease
(5) Schistosomiasis

Answer:
1. (a)
2. (2)

Another variant of the association and relatedness type of question is demonstrated by the following example from a test in public health and preventive medicine:

Directions. Each set of lettered headings below is followed by a list of words or phrases. For each word or phrase blacken the space on the answer sheet under

A if the word or the phrase is associated with (a) *only*
B if the word or the phrase is associated with (b) *only*
C if the word or the phrase is associated with *both* (a) *and* (b)

D if the word or the phrase is associated with *neither* (a) nor (b)

Questions 22–26

(a) Maternal hygiene program
(b) School health program
(c) Both
(d) Neither

22. Periodic physical examination *Answer:* C
23. Audiometer test *Answer:* B
24. Nutritional guidance *Answer:* C
25. Serologic test for syphilis *Answer:* A
26. Immunization against rubella *Answer:* B

Quantitative Values and Comparisons

In general, questions in this category call for an understanding of quantitative values rather than rote memory of the quantities themselves. Medical qualifying test committees have agreed that these examinations should contain a minimum of questions calling for the memorization of absolute quantitative amounts. Actual figures are found only where they are considered of such importance that they should be part of a practicing physician's working knowledge. Knowledge of the comparative significance of quantitative values may be called for by questions such as the following:

Directions. The following paired statements describe two entities that are to be compared in a quantitative sense. On the answer sheet blacken the space under

A if (a) is *greater than* (b)
B if (b) is *greater than* (a)
C if the two are *equal or very nearly equal*

Questions 27–31

27.
(a) The usual therapeutic dose of epinephrine
(b) The usual therapeutic dose of ephedrine
   Answer: B

28.
(a) The inflammability of nitrous oxide–ether mixtures
(b) The inflammability of chloroform–air mixtures *Answer:* A

29.
(a) The susceptibility of premature infants to rickets
(b) The susceptibility of full-term infants to rickets *Answer:* A

30.
(a) Life expectancy with glioblastoma of the occipital lobe
(b) Life expectancy with glioblastoma of the frontal lobe *Answer:* C

31.
(a) The amount of glycogen in the cells of Henle's loop in a diabetic
(b) The amount of glycogen in the cells of Henle's loop in a nondiabetic *Answer:* A

Directions. *Each of the following pairs of phrases describes conditions or quantities that may or may not be related. On the answer sheet blacken the space under*

A if increase in the first is accompanied by increase in the second or if decrease in the first is accompanied by decrease in the second
B if increase in the first is accompanied by decrease in the second or if decrease in the first is accompanied by increase in the second
C if changes in the second are independent of changes in the first

Questions 32–34

32.
(1) Urine volume
(2) Urine specific gravity *Answer:* B

33.
(1) Plasma protein concentration
(2) Colloid osmotic pressure of plasma
Answer: A

34.
(1) Cerebrospinal fluid pressure
(2) Intraocular pressure *Answer:* C

Cause and Effect

A type of question that is especially applicable to some of the more elusive aspects of medicine and calls for an understanding of cause and effect is illustrated below:

Directions. *Each of the following sentences consists of two main parts: a statement and a reason for that statement. On the answer sheet blacken the space under*

A if the statement and the proposed reason are *both true* and are *related* as cause and effect
B if the statement and the proposed reasons are *both true* but are *not related* as cause and effect
C if the statement is *true* but the proposed reason is *false*
D if the statement is *false* but the proposed reason is *an accepted fact or principle*

E if the statement and the proposed reason are *both false*

Directions summarized:

A = True True and related
B = True True and not related
C = True False
D = False True
E = False False

In situations that are described in this type of question, the right answer may sometimes be arrived at through reasoning from an appreciation of the basic principles involved.

Questions 35–39

35. Herpes simplex usually is regarded as an autogenous infection BECAUSE patients given fever therapy frequently develop herpes. *Answer:* A
36. Cow's milk is preferable to breast milk in infant feeding BECAUSE cow's milk has a higher content of calcium. *Answer:* D
37. The corpus luteum of menstruation becomes the corpus luteum of pregnancy BECAUSE progesterone inhibits the activity of the anterior portion of the pituitary gland. *Answer:* B
38. The sinoauricular node serves as the pacemaker BECAUSE after its removal the heart fails to beat. *Answer:* C
39. A higher titer of antibody against the H antigen of the typhoid bacillus is a good index of immunity to typhoid BECAUSE any antibody to an organism can protect against disease caused by that organism. *Answer:* E

A modification of the true-false type of question that calls for careful thought and discrimination is the "multiple true-false" variety. In this question a list of numbered items follows a statement for which several possible answers are given and the candidate is required to select the appropriate response from a list of answers designated by letters:

Question 40

Live virus is used in immunization against:

1. Influenza
2. Poliomyelitis
3. Cholera
4. Smallpox

Answers:
A Only 1, 2, and 3 are correct
B Only 1 and 3 are correct

C Only 2 and 4 are correct
D Only 4 is correct
E All are correct   *Answer:* C

Structure and Function

Diagrams, charts, electrocardiograms, roentgenograms, or photomicrographs may be used to elicit knowledge of structure, function, the course of a clinical situation, or a statistical tabulation. Questions then may be asked in relation to designated elements of the same.

Case Histories

The most characteristic situation that confronts the practicing physician can be simulated by a clinical case history derived from a patient experience. This is followed by a series of questions concerning diagnosis, signs and symptoms, laboratory determinations, treatment, and prognosis. Answering these questions largely depends on arriving at the proper diagnosis; an incorrect diagnosis will lead to incorrect answers about related symptoms, laboratory data, and treatment.

Directions. This section of the test consists of several case histories, each followed by a series of questions. Study each history, select the best answer to each question following it, and blacken the space under the corresponding letter on the answer sheet.

The patient is a 21-year-old white man with a complaint of malaise, cough, and fever. The present illness had its onset 10 days prior to admission with malaise and a nonproductive cough, followed in 24 hours by a temperature varying from 100 to 101 that persisted up to the time of admission. On about the fourth day of illness the cough became more severe, producing scant amounts of white viscid sputum. Three days prior to admission, paroxysms of coughing began, followed sometimes by vomiting. Chilly sensations were noted, but there were no frank shaking chills. Anterior parasternal pain on coughing has been present since the fifth day of illness.

On physical examination the patient's temperature is 101° F; pulse rate 110 beats per minute; respiratory rate 32 per minute; and blood pressure 108 mmHg systolic, 60 mmHg diastolic. The patient is well developed and well nourished, appears to be acutely but not chronically ill, and is dyspneic but not cyanotic.

Positive physical findings are limited to the chest and are as follows:

Vocal and tactile fremitus and resonance are within normal limits. In the left axilla a few fine rales are heard, and the bronchial quality of the sounds is increased, although the intensity is normal.

Hematological findings are reported as follows: White blood count is 3,400 (polymorphonuclears 30%, lymphocytes 62%, monocytes 5%, eosinophils 3%).

Roentgenogram of the chest reveals an increase in the density of the perihilar markings with ill-defined areas of patchy, soft, increased radiodensity at both bases and in the left upper lung field.

Questions 41–45

41. Which one of the following is the most likely diagnosis?
    (a) Tuberculosis
    (b) Pneumococcal pneumonia
    (c) Primary atypical pneumonia
    (d) Coccidioidomycosis
    (e) Bronchopneumonia   *Answer:* (c)
42. Which one of the following is the most likely additional physical finding?
    (a) Splenomegaly
    (b) Signs of meningeal irritation
    (c) Pleural friction rub
    (d) Frequent changes in distribution of chest findings
    (e) Signs of frank lobar consolidation   *Answer:* (d)
43. Which one of the following laboratory findings is consistent with the diagnosis?
    (a) Elevation and further increase of cold agglutinins
    (b) Positive blood culture
    (c) Marked leukocytosis with the beginning of recovery
    (d) Positive sputum examination
    (e) Positive skin test   *Answer:* (a)
44. Which one of the following is the therapy that should be given?
    (a) Bed rest and streptomycin
    (b) Bed rest and penicillin
    (c) Streptomycin and para-aminosalicylic acid
    (d) Bed rest and Aureomycin
    (e) Psychotherapy and physical rehabilitation   *Answer:* (d)
45. Which one of the following is the probable outcome of this disease in this patient if untreated?
    (a) The fever will subside spontaneously by crisis
    (b) Recovery will be gradual, with relapse not unexpected
    (c) Empyema will develop
    (d) Residual fibrosis will appear with healing
    (e) Lung cavitation will not be unexpected   *Answer:* (b)

Rypins' Questions & Answers for Basic Sciences Review, Second Edition, edited by Edward D. Frohlich. J. B. Lippincott Company, Philadelphia © 1993.

CHAPTER

2 Anatomy

J. Robert Troyer, Ph.D.

The John Franklin Huber Professor and Chairman of Anatomy and Cell Biology, Temple University School of Medicine

Neal E. Pratt, Ph.D., PT

Professor of Orthopedic Surgery and Anatomy, Hahnemann University

QUESTIONS

Directions. Select the one statement that most accurately completes the sentence or answers the question. Answers are at the end of the chapter.

1. Which one of the following is true for the oocyte at the time of its ovulation?
   (a) It has completed meiosis II.
   (b) It is a secondary oocyte.
   (c) It is arrested at the dictyotene stage.
   (d) It lacks a zona pellucida.

2. The following characteristics best describe which one of the organs listed below: ciliated cells, goblet cells, mucosal or submucosal glands, and no serosa?
   (a) Duodenum
   (b) Colon
   (c) Uterine tube
   (d) Bronchus

3. Which one of the following occurs in intramembranous ossification?
   (a) Zone of calcification of cartilage
   (b) Zone of cell hypertrophy
   (c) Trabecula formation
   (d) Interstitial growth

4. Select the one correct statement.
   (a) Granulopoiesis occurs mostly in "yellow" bone marrow.
   (b) In neutrophilic development, specific granules are synthesized before azurophilic granules.
   (c) Monocytes are precursors of tissue macrophages.
   (d) Eosinophilic granules contain histamine and heparin.

5. Select the one correct statement.
   (a) Primordial follicles consist of an oocyte surrounded by a stratified cuboidal follicular epithelial layer.
   (b) Glassy membranes are clear follicular cells of degenerating corpora lutea.
   (c) High levels of estrogen occur before the surge of LH at midcycle.
   (d) Many ovarian follicles are located in the medulla of the ovary.

6. Which one of the following statements regarding the adrenal gland is correct?
   (a) The cells of the adrenal medulla receive a dual blood supply from arterioles of the capsule and from direct branches of the suprarenal artery.
   (b) Mineralocorticoid (aldosterone) is secreted by the zona fasciculata.
   (c) The zona glomerulosa is under pituitary control through ACTH.
   (d) Cells of the zona fasciculata contain abundant rough endoplasmic reticulum and secretory granules.

7. Which one of the following "structure–function" pairs is correct?
   (a) Microtubule—low resistance pathway between adjacent cells
   (b) Ribosome—location of steroid synthesis

(c) Inner mitochondrial membrane—site of electron transport system

(d) Golgi apparatus (complex)—involved in mitochondria formation

8. Submucosal glands are present in which one of the following organs?
   (a) Duodenum
   (b) Colon
   (c) Anal canal
   (d) Stomach

9. Inhibition of lysosomal enzymes would most likely decrease hormone secretion by which one of the following?
   (a) Acidophils of the pars distalis
   (b) Chromaffin cells of the adrenal medulla
   (c) Follicular epithelial cells of the thyroid gland
   (d) Oxyphil cells of the parathyroid gland

10. The "specific" granules that mark the development of the three types of granulocytes are first produced in which one of the following cell stages?
    (a) Myeloblast
    (b) Promyelocyte
    (c) Myelocyte
    (d) Metamyelocyte

11. Peripheral blood elements have variable life spans. Which one of the following elements has the longest life span in the circulating blood?
    (a) Basophil
    (b) RBC
    (c) Neutrophil
    (d) Eosinophil

12. Transection of a myelinated motor nerve in the hand would usually result in which one of the following?
    (a) Degeneration of axons all the way back to the spinal cord
    (b) Degeneration of myelin all the way back to the dorsal root ganglion
    (c) Degeneration of most of the Schwann cells of the nerve distal to the lesion site
    (d) Phagocytosis of myelin by Schwann cells

13. Select the one true statement concerning the pancreas.
    (a) Cholecystokinin causes the intercalated ducts to secrete a bicarbonate-rich secretion.
    (b) Insulin, produced by alpha cells of the islets of Langerhans, decreases blood sugar levels.
    (c) Intercalated ducts are involved in regulating the alkalinity of the pancreatic secretion.
    (d) Centroacinar cells secrete protease.

14. Select the one true statement concerning the major salivary glands.
    (a) Striated ducts are found in the parotid and sublingual glands, but not in the submandibular gland.
    (b) Intercalated and striated ducts are interlobular ducts.
    (c) The submandibular gland has more serous demilunes than has the parotid gland.
    (d) The parotid, submandibular, and sublingual glands are mixed seromucous glands.

15. The intercellular "sealing" cement between stratum corneum cells of the epidermis is provided by:
    (a) Membrane-coating granules
    (b) Keratohyaline granules
    (c) Tight junctions between cells in the stratum spinosum
    (d) Macula adherens (desmosomes)

16. Which one of the following is true of the utricle?
    (a) It is a component of the membranous labyrinth.
    (b) It makes direct contact with the stapes.
    (c) It is part of the bony labyrinth.
    (d) It contains a crista.

17. Which one of the following structures contains lymphatic nodules, efferent lymphatic vessels, crypts, and stratified squamous epithelium?
    (a) Peyer's patches
    (b) Appendix
    (c) Palatine tonsil
    (d) Spleen

18. Which one of the following is true of the ciliary body?
    (a) It is largely made up of striated skeletal muscle.
    (b) Occluding junctions are found between ciliary epithelial cells.
    (c) Contraction of the circular muscle flattens the lens.
    (d) It secretes vitreous humor into the posterior chamber.

19. In which one of the following cells would you expect to find an abundance of smooth endoplasmic reticulum and numerous lipid droplets?
    (a) Acidophil of the anterior pituitary
    (b) Goblet cell in the bronchial epithelium
    (c) Cell in the zona fasciculata of the adrenal gland
    (d) Chief cell of the parathyroid gland

20. Which one of the following is true of loose areolar connective tissue?
    (a) It is found in the superficial fascia (hypodermis, subcutaneous tissue).
    (b) It is comprised mostly of a firm ground substance.
    (c) It contains collagenous but no elastic fibers.

(d) It contains fibroblasts that are noted for their lysosomal activity.

21. Cells possessing much smooth endoplasmic reticulum are most likely to:
    (a) Synthesize a proteinaceous secretory product
    (b) Produce steroids
    (c) Phagocytize dying cells
    (d) Be specialized for electrical conductivity

22. Which of the following contains relatively fewer serous-secreting cells than mucous-secreting cells?
    (a) von Ebner's glands
    (b) Parotid gland
    (c) Pancreas
    (d) Sublingual gland

23. Which of the following is *incorrect*?
    (a) Monocytes produce fibrinogen.
    (b) Leukocytes function in inflammatory and immunologic reactions.
    (c) Megakaryocytes give rise to platelets.
    (d) Monocytes, RBCs, granulocytes, and some lymphocytes are produced in the bone marrow.

24. Select the one *incorrect* statement.
    (a) A release of calcium from the terminal cisternae is necessary for muscle contraction.
    (b) In skeletal muscle, a triad consists of a T tubule and two flanking cisternae of sarcoplasmic reticulum.
    (c) Thin actin filaments are components of the I and A bands.
    (d) The cells that make up a neuromuscular spindle are called satellite cells.

25. Which of the following is *incorrect*?
    (a) Gap junctions are found in intercalated disks of cardiac muscle.
    (b) Acetylcholine is released from the motor endplate.
    (c) During contraction of skeletal muscle, the A band shortens.
    (d) Cardiac and skeletal muscles possess T tubules.

26. Which of the following is *least* characteristic of an osteon (haversian system)?
    (a) Blood vessels occupy its central (haversian) canal.
    (b) Osteoclasts are involved in its remodeling.
    (c) Osteoid and osseous tissue are present.
    (d) Circumferential lamellae make up its wall.

27. Which of the following is *not* true of chondrocytes?
    (a) They produce chondromucoprotein.
    (b) Gap junctions occur in canaliculi between chondrocytes.
    (c) They can undergo mitosis.

(d) They are involved in the calcification of cartilage during endochondrial bone formation.

28. Fused, or adjacent, basal laminae are found in all of the following places of gaseous or ionic exchange *except*:
    (a) Lung alveoli
    (b) Placental villi
    (c) Endothelial cells and podocytes of the renal glomerulus
    (d) Liver sinusoids

29. Which one of the following statements is *incorrect*?
    (a) Fenestrated capillaries can be found in the kidney and endocrine organs.
    (b) Venules have relatively thicker walls than arterioles of the same diameter.
    (c) Muscular (medium-sized) arteries have a distinct tunica media containing smooth muscle cells.
    (d) The tunica media of large arteries contain many elastic lamellae.

30. In the last trimester of pregnancy, when oxygen molecules pass through the thinnest part of the blood–placenta barrier, which of the following is the *least* likely to be encountered?
    (a) Syncytial trophoblast
    (b) Basal lamina
    (c) Endothelial cell cytoplasm
    (d) Fetal connective tissue

31. All of the following are true of the cytotrophoblast *except*:
    (a) It produces gonadotropin-releasing hormone.
    (b) It is part of the "placental barrier" in the first trimester of pregnancy.
    (c) It develops from the inner cell mass.
    (d) It gives rise to the syncytial trophoblast.

32. Which of the following is *not* a component of the cornea?
    (a) Bowman's membrane
    (b) An endothelial layer containing melanin
    (c) Stratified squamous nonkeratinized epithelium
    (d) Lamellae of collagenous fibrils

33. Choose the one *incorrect* statement concerning the eye.
    (a) The cornea and sclera are components of the fibrous tunic.
    (b) The canal of Schlemm is involved in drainage of aqueous humor from the anterior chamber.
    (c) The iris is lined by a stratified epithelium on both its anterior and its posterior surfaces.
    (d) The vascular coat (uvea) is comprised of the choroid, the ciliary body, and the iris.

34. Which one of the following statements concerning the lens is *incorrect*?
    (a) It is encapsulated by a basal lamina.
    (b) Its anterior epithelium is simple cuboidal.
    (c) Lens fibers are composed of collagen.
    (d) Zonule fibers (ligaments) attach the lens to the processes of the ciliary body.

35. Which one of the following "structure–function" pairs is *incorrect*?
    (a) Ciliary processes—production of aqueous humor
    (b) Sclera—site of attachment for extraocular muscles
    (c) Lacrimal gland—production of a serous fluid
    (d) Optic disk (papilla)—site of most acute vision

36. Choose the *incorrect* statement concerning the secretory portions of sweat glands.
    (a) The secretory cells are high cuboidal.
    (b) Myoepithelial cells invest the secretory cells.
    (c) The secretory cells secrete by the merocrine mode.
    (d) They are found in the papillary layer of the dermis.

37. All of the following are found in the white pulp of the spleen *except*:
    (a) Central arteries
    (b) Subcapsular sinus
    (c) Reticular cells
    (d) Lymphocytes

38. Which of the following "structure–function" pairs is *least correct*?
    (a) Cytotoxic (killer, T) lymphocytes—production of antibodies
    (b) Kupffer cells of the liver—phagocytosis of red blood cells
    (c) Alveolar macrophages of the lung—defense against particulate matter
    (d) Osteoclasts—resorption of bone

39. All of the following are part of the organ of Corti *except*:
    (a) Microvilli
    (b) Hair cells
    (c) Supporting phalangeal cells
    (d) Otoliths

40. All of the following are part of the placenta *except*:
    (a) Decidua basalis
    (b) Chorionic plate
    (c) Decidua parietalis
    (d) Chorion frondosum

41. All of the following cells produce collagen (procollagen) *except*:
    (a) Osteoblasts
    (b) Chondroblasts
    (c) Fibroblasts
    (d) Mast cells

42. Choose the one *incorrect* statement.
    (a) Blood spaces (lacunae) in the corpus cavernosa of the penis are lined by endothelium.
    (b) Contraction of smooth muscle in the walls of the vas deferens and ductus epididymidis propels spermatozoa into the prostatic urethra during the ejaculatory process.
    (c) During erection, the helicine arteries constrict, forcing blood away from arteriovenous shunts and into the blood spaces of the erectile tissue.
    (d) In the male reproductive tract, stereocilia are long microvilli.

43. Select the *incorrect* statement.
    (a) Schwann cells develop from neural crest.
    (b) Axons contain much rough endoplasmic reticulum and many Golgi elements.
    (c) Schwann cells surround axons of spinal nerves.
    (d) Oligodendroglia form the myelin of axons in the central nervous system.

44. All of the following are true of endochondral bone formation *except*:
    (a) Osteoprogenitor cells (osteogenic tissue) give rise to osteocytes.
    (b) Secondary ossification centers develop in the epiphyseal regions of long bones.
    (c) Growth in length is due to mitosis of osteocytes.
    (d) Bone is laid down on remnants of calcified cartilage.

45. Select the *incorrect* statement.
    (a) The organ of Corti is found in the cochlear duct (scala media).
    (b) Cristae ampullares are found in the semicircular canals.
    (c) The stria vascularis produces perilymph.
    (d) The spiral cochlear ganglion contains bipolar neurons.

46. Which one of the following "stomach secretory cell–secretory product" pairs is *incorrect*?
    (a) Argentaffin (Enteroendocrine, APUD) cell—gastrin
    (b) Chief cell—HCL
    (c) Surface lining cell—mucus
    (d) Parietal cell—gastric intrinsic antipernicious anemia factor

47. Which one of the following does *not* aid in increasing surface area in the small intestine?
    (a) Plicae circulares
    (b) Villi
    (c) Taeniae coli
    (d) Microvilli

48. Choose the one *incorrect* statement.
   (a) The parotid gland consists of serous acini and ducts.
   (b) The sublingual gland is a mixed gland whose mucous alveoli predominate.
   (c) Striated (salivary ducts) are involved in the reabsorption of water and sodium.
   (d) The striated ducts of the pancreas produce bicarbonate.

49. One would normally expect to find calcified cartilage in all of the following locations of a developing long bone *except*:
   (a) Primary ossification center
   (b) Secondary ossification center
   (c) Metaphysis
   (d) Articular surface

50. Choose the one *incorrect* statement concerning spermatogenesis.
   (a) Spermatogonia divide mitotically and give rise to primary spermatocytes.
   (b) Both primary and secondary spermatocytes contain 46 chromosomes.
   (c) Spermatids are located in infoldings of the apices of Sertoli cells.
   (d) Primary and secondary spermatocytes occupy the adluminal compartment of the seminiferous epithelium.

51. All of the following are characteristics of a lactating mammary gland *except*:
   (a) Areola containing skeletal muscle and non-pigmented epithelium
   (b) Pyramidal secretory cells invested by myoepithelial cells
   (c) Proteins secreted in the mammary gland by the merocrine mode
   (d) Lipids secreted in the mammary gland by the apocrine mode

52. Which one of the following is *least* characteristic of a placenta in the first trimester of pregnancy?
   (a) Nucleated red blood corpuscles are found in fetal capillaries.
   (b) Cytotrophoblastic cells form a layer between the syncytial trophoblast and the basal lamina of the trophoblast.
   (c) Fibrinoid material coats the surface of the free villi and chorionic plate.
   (d) Cytotrophoblastic cells produce gonadotropin-releasing hormone (GnRH, LH-RH).

53. Which one of the following "cell–location" pairs is *incorrect*?
   (a) Steroid-producing cell—between seminiferous tubules, in ovarian follicles and corpus luteum

   (b) Mucus-secreting cell—esophagus, stomach, colon
   (c) Fenestrated endothelial cell—glomerulus, sinusoid of bone marrow, alveolar capillaries of the lung
   (d) Cells with (true) cilia—uterine tube, hair cells of crista ampullaris, trachea

54. Select the one *incorrect* statement.
   (a) Hepatocytes at the periphery of the classical liver lobule are subjected to arterial blood before hepatocytes at the center of the lobule.
   (b) The portal triad is in the central region of a portal lobule.
   (c) The gallbladder synthesizes bile and bilirubin.
   (d) Kupffer cells are components of the reticuloendothelial (mononuclear phagocyte) system.

55. All of the following are true of the distal tubule of the nephron *except*:
   (a) Its cells have extensive basal infoldings of the plasma membrane.
   (b) It contains juxtaglomerular cells in its epithelial wall.
   (c) Aldosterone acts on it to bring about the reabsorption of sodium.
   (d) It forms a macula densa where the distal tubule abuts against the afferent glomerular arteriole

56. Choose the one *incorrect* statement.
   (a) Some coated vesicles are involved in receptor-mediated endocytosis.
   (b) Plasma membranes may contain glycoproteins, which have carbohydrate components that help make up the glycocalyx.
   (c) Microtubules are hollow structures composed of actin.
   (d) Ribosomes are essential for the production of lysosomal enzymes.

57. Select the one *incorrect* statement about the suprarenal gland.
   (a) Chromaffin cells secrete when stimulated by preganglionic sympathetic fibers.
   (b) Fenestrated capillaries are located between cords of zona fasciculata cells.
   (c) The epinephrine and norepinephrine-secreting cells of the medulla develop from mesoderm of the urogenital ridge.
   (d) Pigment (lipofuscin) is found in cells of the zona reticularis.

58. All of the following cell types secrete a known hormone or hormone precursor *except*:
   (a) Parafollicular cells of the thyroid gland
   (b) Interstitial cells of Leydig

(c) Oxyphil cells of the parathyroid gland
(d) Neurosecretory neurons in the hypothalamus

59. The surface epithelium lining the lumen of which one of the following organs produces the *least* mucus?
    (a) Esophagus
    (b) Stomach
    (c) Small intestine
    (d) Large intestine

60. All of the following are true statements concerning the uterine tube (oviduct) *except*:
    (a) Some of the ciliated cells may contact the corona radiata investing an ovulated secondary oocyte.
    (b) It is comprised of infundibular, ampullary, isthmus, and interstitial (intramural) regions.
    (c) Cells with 23 chromosomes and cells with 46 chromosomes may be found in its lumen.
    (d) Its smooth muscle layer is thicker in the infundibular region than in the isthmus region.

61. Which one of the following is *least* present in the endometrium during the proliferative (follicular) phase of the menstrual cycle?
    (a) Coiled (corkscrew-shaped) uterine glands
    (b) Mitosis of stromal cells
    (c) Basal (straight) arteries
    (d) Ciliated·cells

62. The pain and temperature pathway originating from receptors of the trunk and extremities:
    (a) Includes central processes of primary (first-order) neurons (neuron I) whose cell bodies are located in the substantia gelatinosa
    (b) Is more widely separated from the medial lemniscus in the medulla than at levels above the medulla
    (c) Includes a third-order neuron (neuron III) whose axons project to the precentral gyrus
    (d) Crosses to the opposite side at closed medulla levels

63. The posterior spinocerebellar tract:
    (a) Is present at all levels of the spinal cord
    (b) Is not present at cervical levels of the spinal cord
    (c) And the cuneocerebellar fibers become components of the inferior cerebellar peduncle
    (d) Is formed of axons of cells of the nucleus proprius

64. Choose the correct statement.
    (a) Cranial nerve VII contains SVE fibers originating in the nucleus ambiguus.
    (b) The facial nerve contains SVA and GSA fibers, whose cell bodies lie in the geniculate ganglion.
    (c) The facial colliculus is formed by the

abducens nerve looping over the facial nucleus.
    (d) The motor nucleus of the facial nerve receives only ipsilateral corticobulbar (upper motor neuron) projections.

65. Which of the following reflexes tests the integrity of the nucleus ambiguus?
    (a) Corneal reflex
    (b) Pupillary light reflex
    (c) Jaw jerk reflex
    (d) Gag reflex

66. Choose the correct statement concerning the motor component of the trigeminal system.
    (a) A unilateral lesion of the trigeminal motor nucleus produces marked paresis of the contralateral muscles of mastication.
    (b) Upper motor neuron (corticobulbar) axons to the trigeminal motor nucleus are mostly crossed.
    (c) The efferent limb of the corneal reflex originates in the trigeminal motor nucleus.
    (d) Facial representation areas in the primary motor cortex are located in that portion of the precentral gyrus that is supplied by the anterior cerebral artery.

67. On examination in an emergency room, a patient is found to have an external (lateral) strabismus of the right eye. The patient's tongue deviates to the left on protrusion, and there are increased deep tendon reflexes of the left arm and leg. A single destructive unilateral lesion that is most consistent with these findings would be in which general area?
    (a) Cerebral cortex
    (b) Basilar pons
    (c) Cerebral peduncle
    (d) Medulla

68. Which one of the following structures has a *direct* projection to lower motor neurons?
    (a) Cerebellum
    (b) Globus pallidus
    (c) Precentral gyrus
    (d) Ventral lateral nucleus of the thalamus

69. If the left subthalamic nucleus were lesioned, along with the immediately adjacent fibers of the internal capsule, which one of the following symptoms would be most likely to occur?
    (a) Spastic paralysis on the left side
    (b) Intention tremor on the right side
    (c) Loss of pain sensation on the left hand
    (d) Hemiballism on the right side

70. Increased activity in which one of the following hypothalamic nuclei would lead to eating?
    (a) Supraoptic
    (b) Lateral

(c) Ventromedial

(d) Preoptic

71. In which one of the following nuclei would descending hypothalamic projections most likely terminate?
    (a) General visceral efferent nucleus
    (b) Special visceral efferent nucleus
    (c) Special somatic afferent nucleus
    (d) Somatic motor nucleus

72. A lesion of which one of the following hypothalamic nuclei would most likely lead to diabetes insipidus?
    (a) Ventromedial
    (b) Lateral hypothalamus
    (c) Paraventricular
    (d) Supraoptic

73. A patient who has difficulty recognizing objects placed in the right hand but who can feel the textures and shapes of the objects most likely has a lesion of the:
    (a) Left postcentral gyrus
    (b) Left parietal lobe unisensory association areas
    (c) Left fasciculus cuneatus at upper cervical cord levels
    (d) Right medial lemniscus in the pons

74. Destruction of the lateral spinothalamic tract at C3 is most likely to result in which one of the following?
    (a) Demyelination of fibers in the area that lies in the postolivary lateral aspect of the medulla
    (b) Damage to cell bodies in the ipsilateral posterior gray horn below the level of the lesion
    (c) Damage to cell bodies of the ipsilateral VPL thalamic nucleus
    (d) Damage to cell bodies in the contralateral dorsal root ganglia below the level of the lesion

75. In examining a patient, you discover the following: no response to pinprick from T9 down on the left; loss of vibratory sense and two-point discrimination from T8 down on the right; deep tendon reflexes present bilaterally; paralysis of the right lower extremity. The lesion most consistent with these findings is:
    (a) Vascular accident involving the anterior spinal artery at T8
    (b) Disruption of the anterior white commissure at T8
    (c) Complete transection of the spinal cord at T9
    (d) Hemisection of the spinal cord at T8

76. You are examining a patient whose right upper limb is carried in a flexed position, whose right lower limb is carried in an extended position, and who does not feel pain in the left arm or leg when struck by a pin. Your patient most likely has a lesion of the:
    (a) Left pyramid of the medulla
    (b) Left base of the pons
    (c) Left posterior limb of the internal capsule
    (d) Right lateral funiculus at a high cervical cord level

77. A thrombosis that cuts off the blood supply to the entire nondominant cortical area supplied by the right middle cerebral artery is most likely to result in:
    (a) Loss of fine voluntary movements of the right extremities
    (b) Loss of two-point touch localization on the right foot
    (c) Inability to identify objects placed in the left hand
    (d) Expressive aphasia

78. Neural crest tissue:
    (a) Gives rise to autonomic ganglia associated with cranial nerves III, VII, IX, and X
    (b) Develops into all peripheral sensory neurons of the cranial nerves
    (c) Gives rise to the sensory nuclei of termination of the brain stem (*e.g.*, spinal nucleus of V)
    (d) Gives rise only to multipolar neurons

79. The cell columns:
    (a) Of the brain stem tend to be more continuous than those of the spinal cord
    (b) Of the brain stem include special somatic afferent nuclei of termination that are present at medullary and pontine levels
    (c) Of the brain stem comprise eight functional components
    (d) Of motor function (nuclei of origin) develop from cells that usually are either dorsal or lateral to the sulcus limitans

80. In the development of the brain stem:
    (a) The cerebellum arises from the rhombic lip of the metencephalon.
    (b) The optic nerve develops as an evagination of the telencephalic portion of the prosencephalon (forebrain).
    (c) The expanding telencephalic hemispheres (cerebrum) fuse with the lateral aspects of the mesencephalon.
    (d) The globus pallidus develops from the diencephalon.

81. A lesion of the entire sensory and motor roots of the left fifth nerve would most likely produce which of the following symptoms?
    (a) Loss of consensual blink upon stimulation of the right cornea
    (b) Paralysis of the left muscles of mastication

(c) Deviation of the jaw to the right upon opening (protrusion)

(d) Loss of sensation of pain, temperature, and touch on the right side of the face

82. A patient has a hoarseness and a uvula that is deviated or points toward the right upon phonation. You conclude that the lesion is most likely located in the:
    (a) Base of the pons
    (b) Cuneate nucleus
    (c) Right vagus nerve
    (d) Left nucleus ambiguus

83. Upon testing, a patient is found to have weakness in rotating the head to the left. A lesion causing this condition is most likely located in the:
    (a) Nucleus ambiguus on the left side
    (b) Left inferior olivary nucleus
    (c) Nucleus solitarius on the right side
    (d) Anterior horn of the right cervical spinal cord

84. A lesion of the right inferior cerebellar peduncle (including the juxtarestiform body) could cause damage to axons that originate from neurons in all of the following *except* the:
    (a) Right accessory cuneate nucleus
    (b) Right posterior horn at the tenth thoracic (T10) level of the cord
    (c) Left inferior olivary nucleus
    (d) Right precentral gyrus

85. The prosencephalon is essential to the development of all of the following structures *except* the:
    (a) Anterior commissure
    (b) Thalamus
    (c) Lamina terminalis
    (d) Cerebral peduncle

86. With the head inclined so that the horizontal semicircular canals are in the horizontal position, all of the following statements are true of the horizontal semicircular canals of the inner ear *except*:
    (a) The right crista ampullaris discharges at the same frequency as the left crista ampullaris when no horizontal movement of the head takes place.
    (b) Past-pointing to the right follows cessation of rotation to the left.
    (c) With cessation of rotation to the right, there is a tendency to fall to the right.
    (d) With cessation of rotation to the right, there is a slow component of nystagmus to the right.

87. Which of the following structures is *not* on the external surface of an intact gross brain?
    (a) Crus cerebri

(b) Mammillary bodies
(c) Cerebellar hemisphere
(d) Facial colliculus

88. Which of the following statements concerning the hypoglossal nucleus or nerve is *false*?
    (a) The nerve exits the lateral surface of the medulla in the postolivary sulcus.
    (b) The nerve contains somatic efferent (SE) fibers.
    (c) The nucleus is supplied by contralateral (crossed) upper motor neuron (UMN) fibers.
    (d) The nucleus is located near the midline in the medulla.

89. A unilateral lesion of the neocerebellum is likely to result in all of the following signs *except*:
    (a) Hypotonia
    (b) Chorea
    (c) Intention tremor
    (d) Asynergia of the limbs

90. Which one of the following "thalamic nucleus–major cortical projection area" pairs is *incorrect*?
    (a) Medial geniculate nucleus—transverse temporal gyri
    (b) Dorsomedial nucleus—occipital lobe
    (c) Ventral posterior lateral nucleus—postcentral gyrus
    (d) Ventral lateral nucleus—motor cortex

91. Which one of the following statements concerning the thalamus is *incorrect*?
    (a) The anterior nucleus projects fibers to the prefrontal cortex.
    (b) Axons from many of its nuclei project to the cerebral cortex via the internal capsule.
    (c) The pulvinar receives sensory information from the geniculate nuclei.
    (d) The globus pallidus projects fibers to the ventral anterior nucleus.

92. A lesion of cranial nerves 10 and 11 just lateral to the medulla might damage axons whose cell bodies are located in all of the following *except*:
    (a) Gray matter of cervical spinal cord
    (b) Nucleus ambiguus
    (c) Nucleus solitarius
    (d) The part of the medulla that develops from the basal plate

93. Choose the *incorrect* statement among the following about the sensory pathways from the face.
    (a) Cell bodies of second-order neurons for the transmission of pain are located in the principal sensory nucleus of V.
    (b) A unilateral brain stem lesion in the pons at the level of the entering trigeminal nerve would result in complete anesthesia of one side of the face.

(c) The ventral secondary ascending tract of V consists of axons that come from cell bodies on the contralateral side.

(d) Ascending tracts conveying tactile information from the face are both crossed and uncrossed.

94. Destruction of which one of the following structures may *not* be followed by the visual defect listed with it?
    (a) Crossing fibers of the optic chiasm—bitemporal heteronymous hemianopsia
    (b) Left optic tract—right homonymous hemianopsia
    (c) Left lingual gyrus—right lower quadrantic anopsia
    (d) Left temporal lobe—right upper quadrantic anopsia

95. Destruction of which one of the following structures is *not* followed by the signs or symptoms listed with it?
    (a) Left abducens nucleus—failure of both eyes to look conjugately to the left
    (b) Left trochlear nucleus—failure of the left eye to look up
    (c) Left abducens nerve—internal strabismus (medial deviation) of the left eye
    (d) Left frontal lobe—initial failure to perform voluntary saccadic eye movements to the right.

96. Which one of the following "structure–function" pairs is *incorrect*?
    (a) Midbrain reticular formation (rostral interstitial nucleus of the MLF)—vertical conjugate gaze
    (b) Paramedian pontine reticular formation—lateral conjugate gaze
    (c) Frontal eye fields—smooth pursuit movements of the eyes
    (d) Brachium of the superior colliculus—pupillary constriction in the light reflex

97. Which one of the following is *not* involved in the reflex that occurs in focusing on a near object after previously focusing on a far object?
    (a) Excitation of cells of the lateral geniculate nucleus
    (b) Contraction of the ciliary muscles and sphincter (constrictor) pupillae muscles in both eyes
    (c) Convergence of the eyes due to excitation of neurons of the Edinger-Westphal nucleus
    (d) Excitation of neurons in the parastriate area (area 18, visual area II)

98. In a lesion of the postcentral gyrus, which of the following is *least* likely to be lost?
    (a) Hearing

(b) Two-point discrimination
(c) Vibratory sensation
(d) Stereognosis

99. An occlusion of the left middle cerebral artery just distal to the anterior communicating artery could cause all of the following *except*:
    (a) Damage to the left lenticular nucleus
    (b) Damage to the left motor cortex
    (c) Deafness on the right side
    (d) Sensory aphasia

100. Which one of the following statements is *incorrect* for ascending (sensory) systems?
    (a) Information from both muscle spindles and Golgi tendon organs is carried by the posterior spinocerebellar tracts.
    (b) Second-order neurons of the two-point touch pathway are located in the medulla.
    (c) Axons from cell bodies in cervical dorsal root ganglia are located in the fasciculus cuneatus, whereas axons from sacral ganglia are in the fasciculus gracilis.
    (d) In the medial lemniscus of the open medulla, projections from the nucleus cuneatus are located more ventrally (anteriorly) than those from the nucleus gracilis.

101. Which of the following is *not* true?
    (a) Ectoderm gives rise to cells in the marginal, mantle, and ependymal layers of the neural tube.
    (b) The motor nuclei of origin develop from the alar plate.
    (c) The roof plates of the medulla and diencephalon are essential for the development of the tela choroidea and choroid plexus.
    (d) The lumen of the neural tube gives rise to ventricles in all parts of the brain stem except the low medulla and mesencephalon.

102. Several weeks after a spinal cord injury, an "upper motor neuron lesion" would likely produce all of the following contralateral findings *except*:
    (a) Weakness (paresis) more pronounced in distal musculature than in proximal musculature of the extremities
    (b) Hyperreflexia of both superficial and deep reflexes
    (c) Hypertonia
    (d) A positive Babinski response

103. A disease that causes destruction of alpha motor neurons can produce all of the following *except*:
    (a) Muscle atrophy
    (b) Muscle weakness (paresis)
    (c) Loss of superficial reflexes
    (d) Exaggerated deep tendon reflexes

104. Which of the following "structure–function" pairs is *incorrect*?

(a) Lateral corticospinal tract—facilitory to antagonists of antigravity muscles

(b) Lateral corticospinal tract—writing your answer to this question

(c) Lateral (medullary) reticulospinal tract—facilitory to antigravity muscles

(d) Vestibulospinal (lateral) tract—facilitory to antigravity muscles

105. Following section of a peripheral nerve, Schwann cells are responsible for all of the following *except*:
(a) Chromatolysis
(b) Neurolemmal tube formation
(c) Phagocytosis of axon remnants
(d) Myelin formation of regenerating axons

106. Which one of the following lesion sites would *least* likely lead to hyporeflexia in the limbs?
(a) Base of pons
(b) Ventral root of spinal nerve
(c) Dorsal root of spinal nerve
(d) Ventral gray horn

107. All of the following are correctly paired *except*:
(a) Inferior salivatory nucleus—submandibular ganglion
(b) Facial nucleus—stapedius muscle
(c) Geniculate ganglion—solitary (gustatory) nucleus
(d) Geniculate ganglion—spinal nucleus of the fifth cranial nerve

108. Failure of the first branchial arches to develop is most likely to lead to absence, or abnormal development, of the:
(a) Taste buds on the posterior one third of the tongue
(b) Stapes
(c) Tongue musculature
(d) Soft palate

109. You are examining a patient whose nasomedial (medial–nasal) processes did *not* develop. Your patient will most likely:
(a) Have a defect of the soft palate
(b) Be lacking upper canine teeth
(c) Have a defect of the nasal septum
(d) Have a unilateral cleft lip on the right side

110. Which one of the following develops directly from the primitive optic vesicle?
(a) Epithelium of the cornea
(b) Choroid
(c) Pigment epithelium of the retina
(d) Lens fibers

111. You are examining a stillborn baby whose neural crest material did not develop, but in whom all other structures from other sources developed normally. If the baby had lived, it would have:
(a) Been able to feel sensations on its fingertips

(b) Been able to maintain normal levels of epinephrine
(c) Had optic nerves
(d) Had postganglionic autonomic neurons

112. Which one of the following develops directly from the mesonephric duct?
(a) Uterus
(b) Seminal vesicle
(c) Nephron
(d) Parenchyma of the prostate gland

113. Which one of the following embryonic structures develops, or gives rise to, the structure (or part of the structure) that follows it?
(a) Primitive streak—artery in the chorion
(b) Ostium primum—foramen ovale
(c) Midgut diverticulum—gallbladder
(d) Urethral (genital) fold—labia minora

114. Which one of the following develops from the trophoblast?
(a) Placenta
(b) Epidermis of the skin
(c) Allantois
(d) Yolk sac

115. Which one of the following develops from the fourth branchial (pharyngeal) arch?
(a) Inferior parathyroid gland
(b) Cricothyroid muscle
(c) Tensor tympani muscle
(d) Greater cornua of the hyoid bone

116. Which of the following develops from both general or stomodeal surface ectoderm and neuroepithelium (from either neural tube or neural crest origin)?
(a) Parenchyma of the hypophysis (pituitary gland)
(b) Eyeball
(c) Both of the above
(d) Neither of the above

117. Which of the following develops from intermediate mesoderm?
(a) Smooth muscle of the gut
(b) Parietal pericardium
(c) Mesonephric duct
(d) Parietal peritoneum

118. Which one of the following is *true* of a complete (internal and external) branchial (cervical) fistula that opens into the tonsillar region (supratonsillar fossa)?
(a) It runs between the glossopharyngeal and vagus nerves.
(b) It runs posterior to the internal and common carotid arteries.
(c) It opens externally into a posterior triangle of the neck just posterior to the sternocleidomastoid muscle.

(d) It opens into the region of the second pharyngeal pouch.

119. Which one of the following is true for the development of the face?
    (a) The nasomedial and maxillary processes normally give rise to the upper lip.
    (b) The nasolateral process does not normally fuse with the maxillary process.
    (c) The frontal prominence forms the medial portion of the upper jaw.
    (d) The upper molar teeth develop out of the nasomedial process.

120. Transposition of the ascending aorta and pulmonary trunk are the result of:
    (a) The bulbar (aortic, truncal, conal) septum forming too much to one side
    (b) Improper spiraling of the bulbar (aortic, truncal, conal) septum
    (c) Failure of the bulbar (aortic, truncal, conal) septum to form
    (d) The entire sixth aortic arch remaining on the right side rather than on the left side

121. The portal vein develops from the:
    (a) Umbilical (allantoic) veins
    (b) New venous channels that form a shunt through the liver
    (c) Vitelline (omphalomesenteric) veins and their anastomoses
    (d) Supracardinal veins and their anastomoses

122. Which of the following primitive structures is followed by a structure that normally develops (at least in part) from it?
    (a) Sinus venous—right ventricle
    (b) Distal right sixth aortic arch—ductus arteriosus
    (c) Dorsal aorta—external carotid artery
    (d) Supracardinal vein—azygos vein

123. Which of the following primitive structures is followed by a structure that normally develops (at least in part) from it?
    (a) Ventral mesogastrium—spleen
    (b) Dorsal mesentery of the duodenum—greater omentum
    (c) Dorsal mesogastrium—transverse mesocolon
    (d) Ventral mesentery of small intestine— mesentery proper of the ileum

124. Which of the following is true for the development of the respiratory system?
    (a) All of the glands of the larynx, trachea, and bronchi develop from entoderm.
    (b) There are four main lobar branches of the right bronchus, but only two of the left.
    (c) The respiratory diverticulum (lung bud) arises from the floor of the pharynx in the last trimester of pregnancy (gestation).

(d) The laryngeal opening is normally closed for a short time when the ectoderm of the roof of the stomodeum grows back over the opening.

125. Which of the following is most likely to result from total failure of the paramesonephric (müllerian) ducts to form?
    (a) Arcuate uterus
    (b) Amenorrhea (lack of a menstrual cycle)
    (c) Absence of the vas deferens
    (d) Bicornuate uterus

126. Which one of the following develops from the first branchial (pharyngeal) arch?
    (a) Posterior belly of the digastric muscle
    (b) Incus
    (c) Styloid process
    (d) Lesser cornua of the hyoid bone

127. You are examining a stillborn whose yolk sac never formed. All other structures developed normally. You will expect to find a(n):
    (a) Bare area of the liver
    (b) Urinary bladder
    (c) Aorta
    (d) Thyroid gland

128. Failure of the right third branchial (pharyngeal) arch to develop is most likely to lead to the absence, or abnormal development, of:
    (a) Some muscles of the soft palate
    (b) The right stylohyoid muscle
    (c) The right subclavian artery
    (d) A portion of the hyoid bone

129. All of the following develop from somites *except*:
    (a) Tongue muscles
    (b) Ribs
    (c) Pharyngeal muscles
    (d) Erector spinae muscle

130. You are autopsying a female stillborn baby whose intermediate mesoderm did not develop but in whom all other structures derived from other embryonic tissue developed normally. If the baby had lived, it would have been missing all of the following *except*:
    (a) Kidneys
    (b) Uterine tubes (oviducts, fallopian tubes)
    (c) Ureters
    (d) Urethrae

131. Which of the following does *not* develop directly from the otic vesicle?
    (a) Middle ear cavity
    (b) Cochlear duct
    (c) Crista ampullaris
    (d) Macula of the utricle

132. All of the following contribute directly to the formation of the interventricular septum *except*:
    (a) Interbulbar (conal) septum

(b) Septum primum
(c) Endocardial cushion
(d) Cardiac muscle

133. Which one of the following embryonic structures does *not* give rise to the adult structure that follows it?
    (a) C5 (5th cervical) sclerotome—part of C4 and C5 vertebrae
    (b) Lumbar rib primordium—transverse process
    (c) Coelomic epithelium—Sertoli cells
    (d) Basal plate—postganglionic autonomic neurons

134. All of the following develop in, or from, an entodermal germ layer *except*:
    (a) Hepatocytes (liver parenchyma)
    (b) Islet cells of the pancreas
    (c) Spleen parenchyma
    (d) Parafollicular (calcitonin-producing) cells of the thyroid gland

135. Which of the following aortic arches is *not* followed by the blood vessel that normally develops (at least in part) from it?
    (a) Right third aortic arch—right internal carotid artery
    (b) Right fourth aortic arch—right subclavian artery
    (c) Right sixth aortic arch—ductus arteriosus
    (d) Left sixth aortic arch—pulmonary artery

136. All of the following occur after penetration of the plasma membrane of a developing ovum by a spermatozoan *except*:
    (a) Release of enzymes from the acrosome
    (b) Formation of a zygote with the diploid number of chromosomes
    (c) Mitotic spindle formation for cleavage
    (d) Completion of the second meiotic (MII) division

137. Which of the following structures does *not* develop from neural ectoderm?
    (a) Pigment layer (epithelium) of the retina
    (b) Rods and cones
    (c) Lens
    (d) Pigment epithelium of the iris

138. The cephalic limb of the midgut gives rise to all of the following *except*:
    (a) Part of the duodenum
    (b) Part of the ileum
    (c) Appendix
    (d) Jejunum

139. The diaphragm develops from all of the following *except*:
    (a) Septum transversum
    (b) Pleuropericardial fold (membrane)
    (c) Pleuroperitoneal fold (membrane)
    (d) Body wall mesoderm

140. All of the following develop from splanchnic mesoderm *except*:
    (a) Muscle of the gut wall
    (b) Superior mesenteric artery
    (c) Endocardium
    (d) Skeletal muscles

141. Which one of the following structures does *not* develop in, or from, the septum primum?
    (a) Ostium primum
    (b) Ostium secundum
    (c) Valve of the foramen ovale
    (d) Foramen ovale

142. All of the following muscles develop from branchial (pharyngeal) arches *except*:
    (a) Stylopharyngeus
    (b) Superior oblique muscle of the eye
    (c) Tensor tympani
    (d) Constrictor pharyngeus

143. Of the following, the most difficult (or impossible) to palpate is the:
    (a) Coracoid process
    (b) Acromioclavicular joint
    (c) Medial border of the scapula
    (d) Lateral angle of the scapula

144. Select the one true statement concerning the cubital fossa.
    (a) The bicipital aponeurosis is superficial to both the brachial artery and the median nerve.
    (b) Its lateral border is formed by the pronator teres muscle.
    (c) The brachial artery passes just lateral to the tendon of the biceps brachii muscle.
    (d) The median nerve passes lateral to the brachial artery.

145. A patient presents with a laceration on the palm just distal to the wrist and an inability to oppose the thumb to the other digits. The structure most likely lacerated is the:
    (a) Tendon of the abductor pollicis longus muscle
    (b) Common digital branch of the median nerve
    (c) Ulnar nerve
    (d) Recurrent (motor, thenar) branch of the median nerve

146. Which of the following lists represents the proper sequence of the indicated structures in the palm of the hand, going from most superficial to deepest?
    (a) Long digital flexor tendons, interossei muscles, lumbrical muscles
    (b) Palmar aponeurosis, long digital flexor tendons, median nerve
    (c) Superficial palmar arterial arch, lumbrical muscles, interossei muscles

(d) Superficial branch of the ulnar nerve, adductor pollicis muscle, median nerve

147. The static deformity (position at rest) resulting from a lesion of the superior trunk of the brachial plexus would logically include all of the following positions *except*:
    (a) Adduction at the shoulder
    (b) Internal rotation at the shoulder
    (c) Extension at the elbow
    (d) Supination of the forearm

148. Loss of function of the musculocutaneous nerve would be accompanied by:
    (a) Weakness in supination of the flexed forearm
    (b) Paralysis of the medial rotators of the arm
    (c) Weakness of the forearm pronators
    (d) Weakness of the abductors of the arm

149. Occlusion of the radial artery just distal to its beginning could logically produce all of the following signs *except*:
    (a) Decreased pulsation in the artery located between the tendons of the flexor carpi radialis and brachioradialis muscles just proximal to the wrist
    (b) Decreased pulsation in the artery passing through the anatomical snuff box
    (c) A marked decrease in the blood flow in the superficial palmar arterial arch
    (d) A marked decrease in the blood flow in the deep palmar arterial arch

150. Which of the following statements regarding the subclavian artery is *incorrect*?
    (a) It is palpable in the posterior cervical triangle.
    (b) It may be compressed by a cervical rib.
    (c) It becomes the axillary artery as it passes the upper border of the pectoralis minor muscle.
    (d) The subclavian vein lies anterior to it.

151. Contraction of the gluteus medius and minimus muscles can be palpated.
    (a) Between the crest of the ilium and the greater trochanter of the femur
    (b) Just superior to the ischial tuberosity
    (c) Inferior to the greater trochanter of the femur
    (d) Just inferior to the anterior inferior spine of the ilium

152. The ischiofemoral ligament is most taut when the femur is:
    (a) Flexed
    (b) Abducted
    (c) Extended
    (d) Medially rotated

153. Which of the following statements comparing the shoulder and hip joints is true?
    (a) Each joint has a strong intra-articular ligament that is a strong support of the joint.
    (b) The acetabular labrum grips the head of the femur; the glenoid labrum does not grip the head of the humerus.
    (c) The tendons of the gluteus medius and minimus muscles blend with the capsule of the hip joint just as the tendons of the rotator cuff muscles blend with the capsule of the shoulder joint.
    (d) The extra-articular ligaments are the major supports for each joint.

154. Select the *one* true statement concerning the posterior thigh.
    (a) None of the hamstring muscles attaches to the femur.
    (b) Innervation of the muscles is provided by both components (common peroneal and tibial) of the sciatic nerve.
    (c) A concentric (shortening) contraction of the hamstring muscles produces simultaneous extension at the hip and knee.
    (d) The blood supply is provided primarily by the posterior femoral artery.

155. The knee joint:
    (a) Permits flexion and extension of the leg, as well as rotation of the leg in flexion or extension
    (b) Is enclosed by a joint capsule whose fibrous and synovial portions are coextensive
    (c) Receives anteroposterior support from intra-articular ligaments and mediolateral support from extracapsular ligaments
    (d) Contains medial and lateral menisci, which are firmly attached to the femoral condyles

156. Extension of the great toe tests all of the following structures *except* the:
    (a) Common peroneal nerve
    (b) Fifth lumbar spinal nerve
    (c) Superficial peroneal nerve
    (d) Extensor hallucis longus muscle

157. Paralysis of the gluteus maximus muscle would most noticeably affect the gait cycle at:
    (a) Heel strike
    (b) Midstance
    (c) Toe off
    (d) Midswing

158. The course of the sciatic nerve is best described as one that passes vertically:
    (a) Between the greater trochanter of the femur and the anterior superior spine of the ilium
    (b) Superior to and in line with the ischial tuberosity
    (c) Medial to the posterior superior spine of the ilium

(d) Between the ischial tuberosity and the greater trochanter of the femur

159. An inability to evert the foot would logically be accompanied by a loss of sensation on which of the following?
(a) The plantar aspect of the foot
(b) The medial border of the foot
(c) The lateral border of the foot
(d) Most of the dorsum of the foot

160. Following blockage of the external iliac artery at its beginning, which of the following potential anastomoses would most logically be used to by-pass the obstruction?
(a) The inferior gluteal and obturator arteries
(b) The medial and lateral circumflex femoral arteries and the ascending branches of the perforating arteries
(c) The iliolumbar and lateral sacral arteries
(d) The superior gluteal and lateral femoral circumflex arteries

161. Which of the following statements regarding the surface projection of the heart is most correct?
(a) The superior border of the heart extends from the second left costal cartilage to the third right costal cartilage.
(b) The right border of the heart extends from the third right costal cartilage to the fifth right costal cartilage.
(c) The inferior border of the heart extends from the fifth right costal cartilage to the fourth left intercostal space 3½ inches (9 cm) from the midline.
(d) The left border of the heart extends from the third left costal cartilage to the fourth left intercostal space 3½ inches (9 cm) from the midline.

162. Which of the following statements regarding the pericardium is most correct?
(a) The parietal layer of serous pericardium is also called the epicardium.
(b) The pericardial cavity is located between the fibrous pericardium and the parietal layer of serous pericardium.
(c) The fibrous layer of the pericardium blends with the adventitia of the great vessels superiorly and the central tendon of the diaphragm inferiorly.
(d) The reflection of the serous pericardium around the large veins bounds the transverse sinus.

163. Which of the following organ positions does *not* correspond to the level indicated?
(a) The transpyloric plane passes through the first part of the duodenum.

(b) The bifurcation of the aorta occurs at the level of the fourth lumbar vertebra.
(c) The transpyloric plane passes through the hilar region of both kidneys.
(d) The tail of the pancreas is at the level of the third lumbar vertebra.

164. When filled with contrast medium and x-rayed, the colon can be identified by which of the following?
(a) Prominent haustra
(b) Teniae coli
(c) Epiploic appendices
(d) Plicae circulares

165. The blood supply to the transverse and descending portions of the colon is provided by branches of which of the following?
(a) Celiac artery
(b) Celiac and superior mesenteric arteries
(c) Superior mesenteric artery
(d) Superior and inferior mesenteric arteries

166. Which of the following is the most posterior part of the stomach?
(a) Fundus
(b) Body
(c) Cardiac orifice
(d) Pylorus

167. The head of the pancreas is most closely related to which of the following?
(a) Second part of the duodenum
(b) Spleen
(c) Left lobe of the liver
(d) Ascending colon

168. The smallest diameter of the pelvis is the distance between the:
(a) Ischial tuberosities
(b) Pubic symphysis and the sacral promontory
(c) Ischial spines
(d) Arcuate lines of the ilia

169. The pudendal nerve is most closely related to which of the following?
(a) Sacral promontory
(b) Ischial spine
(c) Symphysis pubis
(d) Ischial tuberosity

170. The blood supply of the rectum is provided by branches of which of the following?
(a) Inferior mesenteric and obturator arteries
(b) Internal pudendal and external iliac arteries
(c) Internal iliac and inferior mesenteric arteries
(d) Internal and external iliac arteries

171. The ischiorectal fossa:
(a) Is considered part of the pelvis and therefore is superior to the levator ani muscle
(b) Is part of the deep perineal space (pouch)

(c) Has a portion that is located superior to the urogenital diaphragm

(d) Is found totally within the anal triangle of the perineum

172. The external urethral opening in the female is found in which of the following locations?
(a) At the apex of the clitoris
(b) In the vestibule just posterior to the perineal body
(c) In the vestibule between the clitoris and the vaginal opening
(d) Between the external vaginal opening and the perineal body

173. The skin of the perineum is innervated primarily by branches of which of the following?
(a) Pudendal and ilioinguinal nerves
(b) Pelvic splanchnic nerves
(c) Pudendal and obturator nerves
(d) Posterior and lateral femoral cutaneous nerves

174. The thyroid gland:
(a) Has an isthmus that crosses the midline at the level of the fourth cervical vertebra
(b) Receives arterial blood from both the subclavian and axillary systems
(c) Has superior and inferior parathyroid glands embedded in the anterior surfaces of its lateral bodies
(d) Has three sets of veins

175. The vocal cords can be abducted (separated) by the:
(a) Arytenoid (transverse arytenoid) muscle
(b) Lateral cricoarytenoid muscles
(c) Posterior cricoarytenoid muscles
(d) Cricothyroid muscles

176. A tumor in the posterior cranial fossa would be *least* likely to damage which of the nerves listed below?
(a) Hypoglossal nerve
(b) Facial nerve
(c) Optic nerve
(d) Vagus nerve

177. A laterally and anteriorly expanding hypophyseal tumor could logically impinge on nearby structures and produce all of the following *except*:
(a) Auditory deficits
(b) Visual field defects
(c) Compression of the internal carotid artery
(d) Multiple extraocular muscle deficits leading to strabismus (deviation of the eyeball)

178. Which of the following statements concerning the meninges and dural venous sinuses is correct?

(a) The inferior sagittal sinus is formed between the periosteal and meningeal layers of dura.
(b) The falx cerebri separates the cerebellum and occipital lobes of the cerebrum.
(c) The superior sagittal sinus joins the great cerebral vein (of Galen) to form the straight sinus.
(d) The sigmoid sinus is continuous with the internal jugular vein through the jugular foramen.

179. Which of the following statements regarding the orbit is correct?
(a) The ophthalmic artery and vein pass through the optic canal.
(b) Postganglionic fibers from the ciliary ganglion supply the lacrimal gland.
(c) The levator palpebrae superioris is innervated by the frontal nerve.
(d) Increased cerebrospinal fluid pressure could compress the central vein of the retina.

180. The fourth cranial nerve can be tested by:
(a) Elevation of the abducted eye
(b) Adduction of the eye
(c) Depression of the adducted eye
(d) Abduction of the eye

181. All of the following empty into the middle meatus of the nasal cavity *except* the:
(a) Middle ethmoid air cells
(b) Nasolacrimal duct
(c) Maxillary sinus
(d) Frontal sinus

182. Which of the following statements concerning the innervation of the oral cavity is *incorrect*?
(a) The genioglossus muscle is innervated by the mandibular division of the trigeminal nerve.
(b) The intrinsic muscles of the tongue are innervated by the hypoglossal nerve.
(c) The mucosa of the palate is innervated by a branch of the maxillary division of the trigeminal nerve.
(d) The upper teeth are innervated by branches of the maxillary division of the trigeminal nerve.

183. Which of the following middle ear cavity relationships is *incorrect*?
(a) Superiorly, the middle cranial fossa
(b) Inferiorly, the auditory (eustachian) tube
(c) Medially, the inner ear
(d) Posteriorly, the mastoid air cells

Directions. *For each of the following questions answer:*

(a) if only 1, 2, and 3 are correct
(b) if only 1 and 3 are correct

(c) if only 2 and 4 are correct
(d) if only 4 is correct
(e) if all are correct

184. Which of the following statements concerning the retina are correct?
    1. The inner nuclear layer contains the nuclei of rods and cones.
    2. Bipolar cells synapse with rods, cones, and ganglion cells.
    3. Visual pigment (rhodopsin) is transported to rods and cones from the pigment epithelium.
    4. The retina is supplied with oxygen by blood vessels from the choroid layer and from the optic nerve.

185. Which of the following "cell–secretory product" pairs in the pancreas are true?
    1. Beta cell—insulin
    2. Acinar cells—pancreatic enzymes
    3. Alpha cells—glucagon
    4. Centroacinar cells—sodium bicarbonate

186. Perilymph is located in which of the following?
    1. Scala tympani
    2. Cochlear duct
    3. Scala vestibuli
    4. Utricle

187. Which of the following cells contain(s) an abundance of smooth endoplasmic reticulum?
    1. Basophil of the pars distalis
    2. Leydig cell of the testis
    3. Thyroid follicular cell
    4. Granulosa lutein cell

188. Which of the following statements regarding the thyroid gland are true?
    1. Colloid contains thyroglobulin, a storage precursor of the thyroid hormones thyroxine (T4) and triiodothyronine (T3).
    2. The simple epithelium of thyroid follicles is regulated by thyroid-stimulating hormone (TSH).
    3. Portions of thyroglobulin are taken back into the follicle cells by pinocytosis.
    4. Thyroxine and triiodothyronine pass from the basal aspect of follicle cells to the adjacent capillaries.

189. Which of the following statements are true?
    1. The T tubules of skeletal muscle conduct the electrical signal from the surface to the deep portions of the muscle fiber.
    2. Neuromuscular spindles are the sensory receptors of skeletal muscle.
    3. The sarcomere is the contractile unit of striated muscle.
    4. Striated skeletal muscle contains actin and myosin, while smooth muscle has only actin.

190. The following characteristics—stratified squamous epithelium, elastic connective tissue, no muscularis mucosae, and no mucosal or submucosal glands—best describe which of the structures listed below?
    1. True vocal cord (fold)
    2. Rectum/anal canal
    3. Vagina
    4. Lip

191. Which of the following statements are correct?
    1. Parafollicular cells of the thyroid secrete calcitonin.
    2. Chief cells produce parathyroid hormone.
    3. Parathyroid oxyphil cells contain many mitochondria and do not appear until the end of the first decade of life.
    4. The parathyroid gland is under the influence of parathyroid-stimulating hormone (PSH) from the adenohypophysis.

192. Which of the following structures are found in the dermis?
    1. Smooth muscle cells
    2. Fibroblasts
    3. Pacinian corpuscles
    4. Ducts of sweat glands

193. Which of the following "cell–function" pairs are correct?
    1. Syncytial trophoblast—secretion of progesterone and estrogen
    2. Hepatocyte—bile production
    3. Cell of zona fasciculata—synthesis of cortisol (glucocorticoids)
    4. Theca interna cell—produce steroid precursor of estrogen

194. Which of the following statements concerning the male reproductive system are true?
    1. Spermatogonia are separated from primary spermatocytes by tight junctions between adjacent Sertoli cells.
    2. A spermatid contains 23 chromosomes.
    3. The acrosome vesicle contains enzymes and forms the head cap of a spermatozoan.
    4. Sertoli cells produce androgen-binding protein (ABP), which serves to concentrate testosterone needed for spermatogenesis.

195. Which of the following events occur during excitation–contraction coupling in a striated skeletal muscle fiber?
    1. Acetylcholine from the motor endplate causes depolarization of the muscle plasma membrane
    2. I bands shorten.
    3. Calcium is released from the terminal cisternae of the sarcoplasmic reticulum.

4. Crossbridges form between adjacent actin filaments.

196. Which of the following would you expect to find in an alveolus?
    1. Dust cells (alveolar phagocytes)
    2. Simple squamous epithelial cells
    3. Surfactant-producing great alveolar (type II) cells
    4. Goblet cells

197. Which of the organs listed below receives blood through a portal system?
    1. Pituitary
    2. Pancreas
    3. Liver
    4. Bone marrow

198. Lymphocytes may enter a lymph node through which of the following structures?
    1. Central arteries
    2. Postcapillary venules
    3. Pulp arteries
    4. Afferent lymphatic vessels

199. Which of the following statements about the male reproductive system are correct?
    1. Both androgen and follicle-stimulating hormone (FSH) are required for spermatogenesis.
    2. Luteinizing hormone (LH) stimulates Leydig cells to secrete testosterone.
    3. The ciliated cells of the efferent ductules help propel the sperm into the ductus epididymidis.
    4. The seminal vesicle produces an alkaline fluid that is rich in fructose.

200. Which of the following statements are correct?
    1. Replacement of the cells at the surface of the villus occurs by division of the stem cells in the intestinal glands (crypts of Lieberkuhn).
    2. Replacement of tooth enamel does not occur in teeth that have erupted.
    3. Replacement of cells of the epidermis occurs primarily by division of those epithelial cells closest to the basement membrane.
    4. Replacement of degenerating neurons in the central nervous system occurs by the division of the remaining neurons.

201. Which of the following are true of the nephron or its parts? (Do not include the collecting tubule in the definition of nephron.)
    1. It is the principal site of action of antidiuretic hormone (ADH).
    2. Sodium is actively transported by its cells.
    3. It is made up in part of a stratified epithelium.
    4. It is found in the pars convoluta, pars radiata, and medulla.

202. Which of the following cells contain organelles needed for the secretion of a proteinaceous product?
    1. Pyramidal cells of the pancreatic acini
    2. Chief cells of the stomach
    3. Serous-secreting cells of the parotid gland
    4. Fibroblast

203. Which of the following are correct?
    1. Axons in the vestibulocochlear nerve could degenerate due to encroachment by a tumor at the pons-medulla junction (cerebellar–pontine angle tumor).
    2. Neurons located in cochlear nuclei may project (or relay) bilaterally to inferior colliculi.
    3. Axons from the cochlear nuclei may terminate in the superior olivary nucleus.
    4. Axons in cranial nerve VIII have their cell bodies located in vestibular and spiral cochlear ganglia.

204. A patient with a lesion of the entire right lateral funiculus, posterior and anterior horns, and anterior white commissure at the T2 to T4 levels of the spinal cord might be expected to have:
    1. Bilateral loss of pain and temperature sensation in dermatome T4
    2. Degenerated axons going to a thoracic sympathetic ganglion
    3. Contralateral loss of pain and temperature from T3 down
    4. Ipsilateral increased tone in extensors of the lower extremity

205. In which of the following locations are lesions likely to result in sensory and motor defects?
    1. Lateral funiculus of the spinal cord
    2. Medial third of the medulla
    3. Posterior limb of the internal capsule
    4. Tegmentum of the pons

206. A lesion of the entire left cerebral peduncle at superior colliculus levels would probably result in:
    1. Neocerebellar abnormal signs in the right extremities
    2. Ptosis of the left eyelid
    3. External (lateral) strabismus of the left eye
    4. Complete hearing loss in the left ear

207. A lesion involving an entire cerebral peduncle would result in the degeneration of fibers of tracts originating from cell bodies in which of the following areas?
    1. Globus pallidus
    2. Cerebellar nuclei
    3. Cerebral cortex
    4. Dorsal horn of gray matter

208. Which of the following could occur if branches of the indicated vessel are thrombosed?

1. Left posterior cerebral artery—right homonymous hemianopsia
2. Left anterior choroidal artery—right homonymous hemianopsia
3. Anterior spinal artery of cervical spinal cord—flaccid paralysis
4. Left ophthalmic artery—blindness in right eye

209. Which of the following could result from a destructive lesion of the left oculomotor nerve?
    1. Loss of left pupillary constriction when light is shone in the left eye
    2. Loss of left pupillary constriction when light is shone in the right eye
    3. Pupillary dilation (mydriasis) in the left eye
    4. Paralysis of the ciliary muscle in the left eye

210. Which of the following "primary receptive area–function" pairs are correct?
    1. Uncus—olfaction
    2. Lingual gyrus—vision
    3. Postcentral gyrus—two-point touch
    4. Somesthetic area II above lateral fissure—pain

211. A patient with a lesion of the right medial lemniscus and pyramid in the open (upper) medulla might display chromatolysis in which of the following nuclei (disregard transneuronal degeneration)?
    1. Left nucleus cuneatus
    2. Right nucleus gracilis
    3. Right precentral gyrus
    4. Left precentral gyrus

212. Ia fibers terminate upon the:
    1. Accessory cuneate nucleus
    2. Alpha motor neurons of the ventral horn
    3. Clarke's column (nucleus dorsalis)
    4. Dorsal root ganglion

213. The functional components of cranial nerves VII, IX, and X are located in which of the following cell columns?
    1. GVA
    2. GVE
    3. SVA
    4. SVE

214. Which of the following could be observed after a necrosis of the right half of the tegmentum of the pons at the level of the facial colliculus?
    1. Paralysis of the ipsilateral muscles of facial expression
    2. Degeneration of axons in the ipsilateral anterior funiculus of the spinal cord
    3. Degenerated axons in the medulla
    4. Decreased two-point touch modalities in the contralateral upper extremity

215. Which of the following could result from damage to corticobulbar neurons to the seventh nucleus from a lesion in the left motor cerebral cortex?
    1. Ptosis of the right eyelid
    2. Inability to close the right eye
    3. Hyperacusis on the left
    4. Inability to smile symmetrically upon command

216. The pons participates in which of the following functions?
    1. Regulation of posture and movement
    2. Conjugate movements of the eyes
    3. Somatic sensory innervation of the face
    4. Motor innervation of muscles of the face

217. Destruction of which of the following ascending pathways at mesencephalic levels will result in a contralateral loss of sensation?
    1. Lateral spinothalamic tract
    2. Medial lemniscus
    3. Ventral secondary tract of V
    4. Dorsal secondary tract of V

218. The inferior vena cava develops from:
    1. A small portion of the right vitelline vein
    2. The right subcardinal vein
    3. The right sacrocardinal vein
    4. The right umbilical vein

219. The tongue develops from:
    1. Ectoderm
    2. Entoderm
    3. Occipital somites
    4. Lateral lingual swellings

220. In the development of the placenta:
    1. Fetal blood vessels form in the first trimester.
    2. The cytotrophoblast gives rise to the syncytial trophoblast.
    3. The chorion laeve lies adjacent to the decidua capsularis.
    4. The stem villi develop from the decidua basalis.

221. You are examining a stillborn baby whose second branchial arch did not develop. Had the baby lived, you would have expected it to have much trouble:
    1. Hearing
    2. Blinking
    3. Smiling
    4. Chewing

222. In the vertebral canal:
    1. Spinal cord segment T10 lies approximately opposite the T8 vertebral body.
    2. The internal venous plexus is found in the epidural space.
    3. Cerebrospinal fluid fills the space between the arachnoid and the pia mater.
    4. The end of the spinal cord lies opposite the

L1 vertebra, or the disk between vertebrae L1 and L2.

223. An intervertebral foramen:
 1. Is bound posteriorly by the transverse process
 2. Can be reduced in size by a herniated nucleus pulposus, which compresses the spinal nerve of the same number as the vertebrae above the ruptured disk
 3. Transmits nerve fibers that synapse in the dorsal root ganglion
 4. Can be reduced in size by inflammatory processes or bony outgrowths of the zygapophyseal joints

224. The scalene triangle (groove):
 1. Is an interval in the muscular floor of the posterior cervical triangle
 2. Transmits the proximal portion of the brachial plexus and the subclavian artery
 3. Is bounded inferiorly by the first rib
 4. Is narrowed anteroposteriorly by turning of the head to the ipsilateral side

225. Which of the following anatomic landmarks would be useful in defining the borders of the posterior triangle of the neck?
 1. The superior border of the clavicle
 2. The superior border of the trapezius muscle
 3. The posterior border of the sternocleidomastoid muscle
 4. The posterior border of the anterior scalene muscle

226. In the region of the shoulder:
 1. The glenohumeral joint permits 180° of abduction.
 2. The glenohumeral joint is reinforced on all aspects (superiorly, inferiorly, anteriorly, and posteriorly) by muscles of the rotator (musculotendinous) cuff.
 3. The subacromial (subdeltoid) bursa is inferior to the supraspinatus tendon and muscle.
 4. The glenohumeral joint permits flexion, extension, abduction, adduction, and both internal and external rotation.

227. At the wrist:
 1. The ulnar nerve is medial to the ulnar artery.
 2. The ulnar artery is lateral to the tendon of the flexor carpi ulnaris muscle.
 3. The radial artery is lateral to the tendon of the flexor carpi radialis muscle.
 4. The median nerve is in the interval between the tendons of the palmaris longus and flexor carpi radialis muscles.

228. In an ulnar nerve lesion proximal to the elbow:
 1. There would be a sensory deficit involving

the skin on the dorsal aspect of the medial one and a half digits.
 2. There would be a sensory deficit involving the skin on the ventral aspect of the medial one and a half digits.
 3. Thumb adduction would be lost.
 4. Wrist adduction would be lost.

229. In the hand:
 1. The synovial sheath of the tendon of the flexor pollicis longus muscle is usually continuous from the wrist to the thumb.
 2. The carpometacarpal joints of the five digits permit only minimal motion.
 3. The terminal portions of the proper palmar digital nerves pass dorsally to innervate the skin over the dorsum of the terminal phalanges.
 4. The metacarpophalangeal joints permit only flexion and extension.

230. The lumbosacral (lumbar and sacral) plexus:
 1. Is formed within both the abdomen and the pelvis
 2. Is formed partially within the substance of the psoas major muscle
 3. Is found partially on the deep aspect of the piriformis muscle
 4. Has branches that innervate the muscles of the lower abdominal wall

231. In the region of the knee:
 1. The popliteal fossa is bounded above by tendons of the hamstring muscles and below by the two heads of the gastrocnemius muscle.
 2. The deepest structure in the popliteal fossa is the popliteal artery.
 3. The popliteal and femoral vessels are continuous through the adductor hiatus.
 4. The common peroneal nerve passes superficially through the central portion of the popliteal fossa.

232. The longitudinal arch of the foot:
 1. Is divided into medial and lateral portions anteriorly with the calcaneus forming a common component posteriorly
 2. Is highest (most superior) at the level of the talus
 3. Receives medial support primarily from the plantar calcaneonavicular (spring) ligament, which directly supports the head of the talus
 4. Is arranged so that weight is distributed anteriorly to the heads of the metatarsals and posteriorly to the calcaneus

233. During quiet breathing, the lower border of the lung is found at the level of the:
 1. Sixth rib in the midclavicular line
 2. Tenth rib in the midaxillary line

3. Eighth rib in the midaxillary line
4. Twelfth rib in the scapular line

234. The lungs:
1. Receive parasympathetic innervation from the vagus nerves
2. Receive sympathetic innervation from preganglionic nerve cell bodies located in the intermediolateral cell column of upper thoracic spinal cord segments
3. Are innervated by visceral afferents that utilize both the vagal and sympathetic pathways to enter the central nervous system
4. Are drained by lymphatic pathways, both sides of which (left and right) terminate in the thoracic duct

235. A cross section through the thorax at the level of the body of the eighth thoracic vertebra would pass through the:
1. Trachea
2. Middle lobe of the right lung
3. Left main bronchus
4. Left atrium

236. Which of the following statements about the thoracic wall is/are true?
1. The terminal branches of the typical posterior intercostal arteries anastomose with branches of the anterior intercostal arteries.
2. The neurovascular bundle in the intercostal space passes along the superior border of the rib.
3. The internal thoracic artery ends by dividing into superior epigastric and musculophrenic arteries.
4. The sternal angle is at the level of the third costal cartilage.

237. The left coronary artery:
1. Has a branch that commonly anastomoses with the right coronary in the coronary sulcus
2. Has a branch that commonly anastomoses with a branch of the right coronary in the interventricular sulcus
3. Is short in that soon after its origin it bifurcates into the anterior interventricular and circumflex arteries
4. Passes anterior to the pulmonary trunk

238. In the mediastinum:
1. The left brachiocephalic vein passes anterior to the brachiocephalic artery.
2. The ligamentum arteriosum interconnects the aortic arch and the left pulmonary vein.
3. The left recurrent laryngeal nerve passes under the arch of the aorta.
4. The thoracic duct is found between the esophagus and the trachea.

239. The esophagus:
1. Passes through the esophageal hiatus at vertebral level T10
2. Is found between the trachea and the thoracic duct in the superior mediastinum
3. Is typically ventral to the azygos vein in the lower thorax
4. Is adjacent to the right atrium as it passes posterior to the heart

240. Which of the following statements about the formation of the inguinal canal is/are true?
1. The superficial inguinal ring is an opening in the aponeurosis of the external abdominal oblique muscle.
2. The anterior wall of the inguinal canal is formed by the aponeurosis of the external oblique and reinforced laterally by fibers of the internal oblique muscle.
3. The posterior wall is formed partially by the transversalis fascia.
4. The deep inguinal ring is an outpouching of the transversalis fascia and is situated lateral to the inferior epigastric vessels.

241. Which of the following statements concerning the anterior abdominal wall is/are correct?
1. The fibers of the external and internal abdominal oblique muscles are oriented perpendicular to one another.
2. A function of the rectus abdominis muscle is extension of the vertebral column.
3. The muscles are innervated partially by lower intercostal nerves.
4. Contraction of its muscles reduces intraabdominal pressure.

242. The lesser peritoneal sac (omental bursa) is bounded:
1. Anteriorly by the stomach
2. Posteriorly by the ileum
3. Posteriorly by the pancreas
4. Posteriorly by the lesser omentum

243. Which of the following statements relative to the gallbladder is/are true?
1. Its fundus is normally situated on the transpyloric line at the tip of the ninth costal cartilage.
2. It occupies a groove that separates the right and quadrate lobes of the liver.
3. It is related posteriorly to the first part of the duodenum.
4. Its arterial supply is typically derived from the left hepatic artery.

244. The posteroinferior (visceral) surface of the liver is related to the:
1. Right kidney
2. Hepatic flexure of the colon

3. Duodenum
4. Esophagus

245. The common bile duct:
1. Passes anterior to the first part of the duodenum
2. Is situated anterior to the portal vein
3. Opens into the third part of the duodenum
4. Is separated from the inferior vena cava by the epiploic foramen

246. Posterior relationships of both kidneys include the:
1. Diaphragm
2. Psoas major muscle
3. Quadratus lumborum muscle
4. Ninth rib

247. The right suprarenal gland is related to the:
1. Third part of the duodenum
2. Inferior vena cava
3. Transverse colon
4. Right lobe of the liver

248. The normal constrictions of the ureter are found:
1. Where the ureter begins at the junction of the renal pelvis and the ureter
2. Where the ureter passes through the bladder wall
3. Where the ureter crosses the common iliac artery or the pelvic brim
4. Where the ureter passes through the cardinal ligament

249. The superior mesenteric artery:
1. Typically arises from the aorta just inferior to the origin of the gonadal (testicular or ovarian) arteries
2. Supplies the entire duodenum
3. Passes between the pancreas and the second part of the duodenum
4. Supplies the jejunum, appendix, and ascending and transverse portions of the colon

250. Which of the following statements regarding the celiac plexus is/are correct?
1. The sympathetic preganglionic input is provided by the greater and lesser splanchnic nerves.
2. Preganglionic and postganglionic parasympathetic neurons synapse in the celiac ganglia, which are associated with the celiac plexus.
3. The parasympathetic preganglionic input is provided by the vagal trunks.
4. The cell bodies of the visceral afferent neurons that pass through this plexus are found in the celiac ganglia.

251. Parasympathetic fibers that pass through the vagus nerve supply the:
1. Stomach

2. Spleen
3. Ileum
4. Sigmoid colon

252. The celiac nodes receive lymphatic drainage from the:
1. Liver
2. Pancreas
3. Spleen
4. Duodenum

253. In the female pelvis:
1. The ovary is related to the anterior leaflet (layer) of the broad ligament.
2. The suspensory ligament of the ovary transmits the ovarian vessels.
3. The ureter passes superior to the uterine artery at the level of the uterine cervix.
4. The posterior fornix of the vagina is related to the rectouterine pouch (of Douglas).

254. The urinary bladder in the male is:
1. Posterior to the pubic symphysis
2. Anterior to the ampulla of the ductus (vas) deferens
3. Superior to the prostate gland
4. Superior to the seminal vesicles

255. Structures found in the superficial perineal space (pouch) of the male include the:
1. Bulb of the penis
2. Bulbospongiosus muscle
3. Ischiocavernosus muscles
4. Superficial transverse perineus muscle

256. Which of the following statements regarding the pharynx is/are correct?
1. The opening of the auditory tube is located in the lateral wall of the nasopharynx.
2. The soft palate is at the level of separation of the nasopharynx and the oropharynx.
3. The pharynx is continuous with the esophagus at the level of the sixth cervical vertebra.
4. The afferent limb of the gag reflex is cranial nerve X; the efferent limb is cranial nerve IX.

257. Injury of the right mandibular division of the trigeminal nerve as it passes through the foramen ovale could logically produce:
1. Loss of taste on the right anterior two thirds of the tongue
2. Deviation of the soft palate to the left
3. Deviation of the chin to the left when the mouth is opened against resistance
4. Loss of general sensation on the right anterior two thirds of the tongue

258. In the infratemporal fossa:
1. The otic ganglion receives preganglionic parasympathetic fibers from the lesser petrosal nerve.

2. The maxillary artery passes deep to the neck of the mandible.
3. The mandibular division of the trigeminal nerve is deep to the lateral pterygoid muscle.
4. The maxillary artery has branches to the muscles of mastication as well as to the meninges in the middle cranial fossa.

Directions. For each of the following groups of items (259–295) you will be given a series of lettered options. Select the one lettered option that is most closely associated with each item. Each lettered option may be selected once, more than once, or not at all.

Questions 259–263

For each numbered abnormality, select the sign or defect of embryological development that is most closely associated with it.

(a) Elevated levels of alpha fetoprotein in the amniotic sac
(b) Absence of a pleuroperitoneal membrane
(c) Remnant of the yolk (vitelline) stalk
(d) Absence of the dorsal mesogastrium
(e) Absence of a pleuropericardial membrane

259. Umbilical fecal fistula
260. Spina bifida with meningomyelocele
261. Defective spleen development
262. Congenital posterolateral defect of the respiratory diaphragm
263. Absence of the omental bursa (lesser peritoneal sac)

Questions 264–267

For each numbered secretion, select cells from the zones or regions that most likely produce each.

(a) Zona glomerulosa
(b) Zona fasciculata
(c) Zona reticularis
(d) Adrenal medulla
(e) Sertoli cells of seminiferous tubules

264. Epinephrine and norepinephrine
265. Aldosterone
266. Androgen-binding protein
267. Cortisol

Questions 268–271

For each numbered cell, select the characteristic that best characterizes the cell.

(a) Adjacent plasma membranes form small ducts between cells
(b) Basal infoldings of the plasma membrane
(c) Part of the mononuclear phagocyte system
(d) Intracellular or intercellular canaliculi
(e) Canaliculi surrounded by collagen, GAGs, and inorganic salts

268. Parietal cell
269. Cells of striated ducts of salivary glands
270. Kupffer cell
271. Hepatocyte

Questions 272–275

For each numbered group of signs and symptoms, list the artery that, when occluded, would most likely produce it.

(a) Right posterior inferior cerebellar artery
(b) Right posterior cerebral artery
(c) Right anterior cerebral artery
(d) Right superior cerebellar artery
(e) Right anterior spinal artery

272. Paresis in left extremities and paralysis of left lower face
273. Left homonymous hemianopsia
274. Spastic paralysis and numbness of the left lower extremity
275. Spastic paralysis of the left lower extremity and flaccid paralysis of the right upper extremity

Questions 276–279

The numbered signs and symptoms would most likely be the result of damage to which anatomical area?

(a) Right postolivary region of the medulla
(b) Right base of the pons
(c) Right frontal eye field
(d) Hippocampus
(e) Prefrontal lobes

276. Loss of pain and temperature on the left side of the body and right side of the face
277. Loss of conjugate saccadic eye movements to the left
278. Loss of memory
279. Internal strabismus of the right eye

Questions 280–283

For each numbered structure, select the part of the perineum in which it is found.
(a) Deep perineal space

(b) Superficial perineal space
(c) Ischiorectal fossa

280. Pudendal nerve
281. Greater vestibular (Bartholin's) glands
282. Sphincter urethrae muscle
283. Corpus spongiosum

Questions 284–287

For each numbered location, select the nerve that is most vulnerable to injury at that point.

(a) Axillary nerve
(b) Radial nerve
(c) Median nerve
(d) Ulnar nerve

284. Carpal tunnel (canal)
285. Surgical neck of the humerus
286. Supinator muscle
287. Superficial aspect of the wrist—medial side

Questions 288–291

For each numbered region of the skull, select the opening(s) through which it communicates with the orbit.

(a) Anterior and posterior ethmoidal foramina
(b) Inferior orbital fissure
(c) Optic canal
(d) Superior orbital fissure

288. Infratemporal fossa
289. Middle cranial fossa, lateral part
290. Middle cranial fossa, central part
291. Nasal cavity

Questions 292–295

For each of the numbered relationships, select the appropriate organ.

(a) Duodenum, second part
(b) Liver
(c) Left kidney
(d) Spleen

292. Anterior to the stomach
293. Posterior to the tail of the pancreas
294. Lateral (to the right) to the head of the pancreas
295. Posterosuperior to the left colic flexure

1. **b** Meiosis I has just been completed at the time of ovulation. Thus, a secondary oocyte, surrounded by a zona pellucida and corona radiata of follicle cells, ovulates. The dictyotene stage is the arrested stage after the prophase of meiosis I.

2. **d** The duodenum and colon do not have cilia. The uterine tube does not have goblet cells or mucosal or submucosal glands.

3. **c** Zones of calcification and cell hypertrophy of cartilage are characteristic of the epiphyseal plate of endochondral bone formation. Interstitial growth does not occur in the bony matrix. Trabeculae do form in the diploe of flat bones of the skull.

4. **c** Granulopoiesis occurs mostly in red marrow. The promyelocyte of neutrophil development has azurophilic granules; specific granules do not occur until the myelocyte stage. Eosinophilic granules have a lysosomal action and may contain histamine but no heparin; basophils have granules containing heparin and histamine.

5. **c** Primordial follicles possess a simple layer of follicle cells. Glassy membranes are the basement membranes of degenerating follicles. Ovarian follicles are found only in the cortex of the ovary. The theca interna and follicle cells function together in the production of estrogen before ovulation. As the estrogen titer rises, FSH production declines and LH surges.

6. **a** Mineralocorticoid is secreted by the zone glomerulosa. The zone fasciculata and zona reticularis are controlled by ACTH, but the zona glomerulosa is not under pituitary gland control. Cells of the zona fasciculata produce steroids and have much smooth endoplasmic reticulum and lipid inclusions, but not much rough endoplasmic reticulum or secretion granules.

7. **c** Mitrotubules are cytoskeletal organelles and are involved in intracellular transport. Steroid synthesis primarily involves smooth endoplasmic reticulum and mitochondria. Mitochondria arise from existing mitochondria.

8. **a** Brunner's glands of the duodenum are submucosal glands; no other glands of the intestine or stomach are submucosal.

9. **c** Lysosomes in follicular cells of the thyroid gland fuse with endocytotic vesicles of colloid; lysosomal enzymes cleave the thyroxine (T4) and triiodothyronine (T3) from the thyroglobulin. Acido-

phils of the pars distalis and chromaffin cells of the adrenal medulla do not rely on lysosomes for similar cleavage. The function of oxyphils is not known.

10. **c** Myelocytes are characterized as the first cells that possess specific granules. Myeloblasts are early "stem" cells. Promyelocytes have azurophilic granules. Metamyelocytes have specific granules but are not as early as myelocytes.

11. **b** The red blood corpuscle has a life span of about 120 days in the circulating blood. The granulocytes generally have a circulating life span of about 6 to 10 hours.

12. **d** Retrograde degeneration of the axon and myelin occurs only for several internodes. The Schwann cells distal to the lesion site proliferate and form bands of Bungner. Schwann cells phagocytize the degenerating myelin and axons.

13. **c** Secretin promotes secretion by the intercalated ducts and centroacinar cells of a fluid that is rich in bicarbonate. Insulin is produced by beta cells of the islets of Langerhans.

14. **c** All three of the major salivary glands have striated ducts. These ducts and the intercalated ducts are introalobular ducts. The parotid gland secretes only a serous fluid, while the submandibular and sublingual glands are mixed seromucous glands that possess serous acini, mucous alveoli, and serous demilunes.

15. **a** The intercellular "sealing" cement of the stratum corneum is a product of membrane-coating granules. Keratohyaline granules become part of the interfilamentous matrix in the stratum corneum. Macula adherens are localized cell-to-cell junctions that are extremely prominent in the stratum spinosum.

16. **a** The utricle and the saccule are membranous components in the vestibule of the bony labyrinth. The foot plate of the stapes fits in the oval window and is in contact with perilymph of the scala vestibuli. Cristae are located in the ampulla of each semicircular canal.

17. **c** Peyer's patches and the appendix contain aggregations of lymphatic nodules that are covered by simple columnar epithelium. The spleen does not have a stratified epithelium associated with it, nor does it have crypts. The palatine tonsil has crypts lined by a stratified squamous nonkeratinized epithelium.

18. **b** The ciliary body possesses smooth muscle. The occluding junctions between ciliary epithelial cells constitute a barrier between the aqueous humor and the underlying tissues of the ciliary body. Contraction of the circular muscle results in greater convexity of the lens by reduction of the tension on the suspensory zonular ligaments. The ciliary epithelium is involved in the production of aqueous humor.

19. **c** An abundance of smooth endoplasmic reticulum and lipid droplets is characteristic of steroid-secreting cells. Zona fasciculata cells produce steroid glucocorticoid hormones; the acidophils of the anterior pituitary, goblet cells, and chief cells of the parathyroid do not produce steroids.

20. **a** Loose areolar connective tissue is found in superficial fascia and it possesses a viscous ground substance and collagenous, reticular, and elastic fibers. Macrophages are known for their lysosomal activity of phagocytized material. Fibroblasts produce fibers and ground substance.

21. **b** Steroids are produced by cells with much smooth endoplasmic reticulum. Rough endoplasmic reticulum would be characteristic of the synthesis of a proteinaceous secretory product. Phagocytic cells would possess many lysosomes. Cells specialized for conductivity usually have abundant microtubules and rough endoplasmic reticulum.

22. **d** von Ebner's gland, the parotid, and the pancreas are serous-secreting glands. The sublingual gland is a mixed gland with a preponderance of mucous-secreting cells.

23. **a** Monocytes become macrophages. Fibrinogen is produced by hepatocytes.

24. **d** The cells that make up a neuromuscular spindle are called intrafusal fibers. Satellite cells are associated with skeletal muscle fibers and with nerve cell bodies in peripheral ganglia.

25. **c** During contraction the I band shortens, but the A band remains the same length as its myosin myofilaments.

26. **d** Concentric lamellae make up the wall of the osteon. Circumferential lamellae are located at the periphery of the bone.

27. **b** There are no canaliculi in cartilage, since nutrition can take place by diffusion through the matrix. Canaliculi are characteristic of bone tissue.

28. **d** Endothelial cells of liver sinusoids are separated from hepatocytes by the basal lamina–free space of Disse.

29. **b** Venules have thinner walls than arterioles of the same diameter; this is due primarily to the less well-developed tunica media.

30. **d** In the last trimester of pregnancy the fetal capillaries lie adjacent to the syncytial trophoblast and the basal laminae of these two structures fuse in the thinnest portion of the blood–placenta barrier. Thus no fetal connective tissue intervenes between the fetal vessel and the syncytial trophoblast.

31. **c** The cytotrophoblast, as its name implies, develops from the trophoblast. The embryo develops from the inner cell mass.

32. **b** The cornea is colorless and transparent. The endothelial layer does not contain melanin.

33. **c** Although the posterior surface of the iris consists of two layers of epithelial cells, the anterior surface is lined by a discontinuous layer of fibroblasts and pigment cells.

34. **c** Lens fibers are highly differentiated prismatic cells that are derived from epithelial cells of the embryonic lens vesicle.

35. **d** The fovea centralis, where cones predominate, is the site of most acute vision. The optic disk, where no rods and cones exist, is the blind spot.

36. **d** The secretory portions of sweat glands are located deep in the reticular layer of the dermis. The ducts traverse the papillary layer of the dermis to reach the rete pegs of the epidermis.

37. **b** There is no subcapsular sinus in the spleen. The subcapsular sinus receives afferent lymphatic vessels and is a characteristic of lymph nodes.

38. **a** B lymphocytes produce antibodies and are components of the humoral immune response. T lymphocytes initiate cell-mediated cytotoxic immune responses.

39. **d** Otoliths are crystal bodies consisting mostly of calcium carbonate. They are components of the otolithic membrane of the maculae of the utricle and saccule.

40. **c** The fetal part of the placenta is the chorion frondosum, consisting of the chorionic plate and villi. The maternal component of the placenta is the decidua basalis. The decidua parietalis is not part of the placenta, but is a component of the afterbirth.

41. **d** Osteoblasts, chondroblasts, and fibroblasts produce the collagen of bone, cartilage, and connective tissue, respectively. Mast cells produce heparin and histamine.

42. **c** During erection, the smooth muscle in the helicine arteries and trabeculae of the erectile tissue relaxes, thus letting blood flood the lucunae. At the end of erection, the helicine artery smooth muscle contracts, shutting off the blood supply to the lacunae.

43. **b** Rough endoplasmic reticulum is found in the cell bodies and dendrites of neurons, but not in axons or axon hillocks. The Golgi elements are located in the cell bodies of neurons.

44. **c** Growth in length is due to the mitotic division of chondrocytes in the epiphyseal plates (metaphyses). Osteocytes do not divide mitotically, and thus no interstitial growth occurs within bone tissue as it does in cartilage.

45. **c** The stria vascularis lines the lateral wall of the membranous cochlear duct and produces endolymph.

46. **b** Chief cells produce pepsinogen. Hydrochloric acid (HCL) is produced by parietal cells.

47. **c** Taeniae coli are thickenings of the longitudinal muscle of the muscularis externa layer of the colon.

48. **d** There are no striated ducts in the pancreas. Bicarbonate is produced by the intercalated ducts and centroacinar cells of the pancreas.

49. **d** Developing articular surfaces consist of cartilage that is not calcified. Calcified cartilage is usually found where cartilage is being replaced by bone, as in the primary and secondary ossification centers and in the metaphysis.

50. **b** Primary spermatocytes contain 46 chromosomes. When they divide meiotically in meiosis I and become secondary spermatocytes, the number of chromosomes is reduced to 23.

51. **a** The areola of a lactating mammary gland contains pigmented epithelial cells and underlying smooth muscle.

52. **c** Fibrinoid material is characteristic of the third trimester of pregnancy and is usually not present in the first trimester.

53. **c** The steroid cells are Leydig cells, theca interna and membrana granulosa cells of ovarian follicles, and cells of the corpus luteum. Mucosal and submocusal glands of the esophagus, lining cells of the stomach, and goblet cells of the colon secrete mucus. Cilia line the uterine tube and trachea and comprise the kinocilia of crista hair cells. Although glomerular endothelial cells are fenestrated, sinusoids of bone marrow and alveolar capillaries of the lung have no fenestrae.

54. **c** Bile is produced by hepatocytes. Bilirubin is produced by macrophages and is converted to bilirubin glucuronide by the hepatic cells. The gallbladder stores and concentrates bile.

55. **b** Juxtaglomerular cells are components of the wall of the afferent glomerular arteriole where it lies adjacent to the macula densa of the distal tubule of the nephron.

56. **c** Microtubles are made up of rows of tubulin. Some microfilaments are actin myofilaments.

57. **c** The norepinephrine- and epinephrine-secreting cells of the suprarenal medulla develop from neural crest material. Thus they resemble postganglionic sympathetic neurons with respect to their origin, innervation, and secretory products.

58. **c** The function of oxyphil cells of the parathyroid gland is not known. Parafollicular cells produce calcitonin, Leydig cells produce testosterone, and hypothalamic neurosecretory cells produce, for example, antidiuretic hormone.

59. **a** The surface lining of the esophagus is bathed in mucus produced by underlying glands, but does not itself produce mucus. Goblet cells in the lining epithelium of the intestines and the lining epithelial cells of the stomach produce much mucus.

60. **d** The smooth muscle layer of the infundibular region of the uterine tube is much thinner than that of the isthmus, although the lumen of the former is considerably larger than that of the isthmus. Ciliated cells of the uterine tube can come into contact with corona radiata cells of 46 chromosomes that surround secondary oocytes of 23 chromosomes.

61. **a** Coiled (corkscrew-shaped) uterine glands are characteristic of the secretory state of the menstrual cycle. Mitosis occurs and ciliated lining cells are present during the proliferative stage. Basal arteries are present at all stages of the menstrual cycle.

62. **b** The lateral spinothalamic tract is adjacent to the medial lemniscus at pons and mesencephalon levels but is in the postolivary sulcus at medullary levels. First-order neurons are in the dorsal root ganglia. Second-order neurons cross at spinal cord levels. Third-order neurons project to the postcentral gyrus and parietal lobe immediately above the lateral fissure.

63. **c** The posterior spinocerebellar tract is located only at cord levels C1 through L3. It arises from cells in nucleus dorsalis (Clarke's column). This tract and the cuneocerebellar fibers enter the cerebellum via the inferior cerebellar penduncle.

64. **b** The SVE fibers of the facial (VII) nerve originate in the facial motor nucleus. The facial colliculus consists of facial nerve fibers looping over the abducens nucleus. Contralateral upper motor neurons go to all parts of the facial motor nucleus, whereas ipsilateral fibers synapse only with those neurons supplying the upper face.

65. **d** The corneal reflex tests cranial nerves V and VII; the pupillary light reflex tests nerves II and III; and the jaw jerk tests nerve V. The gag reflex tests cranial nerves IX and X; X fibers originate in the nucleus ambiguus.

66. **b** Unilateral lesions of the trigeminal motor nucleus produce ipsilateral paresis. The efferent limb of the corneal reflex originates in the facial motor nucleus. The face is represented in the lateral and lower portions of the precentral gyrus and is supplied by the middle cerebral artery.

67. **c** External strabismus of the right eye is due to destruction of third-nerve fibers, leaving the lateral

rectus muscle supplied by the abducens nerve unopposed. The adjacent corticobulbars, which go to the opposite hypoglossal nucleus, are affected, as are the corticospinals, which end on contralateral anterior horn cells of the spinal cord. Cerebral cortex, basilar pons, and medulla lesions would not affect the right third cranial nerve directly.

68. c The cerebellum and globus pallidus project to brain stem nuclei, which are not motor nuclei of cranial nerves. The ventral lateral nucleus projects to the precentral gyrus. The precentral gyrus may synapse directly on anterior horn cells or motor nuclei of cranial nerves.

69. d A left internal capsule lesion might result in spastic paralysis, but it would be on the right. Such a lesion would spare cerebellar fibers, damage to which alone would cause a right-sided intention tremor. A diminution of pain due to third-order neuron damage in the left internal capsule would occur on the right side. The subthalamic nucleus expresses itself contralaterally, so that hemiballism could occur on the right side.

70. b The supraoptic nucleus produces ADH (vasopressin). Lesions of the ventromedial nucleus produce obesity. The preoptic nucleus is involved in regulation of the release of gonadotropic hormones.

71. a The hypothalamus is the highest subcortical center for the regulation of autonomic activity. Thus, descending fibers from this region will most likely terminate on preganglionic autonomic cell bodies. These are located in nuclei of the general visceral efferent cell column.

72. d The supraoptic nucleus is the primary nucleus producing antidiuretic hormone (ADH), which acts on the collecting tubules of the kidney to facilitate reabsorption of water from the urine. Thus, failure to produce ADH produces diabetes insipidus.

73. b If the postcentral gyrus, left fasciculus cuneatus, or right medial lemniscus within the pons were lesioned, the patient would not feel the texture and shape of an object. This astereognosis is due to damage to the unisensory association areas 5, 7, and 40 in the parietal lobe.

74. a The axons of the lateral spinothalamic tract are located laterally behind the inferior olivary nucleus in the postolivary sulcus. These axons arise from cell bodies in the contralateral posterior gray horn. No damage to contralateral dorsal root ganglia or ipsilateral VPL cells would occur, since it is unlikely that transneuronal degeneration whould take place in this pain pathway.

75. d The paralysis of only one lower extremity rules out transection. Involvement of the posterior and lateral funiculi indicates hemisection; anterior spinal artery and anterior white commissure defects would produce only the pinprick loss.

76. d The limb positions are characteristic of spastic paralysis in which antigravity muscle tone has become predominant. This is indicative of upper motor neuron (corticospinal and medullary reticulospinal or corticoreticular tract) damage. Loss of pain in the left extremities and spasticity in the right extremities indicate that the lesion is in the lateral funiculus, where fibers serving both functions reside. A lesion of the pyramid of the medulla or base of the pons would produce only motor deficits. A lesion of the left internal capsule would result in both motor and sensory deficits on the right.

77. c Thrombosis of the right middle cerebral artery damages the right lateral frontal and parietal lobes, resulting in deficits in motor activity and sensation on the left side. Expressive aphasia is due to lesions of Broca's area in the left frontal lobe.

78. a Neural crest tissue gives rise to postganglionic multipolar parasympathetic neurons in the ganglia of cranial nerves III, VII, IX, and X and to pseudounipolar neurons in the dorsal root ganglia. It gives rise to the peripheral nervous system with the exception of some special sensory neurons (*e.g.*, cranial nerve II).

79. b Vestibular nuclei in the pons and medulla are special somatic afferent nuclei of termination. Cell columns of the brain stem are more discontinuous than those of the spinal cord. There are a maximum of seven functional cell columns. In the brain stem the motor nuclei of origin are medial to the sulcus limitans; in the cord they are in the anterior horn.

80. a In the development of the brain stem, the optic nerve is an outgrowth of the diencephalon. The telencephalon fuses with the diencephalon and gives rise to the globus pallidus.

81. b A left-side lesion of the sensory and motor roots of the trigeminal nerve is expressed on the left side. A loss of consensual blink when the right cornea is stimulated is due to a loss of the left facial nerve (efferent root) or the right trigeminal nerve or spinal nucleus of V.

82. d The larynx and uvula muscles are innervated by the vagus nerve. If the uvula points toward the right, the right uvular muscle is able to contract upon phonation whereas the left uvular muscle is not. Thus, the left vagus or its cell bodies of origin are damaged. These cells are located in the left nucleus ambiguus.

83. d The head is rotated to the left in part by the action of the right sternocleidomastoid muscle, which is innervated by the spinal accessory nerve. This nerve arises from the right anterior horn in the cervical spinal cord.

84. d The inferior cerebellar peduncle contains cuneocerebellar and posterior spinocerebellar fibers from the ipsilateral accessory cuneate and nucleus dorsalis nuclei, respectively. Olivocerebellar axons from the contralateral inferior olivary nucleus also are components of the inferior cerebellar peduncle. The right precentral gyrus sends information to the cerebellum via a pathway that includes the middle cerebellar peduncle.

85. d Only descending fibers of the cerebral peduncle develop from the prosencephalon; the rest of this structure develops in the mesencephalon and at lower brain stem and spinal cord levels. The other three structures are derived from the prosencephalon.

86. b With cessation of rotation to the right, there is past-pointing to the right, a tendency to fall to the right, and a slow component of nystagmus to the right. This is due to an alteration in the normal balance of the frequency of discharge of the left and right cristae ampullares that is produced when endolymph in the left horizontal semicircular canal pushes the microvilli of the hair cells toward the kinocilia and increases the firing frequency of the vestibular nerve.

87. d The facial colliculus is in the tegmentum of the pons and bulges into the fourth ventricle.

88. a The hypoglossal nerve exits from the preolivary sulcus. The hypoglossal nucleus is part of the medially located SE cell column of the medulla, and that portion controlling the genioglossus muscle is supplied only by contralateral upper motor neurons.

89. b Chorea is a basal ganglion disorder. Hypotonia, intention tremor, and asynergia of limbs are due to unilateral neocerebellar lesions.

90. b The dorsomedial nucleus of the thalamus projects to the prefrontal cortex.

91. a The anterior nucleus of the thalamus projects to the cingulate gyrus.

92. c The spinal accessory cell bodies are in the cervical anterior horn cells. The SVE vagal cell bodies are in nucleus ambiguus. GVE and SVE vagal cell bodies develop in the basal plate. The nucleus solitarius develops in the alar plate as a nucleus of termination for afferent GVA and SVA neurons; axons of these neurons stay within the CNS.

93. a First-order neurons for pain synapse on second-order neurons located in the spinal nucleus of V. The principal sensory nucleus of V projects "touch" axons to the ipsilateral and contralateral VPL nucleus of the thalamus. A lesion of incoming pain, temperature, and touch fibers in the trigeminal nerve will result in an ipsilateral anesthesia of the face. The ventral secondary tract of V arises from cell bodies in the contralateral spinal and principal sensory nuclei of V.

94. c Damage to crossing nasal fibers in the optic chiasm results in bitemporal hemianopsia. Homonymous anopsias occur from damage behind the optic chiasm. Fibers from the contralateral nasal and ipsilateral temporal halves of the retina comprise the optic tract; their damage gives a homonymous hemianopsia of the opposite side. Projections from the lower retinal quadrant project to the lingual gyrus; damage to this gives a contralateral upper quadrantic anopsia. Lower retinal projections loop rostrally into the temporal lobe; these represent the upper contralateral quadrant.

95. b The left trochlear nucleus gives rise to axons that form the right trochlear nerve, which intorts the eye when abducted and depresses the eye when adducted. Damage to the abducens nucleus involves cells that go to the ipsilateral lateral rectus and travel through the opposite MLF to stimulate the contralateral oculomotor neurons to the medial rectus muscle. A lesion of the abducens nerve results in internal strabismus due to the unopposed action of the medial rectus muscle. The left frontal eye fields project to the opposite lateral conjugate gaze center and cause saccades to the right when stimulated.

96. c Stimulation of the frontal eye fields produces saccades to the opposite side. The rostral interstitial nucleus of the MLF is the vertical gaze center. The paramedian pontine reticular formation (PPRF) is the lateral conjugate gaze center. The pupillary light reflex involves retinal axons that bypass the lateral geniculate nucleus and course through the brachium of the superior colliculus to synapse in a pretectal nucleus.

97. c The pathway in the near reflex involves lateral geniculate projections to the striate cortex, which in turn projects to the parastriate cortex. Convergence of the eyes is due to contraction of medial rectus muscles supplied by neurons whose cell bodies are in the SE oculomotor nucleus. The Edinger-Westphal nucleus projects to ciliary ganglion neurons, which supply the ciliary and sphincter pupillae muscles, which are needed for accommodation and pupillary constriction, respectively.

98. a The primary receptive area for hearing is in the transverse temporal gyrus. The primary receptive area for two-point touch, vibratory sense, and stereognosis is in the postcentral gyrus.

99. c The middle cerebral artery supplies part of the ipsilateral lenticular nucleus, the motor cortex, and the angular gyrus of the parietal lobe; damage of the latter leads to sensory aphasia. Both the right

and left transverse temporal gyri must be damaged to produce deafness, since projections from each cochlear nucleus are bilateral.

100. **d** Second-order neurons in the nucleus gracilis convey touch and position sense from sacral levels. Axons from these cell bodies make up the ventral portion of the medial lemniscus in the medulla. Ia and Ib fibers from neuromuscular spindles and Golgi tendon organs, respectively, synapse on the nucleus dorsalis; axons from the latter compose the posterior spinocerebellar tract.

101. **b** The motor nuclei of origin arise from the basal plate. Neural ectoderm differentiates into marginal, mantle, and ependymal layers. The roof plates of the diencephalon and telencephalon help form the tela choroidea and choroid plexus of the third and lateral ventricles, respectively. Ventricles occur only in the telencephalon, diencephalon, pons, and upper medulla.

102. **b** There are exaggerated deep tendon reflexes, but the superficial reflexes are lost with an upper motor neuron. Corticospinal tract damage results in a positive Babinski response and a weakness to the distal muscles of the extremity controlling fine movements. The hypertonia is due to accompanying medullary reticulospinal fibers, which ordinarily inhibit antigravity muscle tone.

103. **d** Destruction of alpha motor neurons results in the lower motor neuron syndrome of muscle denervation atrophy; weakness or paralysis, depending on the extent of nerve damage; and loss of superficial reflexes. There are no exaggerated deep tendon reflexes (hyperreflexia), since there is no efferent (motor) limb of the reflex.

104. **c** The lateral (medullary) reticulospinal tract is inhibitory to antigravity muscles. The lateral corticospinal tract is needed for carrying out fine voluntary movements.

105. **a** Schwann cells form the basal laminae needed for neurolemmal tube formation and are essential for myelin formation and phagocytosis of degenerating axons and myelin. Chromatolysis is the result of axon damage and is the dispersal of Nissl (rough ER and free ribosome clusters) in the cell body.

106. **a** A lesion of the base of the pons would destroy corticoreticular fibers regulating the lateral (medullary) reticulospinal tract. This would lead to hyperreflexia of the deep tendon reflexes. Damage to the dorsal root destroys the afferent limb, and damage to the ventral root and anterior gray horn damages the efferent limb of the myotatic reflex; these lesions produce hyporeflexia.

107. **a** The superior salivatory nucleus houses preganglionic neurons that synapse on cells of the submandibular ganglion. Axons from the facial nucleus supply the stapedial muscle. Axons from the geniculate ganglion terminate in the solitary nucleus for taste and in the spinal nucleus of V for exteroception from the posterior ear region.

108. **d** Taste buds from the posterior one third of the tongue arise from the floor of the pharynx at third arch levels. The stapes develops from the second arch. The tongue muscles develop from occipital somites. The tensor veli palatini of the soft palate arises from the first arch and is innervated by the mandibular division of the trigeminal nerve.

109. **c** With both nasomedial processes absent, there could not be a unilateral cleft of the lip; it would be a midline defect involving some of the nasal septum. The palatal defect would be in the primary hard palate. Canine teeth develop from the maxillary process.

110. **c** The pigment epithelium arises from the outer layer of the optic cup; the latter is the indented optic vesicle. The lens fibers and epithelium of the cornea arise from surface ectoderm. The choroid originates from mesenchyme.

111. **c** Since peripheral nerves, autonomic ganglia, and the adrenal medulla are derived from neural crest material, there would be no sensory peripheral neurons or postganglionic autonomic neurons, and there would be reduced epinephrine production. Optic nerves would be present, since they develop from the optic stalk, which is an outgrowth of the diencephalon.

112. **b** The seminal vesicle develops as an outgrowth of the mesonephric duct. The uterus develops directly from the paramesonephric (müllerian) ducts. The nephron develops from metanephrogenic tissue, and the prostate develops from urogenital sinus entoderm.

113. **d** The urethral folds become the labia minora. The primitive streak gives rise to embryonic mesoderm. The arteries of the chorion develop from extraembryonic mesoderm, which develops from the trophoblast. The ostium primum normally disappears when septum primum fuses with the endocardial cushion. The gallbladder develops as an outgrowth of the hepatic diverticulum from the foregut.

114. **a** The fetal component of the placenta develops from the trophoblast. The epidermis develops from ectoderm derived from the inner cell mass. Both the allantois and the yolk sac develop from entoderm.

115. **b** The cricothyroid muscle arises from the fourth pharyngeal arch and is innervated by a nerve of that arch, the external branch of the superior laryngeal off of the vagus nerve. The inferior parathyroid develops from the third pharyngeal pouch, the

tensor tympani muscle from the first pharyngeal arch, and the greater cornua of the hyoid bone from the third pharyngeal arch.

116. **c** The adenohypophysis develops from Rathke's pouch, which evaginates from the stomodeal ectoderm. The neurohypophysis develops from the infundibular outgrowth from the diencephalon. The retina also develops as an optic vesicle outgrowth of the diencephalon. The lens and corneal epithelium develop from surface ectoderm.

117. **c** Intermediate mesoderm gives rise to portions of the urogenital system. Thus, the mesonephric duct arises from intermediate mesoderm. Parietal pericardium and peritoneum originate from somatic mesoderm. Smooth muscle of the gut arises from splanchnic mesoderm. Somatic and splanchnic mesoderm are derived from the lateral mesoderm.

118. **d** A complete fistula opening into the supratonsillar fossil opens internally into the original second pharyngeal pouch. Since the second pharyngeal pouch and branchial cleft are between the second and third arches, the fistula would have to run anterior or rostral to the internal and common carotid arteries, both of which orginate from the third aortic arch in the third branchial arch. The fistula would run rostral to the glossopharyngeal and vagus nerves of the third and fourth branchial arches, respectively. The external openings of branchial fistulas are along the anterior border of the sternocleidomastoid muscle.

119. **a** The nasomedial and maxillary processes fuse to form the upper lip. The nasolateral process fuses with the maxillary process in the region of the nasolacrimal groove. The frontal prominence gets displaced above the fused nasomedial processes and probably gives rise to the bridge of the nose. The upper incisor teeth develop from the nasomedial process; the upper molar teeth arise from the maxillary process.

120. **b** Normally the bulbar septum spirals 180° in its course. If it does not spiral, the ascending aorta will arise from the right ventricle and the pulmonary trunk will arise to the left of the aorta; this constitutes a transposition of the normal vessels. If the bulbar septum forms to one side, there will be a stenosis of one of the vessels. Failure of the bulbar septum to form will produce some form of common truncus. If the right distal sixth aortic arch remains, there will be a ductus arteriosus on the right opening into the right subclavian artery.

121. **c** The portal vein develops mostly from the left vitelline vein, but near the liver it incorporates portions of the right vitelline vein by utilizing several anastomoses between the two vitelline veins. The right umbilical vein disappears; the left

remains as the ligamentum venosum and ligamentum teres of the liver. The ductus venosus develops from new channels that form a shunt through the liver. Supracardinal veins give rise to the azygos system of veins.

122. **d** The right supracardinal vein gives rise to much of the azygos vein; it also utilizes a small proximal portion of the right posterior cardinal vein. The sinus venosus becomes the sinus venarum of the right atrium. The distal right sixth aortic arch normally degenerates. The external carotid artery develops from new channels in the vicinity of the ventral aortic roots.

123. **c** The dorsal mesogastrium gives rise to the greater omentum, and a portion of it fuses with the primitive transverse mesocolon to form the definitive transverse mesocolon. The spleen develops in the dorsal mesogastrium. The dorsal mesentery of the duodenum mostly fuses with the dorsal body wall. The only ventral mesentery of the small intestine becomes the hepatoduodenal ligament of the lesser omentum.

124. **a** All epithelial structures of the larynx, trachea, and bronchi develop from the entodermal respiratory diverticulum (lung bud) of the foregut. There are only three lobar bronchi and three lobes in the right lung. The respiratory diverticulum arises in the fourth embryonic week. The laryngeal opening does close for a short time, but this is due to an epithelial overgrowth that is derived from foregut entoderm.

125. **b** A total absence of the paramesonephric ducts would lead to total absence of the uterus and uterine tubes, and would thus result in amenorrhea. Arcuate uterus and bicornuate uterus indicate improper fusion of paramesonephric ducts in the formation of the fundus and body of the uterus, respectively. Since the uterus develops from the paramesonephric ducts and is present in both of these cases, these abnormalities could not be due to a total absence of the paramesonephric ducts. The vas deferens develops from mesonephric ducts.

126. **b** The incus develops from the mandibular process of the first branchial arch. The posterior belly of the digastric muscle, the styloid process, and the lesser cornua of the hyoid bone all develop from the second branchial arch.

127. **c** The aorta develops from mesoderm. The liver, urinary bladder, and thyroid gland all develop from entoderm. No entoderm would form if there had never been a yolk sac.

128. **d** The greater cornua and body of the hyoid bone develop from the third branchial arch. The soft palate muscles develop from the first and fourth arches. The stylohyoid muscle develops from the

second arch, and a portion of the right subclavian artery develops from the right fourth aortic arch.

129. **c** Pharyngeal muscle is innervated by branches of the glossopharyngeal and vagus nerves, indicating that it develops from mesenchyme of the third and fourth branchial arches. Tongue muscles develop from occipital somites. The ribs develop from the sclerotome of the thoracic somites. The erector spinae muscle develops from the myotomes of multiple somites.

130. **d** The urethrae develop from the entodermal urogenital sinus. The kidney and ureters develop from the ureter bud, which develops as an outgrowth of the mesonephric duct; the kidney also develops from metanephrogenic tissue of the nephrogenic cord. The uterine tubes develop from the paramesonephric ducts. The metanephrogenic tissue and the mesonephric and paramesonephric ducts all arise from intermediate mesoderm.

131. **a** The middle ear cavity develops as an expansion of the first pharyngeal pouch. The otic vesicle gives rise to the membranous labyrinth, which includes the cochlear duct, crista ampullaris, and macula of the utricle.

132. **b** Septum primum is essential for the development of the interatrial septum and the valve of the foramen ovale. The septum membranaceum of the interventricular septum develops from the interbulbar septum and a tubercle of the endocardial cushion. The muscular portion of the interventricular septum develops as cardiac muscle.

133. **d** Postganglionic autonomic neurons develop from neural crest material. The cranial part of the C5 sclerotome contributes to the formation of the C4 vertebra, and the caudal part contributes to the development of the C5 vertebra. The rib primordium of the lumbar vertebra becomes the transverse process. Coelomic epithelium of the genital ridge grows inward to form the Sertoli cells of the testis.

134. **c** The spleen develops from mesoderm of the dorsal mesogastrium. Hepatocytes and islet cells of the pancreas originate as entodermal outgrowths of the foregut. Parafollicular cells arise from the entodermal ultimobranchial body.

135. **c** The ductus arteriosus forms from the distal part of the left sixth aortic arch. The proximal portion of the internal carotid forms from the third aortic arch. The proximal portion of the right subclavian artery develops from the right fourth aortic arch. The proximal portion of the left pulmonary artery develops from the proximal portion of the left sixth aortic arch.

136. **a** Enzymes are released from the acrosome before penetration of the zona pellucida by the spermato-

zoan. A zygote is a fertilized ovum that receives the haploid number of chromosomes from each of the spermatozoan and ovum. Cleavage occurs after a zygote is formed. Penetration of a secondary oocyte by a spermatozoan is essential for the second meiotic division to be completed.

137. **c** The lens develops from a lens placode of general surface ectoderm. The pigment layer and rod and cone layer of the retina, as well as the pigment epithelium of the iris, all develop from the optic vesicle, which originates as an outgrowth of the diencephalon region of the neural tube.

138. **c** The appendix develops from the caudal limb of the midgut. The caudal portion of the duodenum, all but the distal 2 to 3 feet of the ileum, and the entire jejunum arise from the cephalic limb of the midgut.

139. **b** The pleuropericardial fold becomes part of the middle mediastinum. The septum transversum and pleuroperitoneal folds become the central tendon of the diaphragm. The muscle of the diaphragm arises mostly from body wall mesoderm.

140. **d** Skeletal muscles develop from somites, mesenchyme of the pharyngeal pouches, and probably somatic mesoderm. Smooth muscles of the gut wall, the superior mesenteric artery, and the endocardium are all splanchnic structures that develop from splanchnic mesoderm.

141. **d** The foramen ovale develops from the formation of septum secundum. Ostium primum occurs as a temporary foramen between septum primum and the endocardial cushion. Ostium secundum occurs from degeneration of a portion of septum primum. The valve of the foramen ovale is the remains of septum primum after foramen secundum is formed.

142. **b** The superior oblique muscle of the eye develops from eye (preotic) somites. The stylopharyngeus develops from third branchial arch mesenchyme, the tensor tympani from first arch mesenchyme, and the constrictor pharyngeus from fourth arch mesenchyme.

143. **d** Many parts of the scapula are palpable. Exceptions include the superior border (although not always) and the lateral angle.

144. **a** The cubital fossa is defined by the brachioradialis muscle laterally, the pronator teres muscle medially, and an imaginary line interconnecting the medial and lateral humeral epicondyles. The bicipital aponeurosis extends medially from the tendon of the biceps brachii muscle to the investing fascia of the forearm, and passes superficial to the brachial artery and median nerve. The median cubital vein is superficial to the bicipital aponeurosis.

145. d The major muscles responsible for opposition of the thumb are the intrinsic muscles of the thumb, especially the opponens pollicis. The three muscles in the thenar compartment (the flexor pollicis brevis, abductor pollicis brevis, and opponens pollicis) are innervated by the recurrent branch of the median nerve. This nerve branches from the median nerve just distal to the carpal tunnel.

146. c In the palm, the most superficial layer of deep fascia is the palmar aponeurosis. Deeper than that are the digital branches of the median and ulnar nerves, and the superficial palmar arterial arch with its branches; the long digital flexor tendons and the accompanying lumbrical muscles; the deep palmar arterial arch, accompanied by the deep branch of the ulnar nerve; and the metacarpals, with the accompanying interossei muscles.

147. d The superior trunk contains nerve fibers from spinal cord segments C5 and C6 and gives rise to nerves that innervate the intrinsic muscles of the shoulder as well as the anterior compartment of the arm. Loss of the superior trunk results in loss of muscles that abduct and externally rotate the humerus, muscles that flex the forearm, and the major supinator of the forearm, which is the biceps brachii muscle.

148. a The musculocutaneous nerve innervates the muscles (biceps brachii, brachialis, and coracobrachialis) in the anterior compartment of the arm. Loss of these muscles would cause a virtual absence of flexion at the elbow and markedly weakened forearm supination. The supination loss would be most obvious with the forearm flexed because the biceps brachii has the greatest mechanical advantage in that position.

149. c The brachial artery typically bifurcates in the cubital fossa; the radial artery descends through the forearm deep to the brachioradialis muscle. Just proximal to the wrist, the radial artery is just lateral to the tendon of the flexor carpi radialis; it then passes dorsally through the anatomical snuff box toward the first web space, where it passes ventrally between the first and second metacarpals into the palm. In the palm the radial artery gives rise to the deep palmar arterial arch. The superficial palmar arterial arch is formed primarily by the ulnar artery.

150. c The subclavian artery enters the posterior triangle of the neck as it passes through the scalene groove and arches across the lateral aspect of the first rib, it becomes the axillary artery. The subclavian vein is anterior to the subclavian artery throughout its course.

151. a The gluteus medius and minimus muscles occupy the interval between the iliac crest and the greater trochanter of the femur. From a rather wide attachment to the lateral aspect of the iliac wing, the fibers converge toward the greater trochanter of the femur. As a result, contraction of these muscles is best palpated superior to the greater trochanter of the femur.

152. c The ischiofemoral ligament attaches medially to the ischium, which forms the posterior and inferior aspect of the acetabulum. From that point the ligament arches superiorly and laterally above the head or neck of the femur to attach anteriorly to the area of the intertrochanteric line. As the femur is extended, the ligament tightens as it is wrapped around the neck of the femur.

153. b The shoulder has no intra-articular ligament, and the extra-articular ligaments of the shoulder joint provide very limited (if any) support of the joint. The tendons of the rotator cuff muscles blend with the joint capsule of the shoulder and thus provide the major support of the joint. There is no such arrangement in the hip.

154. b Generally, the hamstring muscles extend from the ischial tuberosity to the tibia and fibula and are innervated by the tibial nerve. The exception is the short head of the biceps femoris, which attaches to the femur and is innervated by the common peroneal nerve. Contraction of the hamstring muscles produces hip extension and knee flexion. The major blood supply to the posterior thigh is provided by the perforating branches of the deep femoral artery; there is no posterior femoral artery.

155. c The cruciate ligaments provide the anterioposterior support and the collateral ligaments the mediolateral support. The cruciate ligaments, considered intra-articular in location, are found between the synovial and fibrous portions of the joint capsule. The intercondylar portion of the knee joint is not bathed in synovial fluid; thus, the synovial and fibrous portions of the capsule are not coextensive. The collateral ligaments are very taut when the leg is extended; rotation of the leg is not possible in that position. The menisci are attached to the tibial condyles.

156. c The major segmental innervation of the extensor hallucis longus muscle is in the fifth lumbar spinal nerve; the peripheral innervation is the deep peroneal nerve, which is a branch of the common peroneal nerve. The superficial peroneal nerve innervates the peroneus longus and brevis and most of the skin on the dorsum of the foot.

157. a The gluteus maximus, like many muscles that function in gait, undergoes a lengthening contraction to counteract gravity and thus prevent the antagonistic motion. This muscle is very active at heel strike, preventing flexion at the hip.

158. d After exiting the pelvis through the greater

sciatic foramen and inferior to the piriformis muscle, the sciatic nerve descends about midway between the ischial tuberosity and the greater trochanter of the femur.

159. **d** The superficial peroneal nerve innervates the majority of the skin on the dorsum of the foot as well as the peroneus longus and brevis muscles, the major evertors of the foot.

160. **d** Since the external iliac artery is blocked at its beginning, the alternative flow of blood must connect branches of the internal iliac with branches of the external iliac distal to the obstruction. The superior gluteal and lateral femoral circumflex arteries provide such a connection.

161. **a** The outline of the heart can be projected to the surface of the chest wall by the use of four interconnected points. Each of the first three points is 1 cm to 2 cm from the edge of the sternum and includes the second left costal cartilage, the third right costal cartilage, and the sixth right costal cartilage. Point four is in the fifth intercostal space approximately 8 cm from the midline.

162. **c** The pericardial cavity is between the parietal and visceral layers of serous pericardium, the latter of which is also known as the epicardium. The reflection of the serous pericardium around the great veins bounds the oblique sinus.

163. **d** The neck of the pancreas is at the level of the first lumbar vertebra, and the tail of the pancreas is superior to and to the left of the neck.

164. **a** Although characteristics of the colon, neither the teniae coli nor the epiploic appendices can be visualized by x ray. The haustra, which shape the column of contrast medium, are formed partially by the teniae. The plicae circulares are folds of the small intestine.

165. **d** In addition to supplying the transverse colon, the superior mesenteric artery supplies the ascending colon and most of the small intestine. The inferior mesenteric artery supplies the descending and sigmoid portions of the colon and the upper part of the rectum. The celiac artery supplies the liver, stomach, spleen, pancreas, and proximal portion of the duodenum.

166. **a** The stomach is obliquely oriented, because it extends from the left paravertebral gutter to the right across the midline, and hence is anterior to the vertebral column. The most posterior part is the fundus, the most anterior is the pylorus.

167. **a** The head of the pancreas occupies the concavity formed by the first three parts of the duodenum. The visceral surface of the liver is separated from the pancreas by the stomach; the ascending colon is lateral to the head of the pancreas. The spleen is related to the tail of the pancreas.

168. **c** The plane of the midpelvis is the pelvic plane of least dimensions; its transverse diamater, between the ischial spines, is the smallest diameter of the pelvis.

169. **b** The pudendal nerve arises from the sacral plexus and then exits the pelvis through the greater sciatic foramen. It passes around the ischial spine and through the lesser sciatic foramen into the perineum.

170. **c** The rectum is supplied by the superior, middle, and inferior rectal arteries, which are branches of the inferior mesenteric, internal iliac, and internal pudendal arteries, respectively.

171. **c** The ischiorectal fossa is limited to the perineum and therefore is inferior to the levator ani muscle. Most of this fossa is in the anal triangle, but an extension—the anterior recess—extends into the urogenital triangle superior to the urogenital diaphragm (which contains the deep perineal space).

172. **c** In females the external urethral opening is situated in the vestibule between the clitoris and the vaginal opening. Specifically, it is approximately 1 inch (2.5 cm) posterior to the base of the clitoris.

173. **a** The pelvic splanchnic nerves contain parasympathetic fibers that innervate pelvic viscera as well as the descending colon. The obturator nerve innervates the muscles of the medial thigh as well as cutaneous areas in the distal medial thigh and leg. The posterior and lateral femoral cutaneous nerves innervate the skin of the areas indicated by their names.

174. **d** The isthmus of the thyroid gland is inferior to the cricoid cartilage, which is at the level of the sixth cervical vertebra. The superior and inferior thyroid arteries are branches of the external carotid and subclavian arteries, respectively. The parathyroid glands are related to the posterior aspects of the lateral lobes.

175. **c** Only one muscle, the posterior cricoarytenoid, is capable of abduction of the vocal cords. Both the arytenoid and lateral cricoarytenoid muscles are adductors of the cords; the cricothyroid muscles increase the tension in the vocal cord.

176. **c** The optic nerve does not pass through the posterior cranial fossa. The three other nerves arise from the brain stem in the posterior cranial fossa and are therefore vulnerable to a space-taking lesion in that region.

177. **a** Cranial nerves III, IV, and VI and the internal carotid artery pass through the cavernous sinus, which is lateral to the hypophysis. The optic chiasm and nerves are anterior to the hypophysis. Cranial nerve VIII has an intracranial course that is limited to the posterior cranial fossa and thus is not vulnerable to the tumor described.

178. **d** The inferior sagittal sinus is formed completely within the meningeal layer of dura. It joins the great cerebral vein to form the straight sinus. The falx cerebri separates the two cerebral hemispheres.

179. **d** The ophthalmic artery passes through the optic canal, but the ophthalmic veins are continuous with the cavernous sinus through the superior orbital fissure. Postganglionic parasympathetic fibers from the ciliary ganglion innervate only structures within the eyeball (sphincter pupillae and ciliary muscles). The frontal nerve is a branch of the ophthalmic division of the trigeminal nerve; it innervates skin of the forehead.

180. **c** Independent contraction of the superior oblique muscle produces both abduction and depression. Adduction of the eye virtually negates the superior oblique's ability to produce abduction but maximizes its ability to depress the eye.

181. **b** The nasolacrimal duct opens into the inferior meatus of the nasal cavity. The other sinuses that do not empty into the middle meatus are the posterior ethmoid air cells (superior meatus) and the sphenoid sinus (sphenoethmoidal recess).

182. **a** The genioglossus muscle is innervated by the hypoglossal nerve. The action of this muscle is protrusion of the tongue; protrusion of the tongue is used to test the integrity of the hypoglossal nerve.

183. **b** The auditory tube has bony and cartilaginous portions. The bony portion is posterior, and continuous with the middle ear cavity through the upper aspect of its anterior wall.

184. **c** The nuclei of rods and cones are in the outer nuclear layer. Pigment cells supply vitamin A to the outer segments of the rods and cones, where visual pigments are contained in the membranous discs. The inner layers of the retina are supplied by vessels entering at the optic disk, whereas the outer layers are supplied by capillaries in the choroid layer.

185. **e** The alpha and beta cells of the islets of Langerhans produce glucagon and insulin, respectively. The serous acinar cells produce proteases, amylase, and lipase. Centroacinar cells and the intercalated ducts produce a bicarbonate-rich solution.

186. **b** Perilymph is found in the osseous labyrinth, whereas endolymph is located in the membranous labyrinth. The scala tympani and scala vestibuli are components of the osseous labyrinth and contain perilymph. The cochlear duct and utricle contain endolymph.

187. **c** Smooth endoplasmic reticulum is abundant in the steroid hormone–secreting Leydig and granulosa lutein cells. Basophils of the pars distalis and thyroid follicle cells produce proteinaceous secretions.

188. **e** TSH promotes formation of the lamellipodia, which precede the pinocytotic uptake of colloid by follicle cells. The colloid is broken down by lysosomal enzymes into thyroglobulin, T3, and T4. The free T3 and T4 then cross the basal plasma membrane and enter the fenestrated capillaries.

189. **a** T tubules conduct the electrical signal into the deeper portions of both cardiac and skeletal muscle. Neuromuscular spindles are the receptors for only skeletal muscle. The sarcomere is the contractile unit of skeletal and cardiac muscle. Skeletal, cardiac, and smooth muscle all have actin and myosin.

190. **b** The rectum and lip both contain mucus-secreting cells. The true vocal cord and vagina contain elastic fibers and are lined by stratified squamous epithelium, which is kept moist by glandular secretions from the ventricle and cervix, respectively.

191. **a** There is no parathyroid-stimulating hormone produced by the adenohypophysis. The parathyroid responds to fluctuating levels of calcium in the blood.

192. **e** Arrector pili smooth muscle bundles are associated with hair follicles in the dermis. Pacinian corpuscles are located in the deeper portion of the reticular layer of the dermis. The collagen of the dense fibroelastic connective tissue of the dermis is produced by fibroblasts. Sweat ducts are present.

193. **e** The syncytial trophoblast produces placental progesterone and estrogen, which keep the endometrium a nourishing structure during pregnancy. Hepatocytes produce bile and secrete it into bile canaliculi. Under ACTH stimulation, the zona fasciculata produces cortisol. Theca interna cells of the ovarian follicles produce testosterone or dehydroepiandrosterone, which is converted to estrogen by the granulosa cells of the follicle.

194. **e** Spermatogonia are located in a basal compartment that is separated from an adluminal compartment containing primary and secondary spermatocytes and spermatids. Spermatids, the product of meiosis II, contain 23 chromosomes. The acrosome is a membrane-bound head cap that in essence is a large lysosome. Sertoli cells produce ABP under the stimulation of FSH.

195. **a** Upon depolarization of the muscle membrane by acetylcholine from the motor endplate, the electrical activity passes through T tubules to triads, causing the release of calcium by terminal cisternae. The calcium attaches to troponin, resulting in the uncovering of active sites for the attachment of actin to the cross-bridging heads of myosin. Move-

ment of the cross bridges brings about the movement of actin into the A band, thus shortening the I band.

196. **a** Dust cells move into the alveolar lumen to phagocytize dust particles. The alveolus is lined by simple squamous epithelial type I cells and by surfactant-producing great alveolar type II cells. There are no goblet cells beyond the bronchioles of the conducting portion of the respiratory system.

197. **b** The adenohypophyisis is supplied by a hypophyseal portal system that includes venous trunks between a capillary loop in the pituitary stalk and sinusoid capillaries in the pars distalis. The liver is supplied by a portal vein that empties into the hepatic sinusoids.

198. **c** Lymphocytes enter a lymph node by way of postcapillary venules in the deeper portions of the cortex. They also enter the subcapsular (marginal) sinus through afferent lymphatic vessels. Central and pulp arteries are components of the spleen.

199. **e** FSH is needed for the secretion of androgen-binding protein (ABP), which serves to concentrate testosterone needed for spermatogenesis. LH, efferent ductules, and the seminal vesicle all function as stated.

200. **a** There is a gradient of cell replacement in the small intestine that begins with replacement cells from the intestinal glands that move up the villus to the tip, where old cells are discharged into the intestinal lumen. Since enamel is no longer covered by ameloblasts after the eruption of the tooth, there can be no replacement of enamel. Cells of the stratum germinativum undergo mitosis and replace cells of the stratum corneum of the epidermis that are sloughed off by abrasion. There is no replacement of degenerating neurons by the mitosis of existing neurons.

201. **c** Uriniferous tubules are made up of nephrons and collecting tubules. The collecting tubule is the principal site of ADH action. The nephron is composed only of simple squamous and simple cuboidal epithelia. Sodium is actively transported in the distal tubule. The glomerulus and convoluted parts of the nephron are located in the pars convoluta. The straight portions are in the pars radiata and in the medulla.

202. **e** Pyramidal cells of the pancreas, chief cells of the stomach, and serous parotid cells all produce proteinaceous enzymes. Fibroblasts produce proteoglycans and collagen.

203. **e** The vestibulocochlear nerve emerges from the lateral surface of the brain stem at the pons-medulla junction. The cell bodies of this nerve are located in the vestibular and cochlear ganglia. Axons from the cochlear ganglia synapse on cochlear nuclei, which in turn project fibers bilaterally to the superior olivary nuclei and nuclei of the lateral lemniscus and inferior colliculus.

204. **a** A lesion of the anterior white commissure would result in bilateral loss of pain and temperature in dermatome T4. There would be damage to the preganglionic sympathetic neurons of the intermediolateral cell column. Damage to the lateral spinothalamic tract at T2 to T4 levels would cause contralateral loss of pain from T3 down; crossing pain fibers at the T2 level would ascend to the T1 level before entering the tract. Increased tone due to damage to the lateral reticulospinal tract would not occur because the anterior horn is out.

205. **e** Sensory and motor defects can occur from lesions of the lateral corticospinal, reticulospinal, and spinothalamic tracts of the lateral funiculus; medial lemniscus and pyramids of the medial medulla; corticospinal and thalamocortical projections of the posterior limb of the internal capsule; and medial lemniscus and motor neuclei of the pontine tegmentum.

206. **a** A left cerebral peduncle lesion would damage dentatothalamic fibers from the contralateral neocerebellum. It would produce ptosis by damage to oculomotor fibers to the levator palpebrae superioris muscle, and it would result in external strabismus due to III nerve damage to the medial rectus muscle, thus leaving the lateral rectus muscle unopposed. Since hearing projections are bilateral, there would be only a diminution in hearing in the left ear.

207. **e** A cerebral peduncle lesion would damage pallidorubral, dentatothalamic, corticospinal, corticobulbar, and spinothalamic fibers.

208. **a** The left posterior cerebral artery supplies the left visual receptive area. The left anterior choroidal artery supplies the optic tract. The anterior spinal artery supplies the anteror horn cells of the spinal cord. The left ophthalmic artery supplies the left optic nerve and retina; damage to it leads to blindness in the left eye.

209. **e** Since there is a bilateral pupillary constriction when light is shone in one eye, damage to the left oculomotor nerve would cause loss of the direct response when light was shone in the left eye and loss of the consensual response when light was shone in the right eye. There would be a pupillary dilation due to unopposed action of the sympathetically controlled dilator pupillae muscle when the sphincter pupillae loses its parasympathetic III nerve supply. The ciliary muscle paralysis would also be due to the loss of parasympathetic III nerve fibers.

210. **e** The uncus is a part of the periamygdaloid olfactory primary receptive area. The lingual gyrus and cuneus comprise the visual area; areas 3, 1, and 2 of the postcentral gyrus are for two-point touch and stereognosis; pain fibers project from the VPL nucleus of the thalamus to somesthetic area II.

211. **b** Chromatolysis is a dissolution of Nissl material in the cell body as a result of damage to the neuron. The right medial lemniscus is composed of axons from cell bodies in the left nucleus gracilis and nucleus cuneatus. The pyramid comprises axons from the ipsilateral precentral gyrus. These axons do not cross until the pyramidal decussation at the medulla–spinal cord junction level.

212. **a** Ia fibers from neuromuscular spindles at cervical cord levels ascend in the posterior white column to synapse on the accessory cuneate nucleus. They also synapse on alpha motor neurons in the monosynaptic myotatic reflex (*e.g.,* knee-jerk reflex), and on Clarke's column for the posterior spinocerebellar pathway to the cerebellum. No synapses of any kind occur in the dorsal root ganglia.

213. **e** Nerves VII, IX, and X contain GVE parasympathetic neurons from the superior and inferior salivatory nuclei and dorsal motor nucleus of the vagus. GVA fibers return by these nerves from the major salivary glands and viscera supplied by the vagus. Taste SVA fibers from the tongue and epiglottis are conveyed by these nerves. SVE fibers from the facial motor nucleus and nucleus ambiguus supply, for example, the facial (VII), stylopharyngeus (IX), and pharyngeal (X) muscles.

214. **e** Damage to the tegmentum of the pons would involve the facial motor nucleus supplying ipsilateral facial muscles. Degeneration of axons of the ipsilateral anterior funiculus would occur from damage to cell bodies whose axons comprise the pontine (medial) reticulospinal tract; these fibers descend through the medulla to reach the cord. Damage to the medial lemniscus would result in loss of two-point touch in the contralateral extremities.

215. **d** Since corticobulbar fibers are bilaterally represented to the upper face, damage to only the left cerebral cortex would not prevent the right eye from being closed. Ptosis is due to damage either to the oculomotor nerve supplying levator palpebrae superioris or to sympathetic fibers supplying the superior tarsal muscle. Hyperacusis is usually due to damage to lower motor neurons of the facial nerve. Corticobulbars are crossed only to the facial motor nucleus supplying lower facial muscles; thus, the right corner of the mouth would not be raised during voluntary smiling.

216. **e** Pontine nuclei are part of the corticocerebellar pathway needed for the coordination of movement; the vestibular nuclei and reticulospinal and corticospinal tracts are also concerned with posture and movement. The lateral conjugate gaze center is located in the pontine paramedian reticular formation (PPRF). The spinal nucleus and principal nucleus of V, located in the pontine tegmentum, relay somatic sensory innervation of the face. The motor nuclei of V and VII in the pontine tegmentum innervate masticatory and facial muscles, respectively.

217. **a** The lateral spinothalamic tract is formed of axons that cross the midline at spinal cord levels. Medial lemniscus fibers cross in the decussation of the medial lemniscus at medullary levels. The ventral secondary tract of V arises from the contralateral spinal nucleus of V; its axons cross at medulla and pons levels. The dorsal secondary tract of V arises from the ipsilateral principal sensory nucleus.

218. **a** The most proximal portion of the inferior vena cava develops from a small segment of the right vitelline vein. The right subcardinal vein contributes to that portion that receives the renal veins. The most distal portion of the inferior vena cava develops from the right sacrocardinal vein. The right umbilical vein degenerates in the fetus.

219. **e** The lateral lingual swellings are lined by both ectoderm and entoderm; they form most of the anterior two thirds of the tongue. The root of the tongue is also lined by epithelium derived from entoderm of the floor of the primitive pharynx. Tongue muscle originates from occipital somites.

220. **a** Fetal blood vessels arise in the third week. Cytotrophoblastic cells become incorporated into the syncytial trophoblast. The chorion laeve is the smooth-surfaced chorion that lies adjacent to the decidua capsularis. The stem villi develop from the chorionic plate.

221. **a** The baby would have had trouble hearing, since the stapes would have been absent; blinking, since the orbicularis oculi muscle would have been missing; and smiling, because the facial muscles would have been missing. The muscles of mastication develop from the first branchial arch, so chewing movements would have been possible.

222. **e** Only the uppermost cervical spinal cord segments lie opposite their respectively named vertebrae, and the conus medullaris typically lies opposite the first lumbar vertebrae. The subarachnoid and epidural spaces, the only actual spaces around the spinal cord, contain the cerebrospinal fluid and the internal venous plexus, respectively.

223. **d** At all levels of the vertebral column the intervertebral foramen is formed by pedicles superiorly and inferiorly, by both vertebral bodies and the intervertebral disk anteriorly, and by the zyga-

pophyseal joint (or articular processes) posteriorly. In the cervical and lumbar regions, where the vast majority of herniated intervertebral disks occur, herniation of a disk that involves a single spinal nerve typically affects the nerve that has the same name and number as the vertebrae below the herniated disk.

224. **e** The scalene groove, or triangle, is an opening in the muscular floor of the posterior cervical triangle that transmits the roots (ventral rami) or trunks of the brachial plexus and the subclavian artery. The narrow groove is formed between the anterior and middle scalene muscles and a small segment of the first rib, to which both muscles attach. The more movable attachments of the scalenes are the transverse process of the upper cervical vertebrae. As the head is turned toward the ipsilateral side, the apex of the triangle is moved posteriorly, reducing the anteroposterior dimension of the triangle.

225. **a** The borders of the posterior triangle of the neck—the middle third of the clavicle, the posterior border of the sternocleidomastoid muscle, and the superior border of the trapezius muscle—are all readily palpable. Turning the head to the opposite side and hunching the shoulder make the borders even more obvious.

226. **d** The glenohumeral joint is a ball-and-socket type of joint and thus permits motion in a virtually unlimited number of planes. Full shoulder abduction or flexion (180°), however, necessitates scapular rotation as well as motion at the glenohumeral joint. Although the muscles of the rotator cuff hold the humerus and scapula together, there is none inferior to the joint. The subacromial bursa is superior to the supraspinatus tendon or muscle.

227. **e** On the ventral aspect of the wrist, the medial-to-lateral relationships are the tendon of the flexor carpi ulnaris, ulnar artery, tendons of the flexor digitorum superficialis, tendon of the palmaris longus (if present), median nerve, tendon of the flexor carpi radialis, and radial artery. The ulnar nerve is deep to the tendon of the flexor carpi ulnaris muscle.

228. **a** The ulnar nerve innervates the skin of the medial one and a half digits both dorsally and ventrally; the flexor carpi ulnaris, which helps adduct the wrist; the medial half of the flexor digitorium profundus; the interossei muscles, which abduct and adduct the digits; and the single muscle (adductor pollicis) that adducts the thumb. The branches to these structures or areas arise below the elbow.

229. **b** The carpometacarpal joints of the four medial digits permit very limited motion. The carpometacarpal joint of the thumb, however, permits relatively free motion in the form of the metacarpal

rotation that is necessary for opposition of the thumb. The metacarpophalangeal joints permit abduction and adduction of the digits as well as flexion and extension. Abduction and adduction are relatively free when the proximal phalanx is extended but become increasingly restricted as the proximal phalanx is flexed.

230. **e** The lumbar portion of the plexus is formed within the substance of the psoas major muscle, which is part of the posterior abdominal wall; the sacral portion is in the pelvis on the deep surface of the piriformis muscle. The lumbar portion of the plexus provides muscular and cutaneous branches to the lower abdominal wall.

231. **a** The common peroneal nerve does follow a superficial course through the fossa, but it is laterally placed and follows the tendon of the semitendinosus muscle.

232. **e** Weight is transmitted to the ground through the heads of the metatarsals and the tuberosity of the calcaneus. The major ligamentous support of the longitudinal arch is the medially located spring ligament.

233. **b** The inferior border of the lung is two rib levels above the inferior level of the pleural reflection. Thus, the inferior border of the lung corresponds to the sixth, eighth, and tenth ribs in the midclavicular, midaxillary, and scapular lines, respectively.

234. **a** The synapse between preganglionic and postganglionic sympathetic neurons occurs in the thoracic portion of the sympathetic trunk. Only the lymphatic drainage from the left lung enters the thoracic duct; that from the right lung terminates in the right lymphatic trunk.

235. **c** Both the left atrium and the middle lobe of the right lung would be included in such a cross section. The section would also pass through the junction of the fourth rib with the sternum. The trachea ends at the upper border of the fifth thoracic vertebra, and the left main bronchus branches into its lobar bronci well above the level of this section.

236. **b** The intercostal neurovascular bundle passes along the inferior border of the rib in the upper portion of the intercostal space. The sternal angle is at the level of the second costal cartilage.

237. **a** Typically, the circumflex artery anastomoses with the right coronary artery in the coronary sulcus and the anterior interventricular artery anastomoses with a branch of the right coronary artery in the interventricular sulcus on the diaphragmatic surface of the heart. The left coronary artery passes posterior to the pulmonary trunk.

238. **b** The ligamentum arteriosum interconnects the aortic arch and the left pulmonary artery, and

the thoracic duct is located on the ventral aspect of the thoracic vertebral bodies and posterior to the esophagus.

239. **a** The esophagus is posterior to the left atrium as it passes posterior to the heart.

240. **e** The anterior wall of the inguinal canal is formed entirely by the aponeurosis of the external abdominal oblique muscle; the lateral reinforcement by the internal oblique muscle is variable. The lateral aspect of the posterior wall is formed by the transversalis fascia, and the medial aspect is formed by the conjoined tendon.

241. **b** In addition to being innervated by the lower intercostal nerves, the muscles of the abdominal wall are innervated by the subcostal and iliohypogastric nerves. Contraction of the abdominal muscles produces flexion of the vertebral column and increases intra-abdominal pressure.

242. **b** The lesser peritoneal sac is found between the stomach and lesser omentum anteriorly and the posterior body wall and related structures posteriorly. The retroperitoneal pancreas, left kidney, and left suprarenal gland are posterior boundaries. The lesser sac may extend inferiorly into the greater omentum.

243. **a** The blood supply to the gallbladder is provided by the cystic artery, which is usually a branch of the right hepatic artery.

244. **e** The visceral surface is also related to the stomach, gallbladder, and right suprarenal gland.

245. **c** The common bile duct descends in the free edge of the lesser omentum anterior to the portal vein. It passes posterior to the first part of the duodenum and opens into its second part.

246. **a** The kidneys are more posterior than any abdominal organs and lie against the posterior body wall. The kidney bed is formed by the diaphragm, psoas major muscle, and quadratus lumborum muscle. However, the kidneys lie against the twelfth rib and virtually never extend superiorly to the level of the ninth rib.

247. **c** Like the kidneys, the suprarenal gland is situated against the posterior body wall. The right suprarenal gland is related medially to the inferior vena cava and anteriorly to the right lobe of the liver. Both the third part of the duodenum and the transverse colon are inferior to the right superarenal gland.

248. **a** Although the ureter passes through the cardinal ligament in the female, it is not constricted at that point.

249. **d** The superior mesenteric artery arises from the aorta between the middle suprarenal and renal arteries. The gonadal arteries typically arise inferior to the renal arteries. The superior mesenteric supplies the gastrointestinal tract from the distal part of the duodenum to the splenic flexure of the colon. The artery passes inferior to the pancreas and superior to the third part of the duodenum.

250. **b** The celiac ganglia contain the synapses for sympathetic fibers only. The parasympathetic synapses occur either in or very near the target organs; the visceral afferent cell bodies are located either in vagal ganglia at the base of the skull or in the dorsal root ganglia of spinal nerves.

251. **a** Vagal fibers supply the gastrointestinal tract and associated organs in the abdomen as far distally as the splenic flexure of the large intestine. Since the nerve fibers are distributed by way of periarterial plexuses, there are vagal fibers as far distally as the superior mesenteric plexus. The inferior mesenteric plexus supplies the sigmoid colon.

252. **e** For the most part, lymphatic drainage in the abdomen corresponds to the arterial supply. Therefore, lymph from the organs supplied by the celiac artery will drain through the celiac lymph nodes.

253. **c** The ovarian ligament and the ovary are partially enclosed by the posterior leaflet of the broad ligament, and the ureter passes inferior to the uterine artery at the level of the uterine cervix.

254. **a** Additional posterior relationships include the seminal vesicles, rectum, and rectovesical pouch.

255. **e** The superficial perineal space is limited by the inferior facscia of the urogenital diaphragm and the membranous layer of subcutaneous (Colles') fascia. In addition to the structures indicated, this space contains the crura of the corpora cavernosa and the corpus spongiosum.

256. **a** The sensory limb of the gag reflex is cranial nerve IX; the motor limb is cranial nerve X.

257. **c** The soft palate deviates to the left because of loss of the tensor veli palatini muscle. In addition to the loss of the general sensation on the right anterior two thirds of the tongue, there would also be a loss of general sensation on right lower lip, gums, and teeth. There is no taste loss, because the chorda tympani nerve joins the lingual nerve distal to the foramen ovale. The chin would deviate to the right rather than to the left.

258. **e** The arterial branch of the middle cranial fossa is the middle meningeal artery. The mandibular division of the trigeminal nerve is the deepest structure in the infratemporal fossa.

259. **c** The umbilical fecal fistula is a remnant of the yolk stalk that opens at the umbilical cord.

260. **a** Spina bifida with meningomyelocele is often suspected when there is an elevated level of alpha fetoprotein as detected by amniocentesis.

261. **d** Since the spleen develops in the dorsal meso-

grastrium, there would be defective development of the spleen.

262. **b** Congenital posterolateral defect of the respiratory diaphragm would be due to absence of the pleuroperitoneal membrane contribution to the diaphragm.

263. **d** If the dorsal mesogastrium did not develop, the omental bursa would not have boundaries with the left side of the greater peritoneal cavity. Thus, it would not form.

264. **d** Epinephrine and norepinephrine are produced by the neural crest–derived cells of the adrenal medulla.

265. **a** Aldosterone, which acts on distal convoluted tubules of the kidney, is produced by cells of the zona glomerulosa.

266. **e** Androgen-binding protein is produced by Sertoli cells of the testis. It binds testosterone.

267. **b** Cells of the zona fasciculata produce cortisol. These cells are under the control of ACTH, and they contain much smooth endoplasmic reticulum.

268. **d** Parietal cells produce the ions for Hcl. These ions are assembled into Hcl in the intracellular canaliculi.

269. **d** Cells of the striated ducts of salivary glands reabsorb sodium-utilizing basal striations.

270. **c** Kupffer cells phagocytize red blood cells in the sinusoids of the liver. They are cells of the mononuclear phagocyte system.

271. **a** Hepatocytes form bile canaliculi by the plasma membranes of adjacent cells. The bile canaliculi are separated from the rest of the intercellular space by tight junctions.

272. **b** Paresis in left extremities due to corticospinal damage; paralysis of the left lower face from damage to corticobulbars that supply that portion of the facial nucleus receiving only crossed-fibers. Damage probably in the right cerebral peduncle.

273. **b** Left homonymous hemianopsia from damage to posterior cerebral artery supply to the right cuneus and lingual gyrus of the occipital lobe.

274. **c** Spastic paralysis and numbness of the left lower limb would most likely be from thrombosis of the anterior cerebral artery on the right side, which supplies the paracentral lobule.

275. **e** Spastic paralysis of the left lower extremity and flaccid paralysis of the right upper extremity would indicate upper motor neuron (lateral corticospinals) on the right and lower motor neuron (anterior horn cells) on the right. This is anterior spinal artery damage to lower cervical levels on the right.

276. **a** Loss of pain and temperature on the left side of the body and right side of the face would be due to damage to the spinothalamics and spinal nucleus or tract of V.

277. **c** Loss of conjugate saccadic eye movements to the left would be due to damage to the right frontal eye field.

278. **d** Loss of memory is most likely due to hippocampal damage.

279. **b** Internal strabismus of the right eye is due to damage of the right abducens nerve in the right base of the pons.

280. **c** The pudendal nerve and internal pudendal vessels pass through the pudendal (Alcock's) canal. This canal is formed by the fascia of the obturator internus muscle on the lateral wall of the ischiorectal fossa.

281. **b** The greater vestibular glands, the homologue of the male bulbourethral glands, are found in the superficial perineal space.

282. **a** The muscle of the deep perineal space, in both sexes, is the sphincter urethrae muscle.

283. **b** The corpus spongiosum, which is continuous with the bulb of the penis, is found in the superficial perineal space.

284. **c** The median nerve is the only nerve that passes through the carpal tunnel. The other structures in the tunnel are the tendons of the flexor digitorum superficialis and profundus and flexor pollicis longus, and their synovial sheathes. When pressure in the tunnel increases, the nerve is typically affected the most.

285. **a** The axillary nerve curves horizontally around the posterior aspect of the proximal humerus, the surgical neck of the humerus. The nerve rests on the bone and is vulnerable to injury when the surgical neck is fractured. The radial nerve is related to the midshaft region of the humerus.

286. **b** The deep radial (posterior interosseous) nerve passes through the supinator muscle as the nerve wraps around the neck of the radius. It is vulnerable to injury when the radial neck is fractured or with overuse syndromes of the supinator muscle.

287. **d** The ulnar nerve crosses the medial aspect of the wrist on the medial side. It is superficial and related posteriorly to the strong pisohamate ligament. It is vulnerable to lacerations in that position.

288. **b** The orbit communicates with both the infratemporal and pterygopalatine fossae via the inferior orbital fissure.

289. **d** Cranial nerves III and IV and ophthalmic V and VI pass through the superior orbital fissure to enter the orbit.

290. **c** Both the optic nerve and ophthalmic artery pass through the optic canal.

291. **a** The orbit communicates with both the nasal cavity and ethmoidal air cells via the anterior and posterior ethmoidal foramina.

292. **b** The visceral surface of the liver, predominantly the left lobe, is related to the anterior aspect of the stomach.

293. **c** Even though the pancreas is retroperitoneal, the left kidney is located posterior to its tail.

294. **a** The head of the pancreas occupies the concavity formed by the duodenum; the second part is immediately to the right.

295. **d** The junction of the transverse and descending parts of the colon, the left colic or splenic flexure, typically is related to the anteroinferior aspect of the spleen.

Rypins' Questions & Answers for Basic Sciences Review, Second Edition, edited by Edward D. Frohlich. J. B. Lippincott Company, Philadelphia © 1993.

CHAPTER

3
Physiology

Thomas H. Adair, Ph.D
Professor, Department of Physiology and Biophysics, University of Mississippi Medical Center

Jean-Pierre Montani, M.D.
Associate Professor, Department of Physiology and Biophysics, University of Mississippi School of Medicine

QUESTIONS

Directions. *Choose the best answer.*

1. All of the following have an important role in protein synthesis *except:*
   (a) Ribosomal RNA
   (b) Transfer RNA
   (c) Messenger RNA
   (d) Lysosomes
   (e) Ribosomes

2. The following types of mammalian cells can reproduce other cells of their own type *except* for:
   (a) Capillary endothelial cells
   (b) Red blood cells
   (c) Epithelial cells
   (d) Neurons of the central nervous system
   (e) Red blood cells and CNS neurons

3. Protein molecules enter most cells by which process?
   (a) Phagocytosis
   (b) Opsonization
   (c) Passive diffusion
   (d) Pinocytosis

4. Lysosomes are formed in the:
   (a) Centrioles
   (b) Mitochondria
   (c) Golgi apparatus
   (d) Granular endoplasmic reticulum

5. The formation of proteins on the ribosomes is a process called:
   (a) Transcription
   (b) Translation
   (c) Transduction
   (d) Replication

6. Oxidative phosphorylation occurs in which of the following organelles?
   (a) Lysosome
   (b) Nucleus
   (c) Ribosome
   (d) Mitochondria
   (e) Golgi apparatus

7. The cell membrane is *least* permeable to which of the following?
   (a) Water
   (b) Sodium
   (c) Oxygen
   (d) Ethanol
   (e) Carbon dioxide

8. Which of the following substances use a protein-carrier molecule to traverse the cell membrane?
   (a) Water
   (b) Oxygen
   (c) Glucose
   (d) Alcohol
   (e) Glycerol

9. Transport pathways through cell membranes are highly selective for specific substances *except:*
   (a) Simple diffusion through lipid bilayer
   (b) Simple diffusion through protein channels
   (c) Facilitated diffusion via carrier proteins
   (d) Active transport via carrier proteins

Directions. *For each of the following questions answer:*

(a) if only 1, 2, and 3 are correct
(b) if only 1 and 3 are correct
(c) if only 2 and 4 are correct
(d) if only 4 is correct
(e) if all are correct

10. Pores or throughway channels in the cell membrane:
    1. Can often move laterally within the plane of the membrane
    2. Are limited to the outer layer of the lipid bilayer
    3. Are made of globular proteins
    4. Are impermeable to small hydrophilic molecules

11. The endoplasmic reticulum of the cell:
    1. Often connects with the nuclear membrane
    2. Is involved with protein synthesis
    3. Often has ribosomes attached to the outer surface
    4. Shuttles DNA between the cytoplasm and nucleus

12. Lysosomes:
    1. Contain digestive enzymes
    2. Phagocytize bacteria in many tissues
    3. Participate in the digestion of phagocytized materials
    4. Participate in protein synthesis

Directions. *Choose the best answer.*

Questions 13–15

A normal person weighing 60 kg has an extracellular fluid volume of 12.8 liters, a blood volume of 4.3 liters, a hematocrit of 40%, and 57% of his body weight is water. Answer the following three questions based on this information.

13. The intracellular fluid volume is approximately:
    (a) 17.1 liters
    (b) 19.6 liters
    (c) 21.4 liters
    (d) 23.5 liters
    (e) 25.6 liters

14. The plasma volume is approximately:
    (a) 2.0 liters
    (b) 2.3 liters
    (c) 2.6 liters
    (d) 3.0 liters
    (e) 3.3 liters

15. The interstitial fluid volume is approximately:
    (a) 6.4 liters
    (b) 8.4 liters

(c) 10.2 liters
(d) 11.3 liters
(e) 12.0 liters

Questions 16–25

16. The most important *physiological* function of the lymphatic system is to:
    (a) Transport fluid and proteins away from the interstitium
    (b) Concentrate proteins in the lymph
    (c) Remove particulate materials from the interstitium
    (d) Transport antigenic materials to lymph nodes
    (e) Create negative pressure in the free interstitial fluid

17. Extracellular edema may result from all of the following *except:*
    (a) Increased plasma colloid osmotic pressure
    (b) Lymphatic blockage
    (c) Increased capillary permeability
    (d) Increased capillary pressure
    (e) Increased interstitial fluid colloid osmotic pressure

18. Calculate the *net* pressure difference across the capillary wall given the following conditions:

    Interstitial fluid hydrostatic pressure = –3
    Plasma colloid osmotic pressure = 28 mmHg
    Capillary hydrostatic pressure = 17 mmHg
    Interstitial fluid colloid osmotic pressure = 8 mmHg

    (a) + 1.0 mmHg
    (b) + 0.5 mmHg
    (c) 0 mmHg
    (d) –0.3 mmHg
    (e) –0.5 mmHg

19. Movement across capillary walls of:
    (a) Water occurs mainly by diffusion
    (b) Oxygen occurs mainly by diffusion through membrane pores
    (c) Glucose occurs mainly by pinocytosis
    (d) Proteins occurs to the same extent in all capillary beds
    (e) Lipids is limited to intercellular junctions

20. If the intracellular concentration of a permeable solute is much greater than the extracellular concentration which of the following is *not* true?
    (a) ATP is required to maintain the concentration gradient.
    (b) The solute is transported actively into the cell.
    (c) The solute is sodium.
    (d) The solute diffuses passively out of the cells.

21. Plasma colloid osmotic pressure is greatest when:
    (a) Albumin = 4.5 g/dl; Globulin = 2.5 g/dl; Fibrinogen = 0.3 g/dl
    (b) Albumin = 4.0 g/dl; Globulin = 3.0 g/dl; Fibrinogen = 0.3 g/dl
    (c) Albumin = 5.0 g/dl; Globulin = 2.0 g/dl; Fibrinogen = 0.3 g/dl
    (d) Albumin = 4.5 g/dl; Globulin = 2.0 g/dl; Fibrinogen = 0.8 g/dl
    (e) Albumin = 4.5 g/dl; Globulin = 2.7 g/dl; Fibrinogen = 0.1 g/dl

22. Which of the following changes will *decrease* the rate of diffusion of a substance?
    (a) An increase in the concentration gradient
    (b) An increase in temperature
    (c) An increase in the molecular weight of the substance
    (d) An increase in membrane permeability

23. Which of the following Starling forces tend to move fluid from interstitial spaces into blood capillaries?
    (a) Plasma colloid osmotic pressure
    (b) Capillary hydrostatic pressure
    (c) Subatmospheric interstitial fluid pressure
    (d) Interstitial fluid colloid osmotic pressure

24. Capillary permeability to protein molecules is *highest* in:
    (a) Gut
    (b) Liver
    (c) Brain
    (d) Subcutaneous tissue
    (e) Skeletal muscle

25. Net fluid loss from blood capillaries is attributed mainly to:
    (a) Diffusion
    (b) Filtration
    (c) Absorption

Directions. For each of the following questions answer:

    (a) if only 1, 2, and 3 are correct
    (b) if only 1 and 3 are correct
    (c) if only 2 and 4 are correct
    (d) if only 4 is correct
    (e) if all are correct

26. For lymph to flow, a pressure differential is necessary. This may be contributed to or maintained by:
    1. Muscle contractions
    2. Respiratory movements
    3. Lymphatic valves
    4. Arterial pulsations

27. Increased capillary protein permeability will often cause:
    1. Decreased interstitial fluid protein concentration
    2. Increased lymph flow
    3. Increased capillary pressure
    4. Interstitial edema

28. Which of the following will cause lymph flow to increase?
    1. Increased capillary pressure
    2. Increased permeability of the capillaries
    3. Increased interstitial fluid colloid osmotic pressure
    4. Increased plasma colloid osmotic pressure

Directions. Match the function or disease with the appropriate structure.

    (a) Retina
    (b) Ciliary body
    (c) Choroid plexus
    (d) Arachnoid villi
    (e) Canal of Schlemm

29. Drainage pathway for aqueous humor
30. Production of aqueous humor
31. Absorption of cerebrospinal fluid

Directions. Choose the best answer.

32. Reabsorption of fluid by the renal peritubular capillaries can be increased by:
    (a) Decreased plasma protein concentration
    (b) Decreased efferent arteriolar resistance
    (c) Decreased plasma colloid osmotic pressure
    (d) Efferent arteriolar constriction

33. Glomerular filtration rate can be increased by:
    (a) Increasing arterial blood pressure
    (b) Increasing the plasma protein concentration
    (c) Efferent arteriolar dilation
    (d) Afferent arteriolar constriction

34. The clearance rate for a substance that is freely filtered, but neither secreted nor reabsorbed by the kidney is equal to the:
    (a) Filtration fraction
    (b) Renal plasma flow
    (c) Glomerular filtration rate
    (d) Urinary excretion rate of the substance

35. The plasma clearance of para-aminohippuric acid (PAH) is a measure of renal plasma flow because it is:
    (a) Filtered, reabsorbed, and secreted
    (b) Filtered, but not secreted or reabsorbed
    (c) Filtered and secreted, but not reabsorbed

(d) Filtered and reabsorbed, but not secreted
(e) Secreted and reabsorbed, but not filtered

Questions 36–37

The following test results were obtained on specimens from a person during a 24-hour period:

Urine flow rate: 2.0 ml/min
Urine inulin: 100 mg/100 ml
Plasma inulin: 1.0 mg/100 ml
Urine urea: 220 mmole/liter
Plasma urea: 5 mmole/liter

36. What is the glomerular filtration rate?
(a) 100 ml/min
(b) 125 ml/min
(c) 150 ml/min
(d) 175 ml/min
(e) 200 ml/min
37. What is the urea clearance?
(a) 4.4 ml/min
(b) 22 ml/min
(c) 44 ml/min
(d) 88 ml/min
(e) 440 ml/min

Questions 38–49

38. All of the following are actively reabsorbed from the proximal tubules *except:*
(a) Sodium
(b) Urea
(c) Amino acids
39. Which of the following substances has the lowest rate of reabsorption from the renal tubules?
(a) Urea
(b) Sodium
(c) Glucose
(d) Creatinine
(e) Amino acids
40. Which of the following substances is actively secreted into the renal tubules?
(a) Glucose
(b) Sodium
(c) Chloride
(d) Potassium
(e) Amino acids
41. The acute response to increased extracellular fluid volume involves or is associated with all of the following *except:*
(a) Increased urine osmolarity
(b) Stretch of the two atria
(c) Decreased sympathetic stimulation of kidneys

(d) Decreased secretion of antidiuretic hormone
(e) Increased urine output
42. Increased plasma potassium concentration causes all of the following *except:*
(a) Increased aldosterone release from the adrenal cortex
(b) Increased tubular secretion of potassium
(c) Increased tubular reabsorption of sodium
(d) Increased excretion of potassium in the urine
(e) Decreased plasma sodium concentration
43. A notable effect of ethanol consumption is that it:
(a) Inhibits ADH release
(b) Stimulates ADH release
(c) Inhibits the micturition reflex
(d) Stimulates the micturition reflex
44. Renal compensation for metabolic acidosis involves all of the following *except:*
(a) Increased tubular secretion of hydrogen ions
(b) Activation of the tubular ammonia buffer system
(c) Increased filtration of bicarbonate ions
(d) Increased excretion of hydrogen ions in the urine
45. Respiratory acidosis can be caused by which of the following?
(a) Prolonged diarrhea
(b) Cyanotic heart disease
(c) Ingestion of methanol
(d) Hysterical hyperventilation
(e) Sublethal morphine overdose
46. Respiratory acidosis with metabolic compensation is characterized by which of the following in arterial blood?
(a) Normal Pco_2, low pH, and low HCO_3^-
(b) High Pco_2, normal pH, and high HCO_3^-
(c) High Pco_2, low pH, and normal HCO_3^-
(d) Low Pco_2, normal pH, and high HCO_3^-
(e) Low Pco_2, high pH, and normal HCO_3^-
47. Metabolic acidosis can be caused by which of the following?
(a) Muscular dystrophy
(b) Diabetes mellitus
(c) Hysterical hyperventilation
(d) Prolonged vomiting
48. Metabolic alkalosis can be caused by which of the following?
(a) Exercise
(b) Sublethal morphine overdose
(c) Cyanotic heart disease
(d) Acute hypoxic-hypoxia
(e) Vomiting of gastric contents
49. Metabolic acidosis with respiratory compensation

is characterized by which of the following in arterial blood?

(a) Normal P_{CO_2}, low pH, and low HCO_3^-
(b) Normal P_{CO_2}, normal pH, and low HCo_3^-
(c) Low P_{CO_2}, low pH, and low HCO_3^-
(d) Low P_{CO_2}, low pH, and normal HCO_3^-
(e) Low P_{CO_2}, high pH, and high HCO_3^-

Directions Match the values of pressure listed below with the appropriate hydrostatic and colloid osmotic pressures.

(a) 10 mmHg
(b) 18 mmHg
(c) 28 mmHg
(d) 32 mmHg
(e) 60 mmHg

50. Glomerular capillary pressure
51. Glomerular colloid osmotic pressure
52. Net glomerular filtration pressure
53. Hydrostatic pressure in Bowman's capsule

Directions Choose the best answer.

54. Increased amounts of erythropoietin might be released from the kidney *except* when the:
(a) Arterial PO_2 is normal and the arterial O_2 content is reduced
(b) Arterial PO_2 and arterial O_2 content are reduced
(c) Arterial PO_2 is low and the saturation of hemoglobin with oxygen is much reduced
(d) Tissue PO_2 and renal blood flow are both increased

55. Failure to absorb vitamin B_{12} from the gastrointestinal tract results in a syndrome called:
(a) Pernicious anemia
(b) Hemorrhagic anemia
(c) Polycythemia
(d) Erythremia
(e) Thalassemia

56. The need for vitamin B_{12} and folic acid in the formation of red blood cells is related primarily to their effects on:
(a) Synthesis and release of erythopoietin from the kidney
(b) Absorption of iron from the gut
(c) DNA synthesis in the bone marrow
(d) Hemoglobin formation in the red blood cell

57. Anemia is usually characterized by an increased:
(a) Hematocrit
(b) Blood viscosity
(c) Total peripheral resistance

(d) Exercise performance
(e) Work load on the heart

58. Which condition can lead to anemia characterized by destruction of circulating red blood cells?
(a) Total gastrectomy
(b) Living at high altitude
(c) Bone marrow aplasia
(d) Presence of hemoglobin S

59. Which couple *cannot* be the genetic parents of a child with blood group AB?
(a) Mother AA, father BB
(b) Mother OB, father AA
(c) Mother AB, father OO
(d) Mother OA, father OB
(e) Mother BB, father AB

60. Which of the following substances or cell components can usually be found in a mature red blood cell?
(a) Mitochondria
(b) Ribonucleic acid (RNA)
(c) Adenosine triphosphate (ATP)
(d) Deoxyribonucleic acid (DNA)

61. Which one of the following anticoagulants is preferred by the blood bank for blood storage?
(a) Citrate
(b) Coumarins
(c) Heparin
(d) Oxalate
(e) Anti-vitamin K agents

Directions For each of the following questions answer:

(a) if only 1, 2, and 3 are correct
(b) if only 1 and 3 are correct
(c) if only 2 and 4 are correct
(d) if only 4 is correct
(e) if all are correct

62. In most instances of erythroblastosis fetalis:
1. The fetus is Rh-positive.
2. The mother is Rh-negative.
3. The father is Rh-positive.
4. Many of the fetal red blood cells are nucleated.

63. Anticoagulants that prevent coagulation when placed in a blood sample *outside* the body include:
1. Citrates
2. Oxalate
3. Heparin
4. Coumarins

64. Hemostasis is normally accomplished by or associated with:

1. Polymerization of plasma fibrin molecules
2. Blood coagulation
3. Vascular spasm
4. Formation of a platelet plug

65. Autoimmunity may be involved in the pathogenesis of:
   1. Acute glomerulonephritis
   2. Systemic lupus erythematosus
   3. Myasthenia gravis
   4. Rheumatic heart disease

66. A transfusion reaction may lead to or cause:
   1. Fever
   2. Uremia
   3. Oliguria or anuria
   4. Hemolysis

Directions. For each type of cell listed below, choose the appropriate characteristic or function with which it is usually associated.

(a) Neutrophil
(b) Lymphocyte
(c) Basosphil
(d) Tissue macrophage
(e) Megakaryocyte

67. First line of defense against bacterial invasion from the environment
68. Secretes heparin
69. Fragments from this cell become platelets
70. Produces antibodies

Directions Choose the best answer.

71. The resting membrane potential of a cell is established by or maintained by all of the following *except:*
   (a) The sodium–potassium pump
   (b) Outward movement of sodium ions
   (c) Inward movement of potassium ions
   (d) A net inward movement of positive ions
   (e) Adenosine triphosphate

72. The repolarization of a neuron action potential is associated with all of the following *except:*
   (a) Loss of positive charges from inside the cell
   (b) Outward diffusion of potassium ions
   (c) Return of the membrane potential toward its resting value
   (d) Closure of sodium channels in the cell membrane
   (e) Decreased potassium permeability of the cell membrane

73. Which of the following statements is *not* correct? If the sodium–potassium pump were suddenly poisoned:

(a) The resting membrane potential would become less negative.
(b) No further transmission of nerve impulses could occur.
(c) The intracellular potassium concentration would decrease.
(d) The intracellular sodium concentration would increase.

74. A positive ion will diffuse across a cell membrane:
   (a) Down its electrochemical gradient
   (b) Down its partial pressure gradient
   (c) To the side having greater negativity
   (d) To the side having a lower concentration

75. The sodium–potassium pump is an example of:
   (a) An ion channel
   (b) Vesicular transport
   (c) Facilitated diffusion
   (d) Primary active transport
   (e) Carrier mediated cotransport

76. The threshold for initiation of a neuron action potential is the voltage at which:
   (a) Activation gates close
   (b) Hyperpolarization occurs
   (c) Progressively more sodium channels open
   (d) Acetylcholine is released
   (e) Potassium conductance decreases

77. All of the following substances are found in higher concentrations in the extracellular fluid compared to the intracellular fluid *except:*
   (a) Sodium
   (b) Oxygen
   (c) Potassium
   (d) Calcium

78. Which of the following statements is *not* correct? Release of acetylcholine at the neuromuscular junction:
   (a) Produces an endplate potential
   (b) Increases sodium movement into the muscle fiber
   (c) Always causes the muscle fiber to contract
   (d) Is followed by rapid destruction of acetylcholine

79. In skeletal muscle, the:
   (a) Contraction precedes the action potential.
   (b) Action potential lasts as long as the contraction.
   (c) Action potential lasts longer than the contraction.
   (d) Contraction and action potential begin simultaneously.
   (e) Action potential precedes the contraction.

80. A unique characteristic of smooth muscle is that:
   (a) It can sustain a contraction for prolonged periods.

(b) Calcium is not required for contraction.

(c) Repetitive contractions are not possible.

(d) Myosin filaments are not required.

(e) ATP is required for contraction.

81. A difference between skeletal muscle and cardiac muscle is that:

    (a) Cardiac muscle fibers can hypertrophy.

    (b) Skeletal muscle has shorter action potentials.

    (c) Cardiac muscle requires calcium for contraction.

    (d) Skeletal muscle has actin and myosin filaments.

82. Synaptic vesicles are released at the skeletal muscle neuromuscular junction when:

    (a) The motor endplate hyperpolarizes.

    (b) The skeletal muscle shortens.

    (c) The nerve terminal releases ATP.

    (d) Calcium enters the nerve terminal.

    (e) The motor endplate releases acetylcholine.

83. A difference between skeletal muscle and smooth muscle is that:

    (a) Skeletal muscle fibers are smaller.

    (b) Skeletal muscle fibers can depolarize.

    (c) Smooth muscle fibers lack sarcomeres.

    (d) Smooth muscle fibers lack myosin filaments.

84. After release from the skeletal muscle neuromuscular junction, acetylcholine:

    (a) Enters the sarcoplasmic reticulum

    (b) Causes postsynaptic depolarization

    (c) Suppresses norepinephrine secretion

    (d) Is triggered by acetylcholinesterase

    (e) Activates presynaptic potassium channels

85. The energy for skeletal muscle contraction comes from the:

    (a) Binding of calcium to troponin

    (b) Cleavage of ATP by the myosin head

    (c) Membrane sodium–potassium ATPase pump

    (d) Influx of sodium during the action potential

86. In skeletal muscle, the region near the Z disk is composed mainly of:

    (a) Actin

    (b) Myosin

    (c) Overlapping actin and myosin

87. Which of the following proteins is involved in skeletal muscle contraction but *not* smooth muscle contraction?

    (a) ATPase

    (b) Troponin

    (c) Tropomyosin

    (d) Calmodulin

88. During smooth muscle contraction, calcium ions:

    (a) Bind to troponin

    (b) Do not enter the cell

    (c) Enter the cell from T tubules

    (d) Increase myosin ATPase activity

Directions. *For each of the following questions answer:*

    (a) if only 1, 2, and 3 are correct

    (b) if only 1 and 3 are correct

    (c) if only 2 and 4 are correct

    (d) if only 4 is correct

    (e) if all are correct

89. The strength of contraction of an entire skeletal muscle is dependent on the:

    1. Number of muscle fibers that contract simultaneously

    2. Frequency of contraction of each muscle fiber

    3. Number of active crossbridges in each muscle fiber

    4. Frequency of slow waves

90. The transverse tubules, or T tubules:

    1. Contain intracellular fluid

    2. Conduct depolarizations to the muscle cell interior

    3. Are better developed in thin muscle fibers

    4. Are invaginations of the cell membrane

91. The participation of calcium in the contraction of skeletal muscle is facilitated by or associated with:

    1. Release of calcium from longitudinal tubules

    2. Binding of calcium to the troponin complex

    3. Active transport of calcium into longitudinal tubules

    4. Release of calcium from T tubules

Directions. *Choose the best answer.*

92. The natural rate of rhythmic discharge is greatest in which part of the heart?

    (a) Ventricular myocardium

    (b) Atria

    (c) Sinoatrial node

    (d) Purkinje fibers

    (e) A-V node

93. The velocity of impulse transmission is slowest in the:

    (a) A-V node

    (b) Ventricular myocardium

    (c) Atria

    (d) Purkinje system

    (e) Sinoatrial node

94. Circus movements in the heart can be caused either directly or indirectly by all of the following *except:*

    (a) Increased myocardial conduction velocity

    (b) Decreased myocardial refractory period

    (c) Damage to the Purkinje system

(d) Atrial or ventricular dilation
(e) Chronic mitral stenosis

95. A decrease in the velocity of impulse conduction through the A-V node will usually cause:
(a) The PR interval to increase
(b) The PR interval to decrease
(c) Disappearance of the T wave
(d) Increased heart rate
(e) Atrial fibrillation

96. The rate of conduction of action potentials in Purkinje fibers is about:
(a) 0.2 to 1.1 meters/sec
(b) 1.5 to 4.0 meters/sec
(c) 5.0 to 8.5 meters/sec
(d) 9.0 to 12.5 meters/sec
(e) 15.0 to 18.5 meters/sec

97. The T wave of the normal electrocardiogram is caused by:
(a) Ventricular depolarization
(b) Ventricular repolarization
(c) Atrial repolarization
(d) Atrial depolarization

98. The opening of the A-V valves occurs at about the same time in the cardiac cycle as the:
(a) First heart sound
(b) Beginning of diastole
(c) QRS complex of the electrocardiogram
(d) End of isovolumic contraction

99. A person with a PR interval of 0.23 second indicates:
(a) Atrial flutter
(b) Nothing unusual
(c) Incomplete heart block
(d) Paroxysmal tachycardia

100. The appearance of large QRS complexes between normal beats that are not preceded by P waves indicates:
(a) Atrial flutter
(b) Partial atrioventricular block
(c) Premature ventricular contraction
(d) Increased conduction velocity in Purkinje fibers

101. Which of the following controls the rate of ventricular contraction following complete heart block?
(a) A-V node
(b) An ectopic pacemaker
(c) Internodal pathways
(d) Sinoatrial node

102. A heart murmur that is present during systole suggests:
(a) Aortic stenosis
(b) Mitral stenosis
(c) Aortic insufficiency

103. An ejection fraction of 60% suggests:

(a) Normal ejection
(b) Heart failure
(c) Athletic training

104. Closure of the A-V valves occurs at about the time in the cardiac cycle as the:
(a) First heart sound
(b) Beginning of diastole
(c) End of isovolumic relaxation
(d) T complex in the electrocardiogram

105. Which of the following conditions will often cause an increase in arterial pulse pressure?
(a) Aortic insufficiency
(b) Patent ductus arteriosus
(c) Arteriosclerosis of aorta
(d) Arteriovenous shunt
(e) All of the above

106. In the normal heart, the majority of blood enters the left ventricle:
(a) During early diastole
(b) During isovolumic relaxation
(c) After the aortic valve opens
(d) As a result of atrial contraction

107. Ejection of blood from the left ventricle begins when:
(a) The A-V valves open
(b) The A-V valves close
(c) Left ventricular pressure exceeds left atrial pressure
(d) Left ventricular pressure exceeds aortic pressure

108. Under normal conditions, most of the energy used by cardiac muscle comes from metabolism of:
(a) Lactate
(b) Glucose
(c) Ketoacids
(d) Fatty acids

109. Blood flow through the coronary arteries is markedly attenuated during:
(a) Systole
(b) Diastole
(c) Exercise
(d) Isovolumic relaxation

110. A murmur that occurs throughout systole and diastole indicates:
(a) Aortic stenosis
(b) Aortic regurgitation
(c) Mitral stenosis
(d) Mitral regurgitation
(e) Patent ductus arteriosus

111. The Frank-Starling law of the heart states that:
(a) Cardiac output is controlled entirely by the activity of the heart.
(b) Blood entering the atria is pumped immediately into the ventricles.

(c) The heart can pump a certain amount of blood and no more.

(d) Heart rate controls cardiac output during exercise.

(e) Within physiological limits, the heart pumps all the blood that comes to it.

112. The pressure at one end of an artery is 60 mmHg, the pressure at the other end of the artery is 20 mmHg, and the flow through the artery is 200 ml/min. What is the resistance of the artery expressed in the above units?
    (a) 0.05
    (b) 0.1
    (c) 0.2
    (d) 0.4
    (e) 0.6

113. A resting individual raises a hand and holds it exactly 68 cm above the level of the heart. Arterial pressure at the level of the heart is 100 mmHg. What is the approximate pressure in the larger arteries of the hand?
    (a) 100 mmHg
    (b) 75 mmHg
    (c) 50 mmHg
    (d) 25 mmHg
    (e) 10 mmHg

114. The resistance of a blood vessel is 16 PRU. Doubling the vessel diameter would change the resistance to:
    (a) 10 PRU
    (b) 8 PRU
    (c) 4 PRU
    (d) 2 PRU
    (e) 1 PRU

115. Sympathetic stimulation of which vessels causes the greatest increase in total peripheral resistance?
    (a) Veins
    (b) Venules
    (c) Capillaries
    (d) Arterioles
    (e) Arteries

116. Major blood reservoirs of the body include all of the following *except:*
    (a) Thoracic vena cava
    (b) Liver sinuses
    (c) Major abdominal veins
    (d) Venous plexus of the skin
    (e) Venous sinuses of the spleen

117. Which of the following would *not* be expected to occur during strenuous physical exercise?
    (a) Large increase in pulmonary blood flow
    (b) Large increase in pulmonary arterial pressure
    (c) Large decrease in pulmonary vascular resistance

(d) Pulmonary capillary distention
(e) Pulmonary capillary recruitment

118. Which of the following is most important for mediating angiotensin-induced *long-term* elevation of arterial blood pressure?
    (a) Stimulation of aldosterone secretion
    (b) Constriction of nonrenal peripheral arterioles
    (c) Increased sympathetic stimulation
    (d) Renal effect to decrease sodium and water excretion
    (e) Stimulation of the heart

119. The renal–body fluid volume mechanism for regulating arterial pressure is important for:
    (a) Raising the pressure when a person stands suddenly after having been in a lying position
    (b) Minimizing a decrease in arterial pressure following severe hemorrhage
    (c) Increasing arterial pressure during strenuous physical exercise
    (d) Maintaining arterial pressure at a normal level over a period of weeks, months, or years

120. Which type of heart failure is most likely to be associated with pulmonary edema?
    (a) Heart failure resulting from an arteriovenous fistula
    (b) High cardiac output heart failure
    (c) Left heart failure without right heart failure
    (d) Left heart failure with right heart failure
    (e) Right heart failure without left heart failure

121. Which of the following factors is most important for cardiac output control?
    (a) Metabolic needs of the tissues
    (b) Right atrial pressure
    (c) Mean systemic pressure
    (d) Venous resistance
    (e) Sympathetic nervous system

122. Which of the following factors probably affects myocardial blood flow to the greatest extent under normal conditions?
    (a) Degree of parasympathetic stimulation of coronary vessels
    (b) Rate of release of adenosine from the myocardium
    (c) Degree of sympathetic stimulation of coronary vessels
    (d) Myocardial carbon dioxide concentration
    (e) Rate of release of potassium from the myocardium

123. The most important factor for regulating cerebral blood flow under normal conditions is the:
    (a) Rate of cerebral carbon dioxide formation
    (b) Rate of cerebral oxygen consumption

(c) Degree of sympathetic stimulation of peripheral vasculature
(d) Rate of release of adenosine from the cerebrum
(e) Rate of release of potassium from the cerebrum

124. Which of the following is common to virtually all types of true circulatory shock?
(a) Death occurs regardless of the treatment regimen.
(b) The shock is initiated by hypovolemia.
(c) The tissues fail to receive adequate amounts of nutrients.
(d) A vicious cycle can develop that makes the shock progressively worse.
(e) Both c and d

125. Which of the following types of shock is often associated with an elevated cardiac output?
(a) Septic shock
(b) Neurogenic shock
(c) Traumatic shock
(d) Hemorrhagic shock
(e) Anaphylactic shock

126. Which of the following provides the most powerful mechanism for arterial pressure control at pressures below 60 mmHg?
(a) Baroreceptors
(b) Chemoreceptors
(c) Stress–relaxation
(d) Capillary fluid shift
(e) CNS ischemic response

127. Bulging veins in the neck most likely result from:
(a) Hemolytic anemia
(b) Pulmonary edema
(c) Systemic hypertension
(d) Congestive heart failure
(e) Intermittent claudication

128. An increase in sympathetic stimulation of the peripheral vasculature will most likely:
(a) Decrease venous resistance
(b) Increase venous compliance
(c) Decrease arterial blood flow
(d) Decrease arterial resistance

129. Which of the following types of athletes is most likely to have the highest density of capillaries in the skeletal muscles?
(a) Weight lifter
(b) Sprinter
(c) Marathon runner
(d) Baseball player

130. Which of the following substances causes vasoconstriction?
(a) Adenosine
(b) Angiotensin

(c) Carbon dioxide
(d) Histamine
(e) Hydrogen ion

131. Moderate fluid retention:
(a) Is detrimental in mild heart failure
(b) Is beneficial in mild heart failure
(c) Has no effect in mild heart failure

132. Which of the following vascular beds is vasoconstricted when a person swims?
(a) Coronary
(b) Quadriceps
(c) Kidneys
(d) Brain

133. The maximum rate of oxygen consumption during heavy exercise is limited by the:
(a) Hematocrit
(b) Arterial pH
(c) Tidal volume
(d) Pulmonary ventilation rate
(e) Pumping capacity of the heart

Directions. For each of the following questions answer:

(a) if only 1, 2, and 3 are correct
(b) if only 1 and 3 are correct
(c) if only 2 and 4 are correct
(d) if only 4 is correct
(e) if all are correct

134. Increasing the resistance to fluid filtration through the glomerular membrane for several concurrent weeks would be expected to lead to which of the following in the fully compensated state?
1. Decreased glomerular filtration rate
2. Increased blood volume
3. Decreased sodium and water excretion
4. Increased arterial pressure

135. Hypertension caused by a decreased ability of the kidneys to excrete sodium and water can be caused by which of the following?
1. Pyelonephritis
2. Glomerulonephritis
3. Polycystic kidney disease
4. Arteriosclerotic renal vascular disease

136. The resistance to blood flow varies in direct proportion to the:
1. Length of the blood vessel
2. Hematocrit
3. Blood viscosity
4. Fourth power of the vessel diameter

137. Autoregulation of skeletal muscle blood flow may be mediated to some extent by:
1. Adenosine
2. Carbon dioxide

3. Potassium ions
4. Oxygen availability

138. The increase in skeletal muscle blood flow that occurs during strenuous exercise is caused by or contributed to by:
    1. Sympathetic stimulation of the splanchnic vessels
    2. Increased arterial pressure
    3. Autoregulation of skeletal muscle blood flow
    4. Sympathetic stimulation of skeletal muscle arterioles

139. Cirrhosis of the liver is often associated with which of the following?
    1. Decreased resistance of the portal vasculature
    2. Increased portal venous pressure
    3. Decreased liver lymph flow
    4. Esophageal varicosities

140. Compared with the systemic circulation, the pulmonary circulation is a:
    1. Low-pressure system
    2. Low-flow system
    3. Low-resistance system
    4. High-volume system

141. Increased pressure in the carotid sinus causes:
    1. Reflex slowing of the heart rate
    2. Increased vagal stimulation of the heart
    3. Reflex dilation of the peripheral blood vessels
    4. Increased sympathetic stimulation of the heart

142. A patent ductus arteriosus in the newborn is:
    1. A typical right-to-left shunt
    2. Distinguished by poor oxygenation of the arterial blood
    3. Usually associated with an intraventricular septal defect
    4. An open vessel connecting the aorta to the pulmonary artery

143. Second-degree incomplete heart block is characterized by:
    1. Prolonged PR interval
    2. PR interval of 0.16
    3. More P waves than QRS complexes
    4. More QRS complexes than P waves

Directions. For each type of blood vessel listed below, choose the characteristic with which it is usually associated.

(a) Arteries
(b) Arterioles
(c) Capillaries
(d) Venules
(e) Veins

144. Slowest velocity of blood flow
145. Lowest hydrostatic pressure
146. Least resistance to blood flow
147. Largest surface area

Directions. Choose the best answer.

148. A major function of surfactant is to increase:
    (a) Pulmonary compliance
    (b) Alveolar surface tension
    (c) The work of breathing
    (d) The tendency of the lungs to collapse

149. Muscles of inspiration include which of the following?
    (a) Diaphragm and internal intercostals
    (b) Diaphragm and abdominal muscles
    (c) Abdominal muscles and external intercostals
    (d) Diaphragm and external intercostals
    (e) Internal and external intercostals

150. A swimmer breathing through a snorkel has a respiration rate of 10/min, a tidal volume of 550 ml, and an effective anatomic dead space of 250 ml. What is the alveolar ventilation rate?
    (a) 2,500 ml/min
    (b) 3,000 ml/min
    (c) 3,500 ml/min
    (d) 4,000 ml/min
    (e) 4,500 ml/min

151. Which of the following would cause the greatest increase in alveolar ventilation of the swimmer in Question 150?
    (a) A twofold increase in respiration rate
    (b) A twofold increase in tidal volume
    (c) A twofold increase in respiration rate and a shorter snorkel
    (d) A twofold increase in tidal volume and a shorter snorkel

152. The tidal volume can never become greater than the:
    (a) Anatomic dead space
    (b) Vital capacity
    (c) Functional residual capacity
    (d) Residual volume
    (e) Inspiratory capacity

153. The partial pressure of oxygen in the arterial blood is normally lower than that of the alveolar gas primarily because:
    (a) The lungs use oxygen.
    (b) Blood moves through the lungs too fast.
    (c) Oxygen requires a pressure gradient to diffuse into blood.
    (d) Some portions of the lungs are ventilated but not perfused.
    (e) Some portions of the lungs are perfused but not ventilated.

154. Oxygen tension is *greatest* in which of the following blood vessels?
  (a) Aorta
  (b) Pulmonary artery
  (c) Pulmonary venules
  (d) Coronary artery
  (e) Coronary vein

155. During rest, oxygen tension is *lowest* in which of the following blood vessels?
  (a) Aorta
  (b) Pulmonary artery
  (c) Pulmonary vein
  (d) Coronary artery
  (e) Coronary vein

156. A SCUBA diver at a depth of 66 feet (~20 meters) has a minute respiratory volume of 10 liters per minute. Expressed as a sea level equivalent, the rate of air use from the tank is:
  (a) 5 liters per minute
  (b) 10 liters per minute
  (c) 20 liters per minute
  (d) 30 liters per minute

157. In which of the following conditions would oxygen therapy be *least* beneficial?
  (a) Pneumonia
  (b) Anemia
  (c) Emphysema
  (d) Pulmonary edema

158. The majority of carbon dioxide is carried in the blood as:
  (a) Bicarbonate ions
  (b) Carbonic anhydrase
  (c) CO_2 bound to hemoglobin
  (d) CO_2 bound to plasma proteins
  (e) Dissolved CO_2

Directions. For each of the following questions answer:

  (a) if only 1, 2, and 3 are correct
  (b) if only 1 and 3 are correct
  (c) if only 2 and 4 are correct
  (d) if only 4 is correct
  (e) if all are correct

159. Carbon dioxide is carried in the blood:
  1. As carbamino compounds
  2. As dissolved gas
  3. As bicarbonate
  4. In combination with hemoglobin

160. The Hering-Breuer inflation reflex:
  1. Functions as a protective mechanism
  2. Involves pulmonary stretch receptors
  3. Involves inhibition of the inspiratory center
  4. Protects against underinflation of the lungs

161. Increasing alveolar ventilation about threefold during resting conditions:
  1. Decreases significantly the arterial CO_2 content
  2. Increases the arterial pH
  3. Can lead to dizziness
  4. Increases significantly the arterial O_2 content

162. An abnormally low arterial oxygen tension is often caused by:
  1. Too little hemoglobin in the blood
  2. Obstruction of the respiratory passageways
  3. Decreased hematocrit
  4. Pulmonary edema

163. High-altitude acclimatization may be facilitated by:
  1. Increased production of red blood cells
  2. Increased alveolar ventilation
  3. Growth of new blood vessels
  4. Growth of new skeletal muscle fibers

164. Decompression sickness:
  1. Results from nitrogen bubbles in the body fluids
  2. Can be prevented by rapid decompression
  3. Is characterized by pain and sometimes paralysis
  4. Can occur if one descends a mountain too rapidly

Directions. Match the values of pressure listed below with the appropriate arterial and venous gases.

  (a) 20 mmHg
  (b) 40 mmHg
  (c) 45 mmHg
  (d) 95 mmHg
  (e) 569 mmHg

165. Arterial P_{O_2}
166. Venous P_{CO_2}
167. Arterial P_{CO_2} and venous P_{O_2}

Directions. Choose the best answer.

168. Excitatory synaptic transmitter substances cause which ions preferentially to move through the postsynaptic membrane of a typical neuron?
  (a) Magnesium ions
  (b) Calcium ions
  (c) Potassium ions
  (d) Chloride ions
  (e) Sodium ions

169. What transmitter substance is released by the spinal nerve endings of the neurons whose cell bodies are located in the raphe magnus nucleus?

(a) Endorphin
(b) Substance P
(c) Glycine
(d) Serotonin
(e) Enkephalin

170. What type of neuronal circuit is typified by the nervous control of muscular activity?
(a) Diverging circuit
(b) Converging circuit
(c) Integrative circuit
(d) Reverberating circuit
(e) Parallel circuit

171. The neuronal circuit with the greatest potential for producing a long-lasting output is the:
(a) Diverging circuit with multiple inputs
(b) Converging circuit with multiple outputs
(c) Reverberating circuit
(d) Integrative circuit
(e) Parallel circuit

172. Pushing on the footpads of an animal with a transected spinal cord causes the foot to:
(a) Move anteriorly
(b) Move posteriorly
(c) Be withdrawn
(d) Thrust downward
(e) Move laterally

173. Which sensory system might be more important for maintaining a person's balance when the person is running against the wind compared to when the person is running with the wind?
(a) Vestibular apparatus
(b) Proprioceptors of the neck
(c) Exteroceptive system
(d) Ears
(e) Eyes

174. Damage to which of the following structures is the usual cause of Parkinson's disease?
(a) Subthalamus nucleus
(b) Putamen
(c) Substantia nigra
(d) Globus pallidus
(e) Caudate nucleus

175. Which portion of the brain is most likely to be malfunctioning when the voluntary movements of a person are jerky but there is no tremor when the person is resting?
(a) Cerebellum
(b) Basal ganglia
(c) Hypothalamus
(d) Premotor cortex
(e) Reticular formation

176. Widespread discharge of the sympathetic nervous system will *not* cause:
(a) Dilation of the pupils of the eyes
(b) Increased heart rate
(c) Decreased blood glucose concentration
(d) Increased basal metabolic rate
(e) Increased myocardial contractility

177. The fluid that cushions the brain in the cranium is:
(a) Aqueous humor
(b) Vitreous humor
(c) Intraocular fluid
(d) Cerebrospinal fluid

178. The conduction velocity of the action potential is fastest in which of the following types of axons?
(a) Large diameter, unmyelinated fibers
(b) Large diameter, myelinated fibers
(c) Small diameter, unmyelinated fibers
(d) Small diameter, myelinated fibers

179. From which region of the central nervous system do emotions and complex behaviors arise?
(a) Cerebellum
(b) Spinal cord
(c) Basal ganglia
(d) Limbic system
(e) Reticular activating system

180. Which of the following is a characteristic result of sympathetic stimulation?
(a) Sweating
(b) Pupillary constriction
(c) Slowing of the heart
(d) Increased peristalsis
(e) Fall in blood pressure

181. Smooth muscle cells are innervated by:
(a) Interneurons
(b) Alpha motor neurons
(c) Gamma motor neurons
(d) Postganglionic autonomic neurons
(e) Preganglionic autonomic neurons

182. Which neurons of the autonomic nervous system usually *do not* release acetylcholine?
(a) Preganglionic sympathetic neurons
(b) Postganglionic sympathetic neurons
(c) Preganglionic parasympathetic neurons
(d) Postganglionic parasympathetic neurons

183. At which site does a typical motor neuron receive *most* synapses?
(a) Soma
(b) Dendrites
(c) Axon
(d) Axon hillock
(e) Synaptic terminal

184. When the core temperature is below the hypothalamic set-point temperature,
(a) Sweating occurs.
(b) Pilorelaxation occurs.
(c) Heat production increases.
(d) Blood flow to skin increases.

185. Which of the following is thought to participate in the storage of memories?
    (a) Myelin
    (b) Synapses
    (c) Glial DNA
    (d) Neuronal DNA
    (e) Neuronal RNA

186. Which of the following is consistent with the condition of *retrograde amnesia?*
    (a) A loss of only recent memories
    (b) A loss of only very old memories
    (c) An inability to consolidate memories
    (d) An inability to retrieve stored memories
    (e) An inability to store memories

187. At which site on a motor neuron are action potentials most likely to be initiated?
    (a) Soma
    (b) Dendrites
    (c) Axon
    (d) Axon hillock
    (e) Synaptic terminal

188. Which of the following is a characteristic result of parasympathetic stimulation?
    (a) Dry mouth
    (b) Profuse sweating
    (c) Hypertension
    (d) Slowing of the heart

189. The flexor reflex is integrated in the:
    (a) Thalamus
    (b) Spinal cord
    (c) Reticular formation
    (d) Primary motor cortex

Directions. *For each type of sensory receptor listed below, choose the function with which it is usually associated.*

    (a) Meissner's corpuscle
    (b) Joint receptor
    (c) Pacinian corpuscle
    (d) Golgi tendon apparatus
    (e) Muscle spindle

190. Detects the degree of tension in the muscles
191. Detects the rate of change of muscle length
192. Detects rapid changes in mechanical deformation
193. Responds specifically to light touch

Directions. *For each of the following questions answer:*

    (a) if only 1, 2, and 3 are correct
    (b) if only 1 and 3 are correct
    (c) if only 2 and 4 are correct
    (d) if only 4 is correct
    (e) if all are correct

194. What are some of the modalities of sensation that are detected by free nerve endings?
    1. Crude touch
    2. Pain
    3. Tickle sensations
    4. Itch sensations

195. Stimulation of visceral pain can result from:
    1. Overdistention of tissues
    2. Chemical irritation of tissues
    3. Smooth muscle spasm
    4. Tissue ischemia

196. The macula of the utricle:
    1. Is a type of receptor organ
    2. Is stimulated by movement of the otoliths
    3. Helps maintain equilibrium in the upright position
    4. Is nonfunctional in persons with hearing deficits

197. Damage to Wernicke's area in the dominant hemisphere is likely to make a person unable to:
    1. Hear high-frequency sounds
    2. Perform complex mathematical functions
    3. Read words
    4. Interpret the meaning of a sentence

198. The nerve fibers of the pyramidal tract:
    1. Carry sensory information to the pyramidal cells
    2. Usually synapse with interneurons in the spinal cord
    3. Originate in the cerebellum
    4. Most often cross to the contralateral side

199. Supraspinal motor centers include which of the following?
    1. Brain stem
    2. Cerebellum
    3. Basal ganglia
    4. Motor cortex

200. The sympathetic and parasympathetic nervous systems have opposite effects on the:
    1. Urinary bladder
    2. Gastrointestinal tract
    3. Pupils of the eyes
    4. Heart

Directions. *Choose the best answer.*

201. What is the color of a monochromatic light that stimulates the red cones about twice as much as the green cones?
    (a) Green
    (b) Orange
    (c) Red
    (d) Yellow
    (e) Blue

202. Why is a sudden loud sound more likely to damage the cochlea than a loud sound that develops slowly?
    (a) The basilar fibers are sensitive to sudden sounds but adapt to slowly developing sounds.
    (b) A sudden sound carries more energy.
    (c) The tympanic membrane becomes flaccid as a sound becomes louder.
    (d) There is a latent period before the attenuation reflex can occur.
    (e) The fluid pressure in the scala tympani decreases as a sound becomes louder.

203. Which of the following taste buds help protect against the ingestion of certain plant poisons?
    (a) Sweet taste buds
    (b) Bitter taste buds
    (c) Sour taste buds
    (d) Salt taste buds

Directions. *For each of the following questions answer:*

(a) if only 1, 2, and 3 are correct
(b) if only 1 and 3 are correct
(c) if only 2 and 4 are correct
(d) if only 4 is correct
(e) if all are correct

204. Contraction of the ciliary muscle of the eye:
    1. Reduces tension on the ligaments of the eye
    2. Allows the lens to thicken
    3. Increases the curvature of the lens
    4. Causes the pupil to dilate

205. Which of the following occur(s) during light adaptation?
    1. The quantity of rhodopsin in the rods decreases.
    2. The eyes adapt fully within a few seconds.
    3. The rate of formation of retinal and scotopsin increases.
    4. The pupillary constrictor increases the pupillary aperture.

206. The pupillary light reflex might be abolished by discrete damage to the:
    1. Third cranial nerve
    2. Pretectal nuclei
    3. Optic nerve
    4. Fovea centralis

207. A person is found to have depressed hearing at all frequencies of sound when tested by air conduction but to have normal bone conduction for all frequencies. What are the possible causes of deafness?
    1. Destruction of the cochlea
    2. Fibrosis causing fixation of the ossicles

3. Lesion of the auditory nerve
4. Missing tympanic membrane

208. Visual acuity is greatest in the retinal fovea because:
    1. Only cones are present in the fovea.
    2. Each foveal cone has its own optic nerve fiber.
    3. Blood vessels and ganglion cells do not cover foveal cones.
    4. The fovea has a greater surface area than the surrounding retina.

Directions. *Choose the best answer.*

209. The process of swallowing involves all of the following *except:*
    (a) Closure of the glottis
    (b) Involuntary relaxation of the upper esophageal sphincter
    (c) Involuntary movements of the tongue against the palate
    (d) Esophageal peristalsis
    (e) Transmission of action potentials from the pharyngeal region to the brain stem

210. Peristalsis may be initiated by or affected directly by all of the following *except:*
    (a) Inhibitors of striated muscle contraction
    (b) The myenteric plexus
    (c) Distention of the gut wall
    (d) Irritation of the mucosa
    (e) The composition of the chyme

211. The stomach secretes all of the following *except:*
    (a) Gastrin
    (b) Hydrochloric acid
    (c) Pepsin
    (d) A gastrotrophic hormone
    (e) Chyme

212. Which of the following substances causes the gallbladder to contract?
    (a) Secretin
    (b) Cholecystokinin
    (c) Vasoactive intestinal polypeptide
    (d) Gastrin inhibitory polypeptide

213. Which ion is most closely associated with fluid *secretion?*
    (a) Chloride
    (b) Sodium
    (c) Potassium
    (d) Bicarbonate
    (e) Phosphate

214. Which ion is most closely associated with fluid *absorption?*
    (a) Chloride
    (b) Sodium
    (c) Potassium

(d) Bicarbonate
(e) Phosphate

215. Gallstones are composed mainly of:
(a) Calcium
(b) Lecithin
(c) Bile salts
(d) Cholesterol
(e) Bilirubin

216. The breakdown of complex foodstuffs is accomplished by which of the following chemical reactions?
(a) Reduction
(b) Hydrolysis
(c) Oxidation
(d) Dehydration
(e) Neutralization

217. Complex starches are mainly digested by enzymes secreted from the:
(a) Stomach
(b) Salivary glands
(c) Small intestine
(d) Pancreas
(e) Large intestine

218. Pepsinogen is activated by:
(a) Trypsin
(b) Gastrin
(c) Acid *p*H
(d) Chymotrypsin
(e) Cholecystokinin

219. Which process transports amino acids across the luminal surface of the epithelia that lines the small intestine?
(a) Simple diffusion
(b) Primary active transport
(c) Cotransport with the sodium ion
(d) Cotransport with the chloride ion

Directions. *For each of the following questions answer:*

(a) if only 1, 2, and 3 are correct
(b) if only 1 and 3 are correct
(c) if only 2 and 4 are correct
(d) if only 4 is correct
(e) if all are correct

220. Which of the following statements about cholecystokinin is true?
1. It is released mainly in response to the presence of fat and proteins in the chyme.
2. It stimulates the secretion of pancreatic enzymes.
3. It inhibits gastric emptying.
4. It helps regulate contraction of the gallbladder.

221. The stomach does not digest itself because the:

1. Gastric mucosa is protected by a thick layer of mucus.
2. Gastric mucosal cells are not digestible.
3. Gastric mucosal cells transport hydrogen ions out of the gastric mucosa.
4. Hydrogen ions are completely neutralized by food.

222. Mucus is secreted by the:
1. Stomach
2. Duodenum
3. Ileum
4. Large intestine

223. Secretin functions to:
1. Inhibit gastric acid secretion
2. Inhibit gastric emptying
3. Stimulate the release of pancreatic bicarbonate
4. Stimulate intestinal motility

224. Emptying of the stomach is inhibited by which of the following?
1. Acid chyme in the duodenum
2. Hyperosmolar chyme in the duodenum
3. Irritation of the duodenal mucosa
4. Fatty acids in the chyme of the duodenum

Directions. *Choose the best answer.*

225. The only available mechanism of heat loss from the body when the environmental temperature is greater than the body temperature is:
(a) Radiation
(b) Conduction
(c) Convection
(d) Forced convection
(e) Evaporation

226. When *excess* amounts of carbohydrates or proteins are consumed, they are stored in the body as:
(a) Glucose
(b) Glycogen
(c) Protein
(d) Triglycerides
(e) Cholesterol

227. Stored fat is usually transported from one part of the body to another in the form of:
(a) Triglycerides
(b) Free fatty acids
(c) Glycerol
(d) Neutral fat
(e) Cholesterol

228. The essential amino acids:
(a) Are all found in all dietary proteins
(b) Can be formed in the body
(c) Must be present in the diet
(d) Are necessary to provide adequate amounts of ATP

Directions. *For each of the following questions answer:*

(a) if only 1, 2, and 3 are correct
(b) if only 1 and 3 are correct
(c) if only 2 and 4 are correct
(d) if only 4 is correct
(e) if all are correct

229. When the core temperature of the body falls below the hypothalamic set-point temperature:
1. The blood vessels of the skin constrict.
2. Heat production increases within minutes.
3. The basal metabolic rate increases.
4. The person feels hot.

230. During the course of febrile illness, shivering is usually associated with which of the following?
1. A recent increase in the hypothalamic set-point temperature
2. A recent reduction in the hypothalamic set-point temperature
3. Rising body temperature
4. Falling body temperature

231. When the core temperature of a person increases to 106° F to 108° F (41–42° C):
1. The person may become poikilothermic.
2. The central nervous system may begin to malfunction.
3. Heat production is increased.
4. Sweating may not occur.

232. The final products of carbohydrate digestion include:
1. Glucose
2. Fructose
3. Galactose
4. Sucrose

233. Creatine phosphate is important for intracellular energetics because:
1. It is much more abundant than ATP.
2. It can energize directly all intracellular reactions.
3. It can transfer energy interchangeably with ATP.
4. Enough is stored to support anaerobic metabolism for hours.

Directions. *Choose the best answer.*

234. Blockage of the hypothalamic–hypophyseal venous portal system would be expected to cause increased secretion of:
(a) Growth hormone
(b) Adrenocorticotropic hormone
(c) Thyroid-stimulating hormone
(d) Prolactin
(e) Follicle-stimulating hormone

235. High plasma levels of thyroxine can lead to all of the following *except:*
(a) Increased cardiac output
(b) Increased plasma triglyceride concentration
(c) Increased heart rate
(d) Decreased body weight
(e) Increased metabolic rate

236. Thyroid-stimulating hormone stimulates thyroid function in many ways, but it does *not* increase:
(a) Synthesis of thyroxine-binding globulin
(b) Rate of synthesis of thyroglobulin
(c) Iodine uptake from the blood
(d) Iodination of tyrosine
(e) Size of the thyroid gland

237. Cortisol can cause all of the following *except:*
(a) Inflammation to be suppressed
(b) Fat to be used for energy
(c) Lysosomal membranes to become unstable
(d) The blood glucose concentration to increase
(e) Proteins to be degraded in many tissues

238. Insulin acts directly on all of the following tissues to cause glucose storage with the *exception* of:
(a) Red blood cells
(b) Skeletal muscle
(c) Brain
(d) Liver
(e) Both a and c

239. Growth hormone increases all of the following *except:*
(a) Blood glucose concentration
(b) Blood free fatty acid concentration
(c) Protein synthesis
(d) Storage of proteins in cells
(e) Metabolism of carbohydrates

240. Glucagon:
(a) Is secreted by beta cells of the islets of Langerhans
(b) Helps correct hyperglycemia
(c) Is secreted by alpha cells of the islets of Langerhans
(d) Promotes glycogen storage by the liver
(e) Decreases gluconeogenesis

241. All of the following hormones mediate their major effects without actually entering the target cell *except:*
(a) Cortisol
(b) Insulin
(c) Growth hormone
(d) Glucagon
(e) Parathyroid hormone

242. In Addison's disease, one would expect:
(a) Hypertension
(b) Increased metabolic rate

A N S W E R S

1. **d** The lysosomes contain enzymes that are used by the cell for digestive purposes.

2. **e** The mature red blood cell cannot replicate because it does not have a nucleus. Neurons in the mammalian central nervous system cannot replicate; however, the cell processes can grow back to form new synapses after they have been severed.

3. **d** Pinocytosis means imbibition of liquids by cells. It is a receptor-mediated, energy-requiring process that is especially important for transporting protein molecules through the brush border of the proximal tubular epithelium, where about 30 g of plasma protein are absorbed each day. Phagocytosis means the ingestion of large particles, such as bacteria, cells, and portions of degenerating tissue. Unlike pinocytosis, only certain cells have the capability of phagocytosis.

4. **c** The Golgi apparatus forms lysosomes as well as secretory vesicles that contain especially the protein substances that are to be secreted by the cell. The endoplasmic reticulum and Golgi apparatus are formed primarily of lipid bilayer membranes, and their walls are packed with protein enzymes that catalyze the synthesis of many of the substances required by the cell.

5. **b** Transcription is the process by which genetic information contained in the DNA is transferred to RNA as a complementary sequence of bases.

6. **d** The mitochondria are often called the "powerhouses" of the cell because as much as 95% of the ATP used by a cell is formed in the mitochondria by oxidative phosphorylation.

7. **b** Lipid soluble substances such as oxygen, ethanol, and carbon dioxide can dissolve directly in the lipid bilayer and diffuse rapidly through the cell membrane. Although water is highly insoluble in the membrane lipids, it penetrates the cell membrane very rapidly, moving through the protein channels as well as directly through the lipid bilayer. Charged molecules such as sodium, potassium, and chloride penetrate the lipid bilayer about one million times less rapidly than does water.

8. **c** Glucose and amino acids cross cell membranes by facilitated diffusion, which is also called carrier-mediated diffusion. In the case of glucose, the carrier molecule can also transport several other monosaccharides that have structures similar to glucose, including mannose, galactose, xylose, and arabinose.

9. **a**

10. **b** Globular proteins in the cell membrane are believed to form aqueous channels, or pores, that span the entire lipid bilayer, thus allowing water and other small molecules, mainly ions, to diffuse through the cell membrane. The lipid bilayer is believed to be fluid and thereby to permit the protein pores to move laterally in the plane of the membrane if they are not restrained by interactions with additional proteins in the underlying cytoplasm.

11. **a** The large surface area of the endoplasmic reticulum and the many associated enzymes provide the machinery for many metabolic functions of the cell. The granular endoplasmic reticulum has many ribosomes attached that function in the synthesis of proteins. Electron micrographs show that the internal portion of the endoplasmic reticulum is connected with the space between the two membranes of the double nuclear membrane.

12. **b** The cell phagocytizes bacteria and other particulate substances, and digestive enzymes from lysosomes digest the phagocytized particles.

13. **c** The total body water is equal to 60 kg × 0.57, or 34.2 liters. The intracellular fluid volume is equal to the total body water minus the extracellular fluid volume, or 34.2 − 12.8 = 21.4 liters.

14. **c** Because 60% of the blood volume is plasma (hematocrit = 40%), the plasma volume is equal to 4.3 × 0.6 or 2.6 liters.

15. **c** The interstitial fluid volume is equal to the extracellular fluid volume (12.8 liters) minus the plasma volume (2.6 liters).

16. **a** The lymphatic system performs all of the functions listed as answers, but removal of fluid and proteins (especially proteins) is the most important *physiological* function. In the absence of the lymphatic system, the interstitial fluid protein concentration would increase greatly, causing widespread extracellular edema.

17. **a** Increased plasma colloid osmotic pressure would decrease, at least transiently, the loss of fluid into the interstitial spaces.

18. **c** The net pressure difference across a capillary wall is the transcapillary colloid osmotic pressure gradient minus the transcapillary hydrostatic pressure gradient. Therefore, in the example, (17 + 3) − (28 − 8) = 0 mmHg.

19. **a** Oxygen is lipid soluble and can therefore move

by diffusion through all portions of the lipid capillary wall. Glucose moves primarily through aqueous pores in the capillary wall. The movement of proteins across capillary walls is greatest in liver, where large gaps exist between endothelial cells, and is lowest in brain, where adjacent endothelial cells form very tight junctions.

20. **c** The intracellular sodium concentration is much lower than the extracellular concentration.

21. **c** Colloid osmotic pressure is proportional to the number of protein molecules in solution. The average molecular weights of the proteins are as follows: albumin, 69,000; globulins, 140,000; fibrinogen, 400,000. Therefore, even though all the plasma samples have protein concentrations equal to 7.3 g/dl, the sample with the most albumin has the greatest number of molecules and, therefore, the highest colloid osmotic pressure. Furthermore, the colloid osmotic pressure of C > E > A > D > B.

22. **c** The rate of diffusion of a substance is proportional to the difference in concentration of the diffusing substance between the two sides of the membrane, the pressure difference across the membrane, the temperature of the solution, the permeability of the membrane, and, in the case of ions, the electrical potential difference between the two sides of the membrane.

23. **a** When the interstitial fluid hydrostatic pressure is negative, that is subatmospheric, only the plasma colloid osmotic pressure promotes fluid transfer into blood capillaries. However, during the edematous state the interstitial fluid pressure can become positive, and thus oppose fluid loss from capillaries. Interstitial fluid hydrostatic pressure is thought to be subatmospheric during normal conditions in such tissues as skin, subcutis, skeletal muscle, and lung; positive pressures are virtually always found in brain, kidney, heart, and liver.

24. **b** The liver capillaries have wide gaps between adjacent endothelial cells and a discontinuous basement membrane allowing plasma proteins to move easily back and forth between the blood and interstitial spaces. The relative permeabilities of the different capillary beds to protein molecules are the following: liver > gut > subcutis > skeletal muscle > brain.

25. **b** It is important to distinguish between filtration and diffusion through the capillary wall. Diffusion occurs in both directions, whereas filtration is the net movement of fluid out of the capillaries. The rate of diffusion of water through all the capillary membranes of the entire body is about 240,000 ml/min, whereas the rate of filtration at the arterial ends of all the capillaries is only about 16 ml/min.

26. **e** Any bodily movement that compresses a lymph vessel will cause lymph to flow forward toward the venous system because the lymph vessels contain one-way valves. Also, the lymph vessels have smooth muscle cells in their walls that contract rhythmically, causing lymph to flow.

27. **c** Increased capillary permeability may be associated with bacterial infections, burns, anaphylaxis, and many other pathologic states. When capillary permeability increases, extra amounts of plasma proteins may pour into the interstitium, causing interstitial edema, increased lymph flow, increased interstitial fluid hydrostatic pressure, and increased interstitial fluid colloid osmotic pressure.

28. **a** Factors that promote fluid loss from capillaries cause lymph flow to increase because the lymphatic vascular system transports the extravasated fluid back to the blood vascular system.

29. **e** Aqueous humor produced by the ciliary processes eventually enters the canal of Schlemm, which empties into extraocular veins.

30. **b** Aqueous humor is secreted by the processes of the ciliary body at an average rate of 2 to 3 microliters each minute. The epithelium of the ciliary processes is believed to secrete sodium, chloride, and bicarbonate into the spaces between the cells. In turn, the ions cause osmosis of water into these spaces, and the fluid then moves out of the spaces and onto the surfaces of the ciliary processes.

31. **d** The endothelial cells covering the arachnoid villi have large vesicular pores directly through the bodies of the cells. Cerebrospinal fluid, protein molecules, and even red blood cells move through these pores and into the venous blood.

32. **d** Constriction of the efferent arterioles increases the efferent arteriolar resistance; this decreases peritubular capillary pressure, allowing greater amounts of fluid to be reabsorbed by the peritubular capillaries. Decreasing the plasma colloid osmotic pressure or protein concentration would decrease reabsorption of fluid.

33. **a** Increasing arterial blood pressure will cause glomerular capillary pressure to increase slightly, thus causing a slight increase in glomerular filtration rate. Efferent arteriolar dilation and afferent arteriolar constriction both tend to decrease glomerular capillary pressure.

34. **c** If a substance passes through the glomerular membrane with perfect ease, the glomerular filtrate contains virtually the same concentration of the substance as does the plasma, and if the substance is neither secreted nor reabsorbed by the tubules, all of the filtered substance continues on into the urine. Therefore, the plasma clearance of the substance is equal to the glomerular filtration rate.

Inulin clearance is commonly used as a measure of glomerular filtration rate because it is freely filtered, but neither secreted nor reabsorbed by the kidney tubules.

35. **c** Para-aminohippuric acid (PAH), like inulin, passes freely through the glomerular membrane. However, most of the PAH remaining in the plasma is then secreted into the tubules by the proximal tubular epithelium. Because about 90% of the PAH is removed from the plasma during a single pass through the kidneys, the plasma clearance of PAH is a measure of the plasma flow through the kidneys.

36. **e** The glomerular filtration rate is equal to the inulin clearance because inulin, a low-molecular-weight polysaccharide, is filtered freely into Bowman's capsule but is not reabsorbed or secreted. The clearance (C) of any substance can be calculated as follows: $C = (U \times V)/P$, where U and P are the urine and plasma concentrations of the substance, respectively, and V is the urine flow rate. Thus, glomerular filtration rate = $(1.0 \times 2.0)/0.01 = 200$ ml/min.

37. **d** Urea clearance = $(0.220 \times 2.0)/0.005 = 88$ ml/min.

38. **b** Active reabsorption of solute in the proximal tubule creates an osmotic gradient for passive reabsorption of water. This reabsorption of water increases the tubular concentration of any solute not being reabsorbed as fast as the water. In turn, the concentration of urea in the tubular fluid becomes greater than that of the peritubular fluid, and small amounts of urea then diffuse passively down the concentration gradient into the peritubular fluid.

39. **d** Only small amounts of urea are reabsorbed and no creatinine is reabsorbed during transit through the tubules even though more than 99% of the water is reabsorbed. Therefore, creatinine and urea, as well as uric acid and other end products of metabolism, are highly concentrated in the urine.

40. **d** The epithelial cells of the late distal tubules and cortical collecting ducts have the unique capability of secreting large amounts of potassium into the tubular fluid.

41. **a** Decreased antidiuretic hormone causes decreased reabsorption of water from the collecting ducts, and this decreases the osmolarity of the urine.

42. **e** Although aldosterone increases the *quantity* of sodium in the extracellular fluid, the increased reabsorption of water along with the sodium usually prevents the sodium concentration from rising more than a few milliequivalents.

43. **a** Alcohol causes diuresis by inhibiting the secretion of antidiuretic hormone from the posterior pituitary gland.

44. **c** Less than normal amounts of bicarbonate ions are filtered during metabolic acidosis because the plasma bicarbonate ion concentration is lower than normal. This decreased filtration of bicarbonate ions is an important component of the renal compensation for metabolic acidosis.

45. **e** Any factor that decreases the rate of pulmonary ventilation increases the concentration of dissolved carbon dioxide in the extracellular fluid. Increases in dissolved carbon dioxide lead to increased carbonic acid and hydrogen ions, thus resulting in acidosis.

46. **b** If a person develops respiratory acidosis that lasts for a long time, the kidneys will secrete an excess of hydrogen ions, resulting in an increase in sodium bicarbonate in the extracellular fluids.

47. **b** In untreated diabetes mellitus, there is an excess of free fatty acids in the plasma because of increased hydrolysis of stored triglycerides, which leads to an increased hepatic oxidation of fatty acids and thus the formation of acetoacetic acid. The concentration of this acid often rises very high and causes severe acidosis.

48. **e** Vomiting of the gastric contents alone would obviously cause loss of acid because the stomach secretions are highly acidic. However, vomiting of contents from deeper in the gastrointestinal tract can lead to loss of alkaline contents and result in acidosis.

49. **c** The high hydrogen ion concentration in metabolic acidosis causes increased pulmonary ventilation, which removes carbon dioxide from the body fluids and leads to a reduction in the hydrogen ion concentration. However, the respiratory system cannot fully compensate for metabolic acidosis; thus respiratory compensation is characterized by low levels of carbon dioxide and sodium bicarbonate as well as low *p*H in the extracellular fluids.

50. **e** The glomerular capillary pressure (60 mmHg) is much higher than capillary pressure elsewhere in the body. This is possible because the glomerulus has an efferent arteriole that is partially constricted most of the time.

51. **d** Although the plasma colloid osmotic pressure averages about 28 mmHg in most tissues of the body, it is slightly greater (32 mmHg) in the glomerular capillaries because large amounts of fluid are filtered continuously into Bowman's capsule, and this concentrates the proteins in the plasma.

52. **a** The net glomerular filtration pressure is $60 - 32 - 18 = 10$ mmHg.

53. **b** The hydrostatic pressure in Bowman's capsule has been measured directly using glass micropipettes.

54. **d** Any condition that sufficiently decreases the

renal microvascular or tissue Po_2 will cause increased amounts of erythropoietin to be released from the kidneys. Such conditions include anemia and carbon monoxide poisoning, in which arterial Po_2 is normal and arterial O_2 content is reduced; hypoxemia, in which the hemoglobin is not fully saturated and arterial Po_2 and arterial O_2 content are low; and others.

55. **a** Pernicious anemia is caused by a vitamin B_{12} deficiency. This usually results from a failure to absorb vitamin B_{12} from the gastrointestinal tract, rather than from lack of vitamin B_{12} in the diet.

56. **c** Both vitamin B_{12} and folic acid are required for DNA synthesis in all cells, and because tissues producing red blood cells grow more rapidly than most other tissues, deficiencies in these vitamins inhibit especially the rate of production of red blood cells.

57. **e** In anemia, the total peripheral resistance is decreased by two factors: a reduced viscosity of the blood and vasodilation resulting from decreased oxygenation of the tissues. The increase in cardiac output caused by the decrease in peripheral resistance can provide the tissues with adequate amounts of oxygen during resting conditions; however, when an anemic person begins to exercise, the heart may not be capable of pumping the extra amounts of blood needed by the tissues.

58. **d** Hemoglobin S is an abnormal type of hemoglobin, caused by abnormal composition of the beta chains. When hemoglobin S is exposed to low concentrations of oxygen, it precipitates into long crystals inside the red blood cell, causing the cell to be shaped like a sickle rather than a biconcave disk. The red blood cells become very fragile so that they rupture during passage through the microcirculation, especially in the spleen. The life span of the cells is so short that serious anemia results, and the condition is called sickle-cell anemia.

59. **c** The O-A-B blood groups are determined by two genes, one on each pair of chromosomes. Because one gene comes from each parent, a mother with blood group AB and father with blood group OO can produce offspring with blood groups OB or OA, but not AB.

60. **c** Mature red blood cells of mammals do not have a nucleus, mitochondria, or endoplasmic reticulum; however, they do contain enzymes that are capable of metabolizing glucose and forming small amounts of adenosine triphosphate (ATP) that serve the red blood cells in several important ways.

61. **a** The citrate ion combines with calcium in the blood to form an un-ionized calcium compound. The lack of ionic calcium prevents coagulation. Following a single transfusion, the citrate ion is removed from the blood within a few minutes by the liver without any dire consequences. Oxalate anticoagulants work in a similar manner, but oxalate is toxic to the body.

62. **e** In most instances of erythroblastosis fetalis the mother is Rh-negative, and the father is Rh-positive. The baby has inherited the Rh-positive characteristic from the father, and the mother has developed anti-Rh agglutinins that have diffused through the placenta into the fetus to cause red-blood-cell agglutination. Erythroblasts are nucleated erythrocytes.

63. **a** A coumarin, such as Warfarin, will not prevent coagulation of a blood sample outside the body, but it does prevent coagulation of blood in the body. Warfarin causes this effect by competing with vitamin K for reactive sites in the enzymatic processes for formation of prothrombin as well as Factors VII, IX, and X in the liver.

64. **e** When a vessel is severed, the wall of the vessel contracts or spasms immediately, and this decreases the loss of blood from the injured vessel.

65. **e**

66. **e** A transfusion reaction usually causes hemolysis with release of large amounts of hemoglobin into the plasma. Because the hemoglobin can enter the renal tubules through the normal glomerular membrane, the tubular load of hemoglobin increases greatly. When the tubular load of hemoglobin surpasses the reabsorption capabilities of the proximal tubules, the excess hemoglobin often precipitates in the nephron, causing oliguria or anuria with subsequent uremia. The untreated patient may die a week of two later from uremia, rather than from the acute effects of the transfusion reaction.

67. **d** Macrophages most often provide the first line of defense against exogenous bacterial invasion *from the environment* because macrophages reside in great abundance in the tissues most likely to be exposed to bacteria, such as the lung alveoli and subcutaneous tissues. When other tissues of the body become infected, the concentration of neutrophils increases rapidly; then, several days later, the macrophages begin to replace the neutrophils.

68. **c**

69. **e** When a megakaryocyte matures, the cytoplasm begins to fragment, forming as many as 5,000 platelets.

70. **b**

71. **d** The opposite is true. The rate of sodium movement out of the cell exceeds the rate of potassium movement into the cell. This produces a net loss of intracellular positive charges, and the inside of the cell becomes negative with respect to the extracellular fluid.

72. **e** The potassium permeability of the cell mem-

brane increases, allowing rapid loss of potassium ions to the exterior.

73. **b** Nerve metabolism can be blocked for minutes to hours without greatly affecting the transmission of nerve impulses. This is because the action potential is a physical phenomenon dependent only on ionic gradients across the cell membrane, and only a minute number of ions move across the cell membrane with each action potential.

74. **a** Small ions, such as sodium, potassium, and chloride, diffuse across a cell membrane in accordance with both chemical and electrical gradients. Let us assume that a cell contains only potassium ions and that the concentration of potassium is the same on both sides of the cell membrane. When a negative charge is applied to the inside of the cell, the positively charged potassium ions will continue to diffuse into the cell, even against a potassium concentration gradient, until electrochemical balance is achieved. The electrical potential that prevents net diffusion of an ion in either direction through a cell membrane is called the *Nernst potential* for that ion.

75. **d** In primary active transport, the energy required to transport a substance against its electrochemical gradient is derived directly from ATP or another high-energy phosphate compound. The sodium–potassium pump transports sodium ions out of the cell at the same time that potassium ions are transported into the cell, and is responsible for maintaining the sodium and potassium concentration differences across the cell membrane as well as for establishing a negative electrical potential inside the cells. The pump is present in all living cells of the body.

76. **c** Any event that leads to the opening of sodium channels can lead to the development of an action potential if the rising voltage itself is sufficient to cause still more voltage-gated sodium channels to open and thus a positive-feedback vicious cycle to begin. A sudden increase in membrane potential from a typical resting value of –90 mV to a typical threshold value of –65 mV will usually initiate an action potential in a motor neuron.

77. **c**

78. **c** When insufficient amounts of acetylcholine are released, the endplate potential may be too small to initiate an action potential, in which case the muscle fiber will not contract.

79. **e** The contraction of a muscle fiber begins a few milliseconds after the upstroke of the action potential, and it usually lasts about 100 times longer than the action potential.

80. **a** The unique ability of smooth muscle to contract continuously for prolonged periods provides what

is called *tone* in blood vessels, intestines, lymph vessels, and so forth.

81. **b** The skeletal muscle action potential lasts for only about 1 to 5 msec, whereas the action potential of ventricular muscle lasts for about 200 msec. The fibers in both types of muscle can hypertrophy and they both contain actin and myosin filaments. Also, cardiac muscle fibers, but not skeletal muscle fibers, are innervated by the autonomic nervous system.

82. **d** When an action potential spreads over the terminal end of a motor neuron, voltage-gated calcium channels open, allowing calcium ions to diffuse into the neuron terminal. The calcium ions cause acetylcholine vesicles within the neuron terminal to fuse with the neural membrane and empty their contents into the synaptic trough by the process of exocytosis.

83. **c** Smooth muscle contains both actin and myosin filaments but their physical organization is different to that of skeletal muscle. Instead of being arranged in sarcomeres, the actin filaments radiate from "dense bodies" that are either attached to the cell membrane or held in place within the cell by a scaffold of structural proteins. The actin filaments radiating from two dense bodies overlap a single myosin filament located midway between the dense bodies so that when contraction occurs the dense bodies move toward each other.

84. **b** When acetylcholine is released into the synaptic trough it attaches to acetylcholine-gated ion channels on the postsynaptic membrane, causing them to open. The net effect of opening the channels is to allow large numbers of sodium ions to pour inside the fiber. This creates a local potential inside the fiber that initiates an action potential at the muscle membrane.

85. **b** The myosin head functions as an ATPase enzyme, allowing it to cleave ATP and to use the energy derived from the high-energy phosphate bond to energize the contraction process.

86. **a** The ends of the actin filaments are attached to the Z disks, and they extend in both directions to interdigitate with the myosin filaments. The Z disk passes from myofibril to myofibril, attaching the myofibrils together all the way across a muscle fiber. The portion of a myofibril that lies between two Z disks is called a sarcomere.

87. **b** The mechanism of smooth muscle contraction is quite different to that of skeletal muscle. In the place of troponin, the smooth muscle contains another regulatory protein, called *calmodulin*. When calmodulin reacts with calcium ions, it initiates contraction by activating myosin crossbridges.

88. **d** When calcium ions bind to calmodulin, the cal-

modulin-calcium combination then joins with and activates myosin kinase, a phosphorylating enzyme. A portion of the myosin head becomes phosphorylated in response to the myosin kinase, allowing the head to bind with the actin filament. The smooth muscle membrane contains many voltage-gated calcium channels, but very few voltage-gated sodium channels. Thus, unlike skeletal muscle, the flow of calcium ions into the interior of the smooth muscle cell is mainly responsible for the generation of action potentials. However, it is also true that smooth muscle contraction is very often initiated not by action potentials but by factors that act directly on the contractile machinery.

89. **a** Slow waves are rhythmical changes in membrane potential that can sometimes initiate action potentials in smooth muscle.

90. **c** Because the T tubules are invaginations of the outer cell membrane, their interior is open to the extracellular fluid. They function to transmit depolarizations rapidly to the depths of the cell interior, and they appear to be especially well developed in thick muscle fibers.

91. **a** The sarcoplasmic reticulum is composed of longitudinal tubules that terminate in large chambers called terminal cisternae. When an action potential of an adjacent T tubule causes current to flow through the cisternae, calcium is released from the cisternae and longitudinal tubules. The calcium ions then diffuse to adjacent myofibrils, where they bind strongly with troponin; this in turn elicits the muscle contraction. The muscle contraction will continue as long as the calcium ions remain in high concentration in the sarcoplasmic fluid. But a continually active calcium pump located in the walls of the sarcoplasmic reticulum pumps calcium ions out of the sarcoplasmic fluid, returning it to the vesicular cavities of the reticulum.

92. **c** The sinoatrial node, or S-A node, has the highest rate of automatic discharge of any tissue in the heart; this makes the S-A node the pacemaker of the heart because it excites other potentially self-excitatory tissues before self-excitation can actually occur.

93. **a** Impulse transmission through the A-V node is slower than through the ventricular myocardium, atria, Purkinje system, and sinoatrial node. This slow velocity delays the impulse from reaching the ventricles, so that the atria contract 0.1 to 0.2 second ahead of the ventricles.

94. **a** One definition of circus movement is the continuous movement of an impulse around the heart. When the impulse arrives back at the starting point, the tissue is reexcited, causing another impulse to travel around the heart because the tissue is not in a refractory state. Therefore, almost any factor that increases the path length around the atria or ventricles, or decreases the refractory period of the heart tissue, can promote circus movement.

95. **a** Damage to the A-V node resulting from ischemia or inflammation may increase the PR interval from a normal value of about 0.16 second to as much as 0.25 to 0.40 second. If conduction through the A-V node becomes severely impaired, complete block of impulses may occur, in which case the atria and ventricles will beat independently.

96. **b** The rate of conduction of action potentials in Purkinje fibers is about six times greater than the velocity in normal cardiac muscle.

97. **b** The T wave in the normal electrocardiogram is an upward deflection representing ventricular repolarization and occurs during the latter half of ventricular systole.

98. **b** At the end of systole, the ventricular muscle relaxes, allowing the ventricular pressure to decrease greatly. When the ventricular pressure falls below the atrial pressure, the A-V valves open, and blood from the atria flows into the ventricles.

99. **c** The duration of time between the beginning of the P wave and the beginning of the QRS complex is the interval between the beginning of atrial depolarization and the beginning of ventricular depolarization. This interval, called the PR interval, is approximately 0.16 second during normal, resting conditions. If the PR interval increases above approximately 0.20 second in a heart beating at a normal rate, the patient is said to have *first-degree incomplete heart block.*

100. **c** Premature ventricular contractions (PVCs) usually result from *ectopic foci* in the heart that emit abnormal impulses during the cardiac cycle. Although some PVCs originate from cigarettes, coffee, or emotional stress, a large share of PVCs originate from infarcted or ischemic areas of the heart.

101. **b** Ectopic pacemakers frequently develop in the Purkinje system when the transmission of impulses from the S-A node is blocked along the conduction pathway to the ventricular muscle, causing the atria to beat at a normal rate, and the ventricles to beat at a much lower rate, somewhere between 15 and 40 beats per minute.

102. **a** In aortic stenosis, the blood is expelled through only a small opening in the aortic valve, causing the ventricular pressure to become extremely high, sometimes as high as 300 mmHg. The blood is thus ejected from the ventricle at a tremendous velocity, causing severe turbulence of the blood and vibration of the walls of the aorta. Also, mitral insufficiency means backward flow through the

mitral valve, which can occur only during systole when the pressure in the ventricle is higher than the pressure in the atrium.

103. **a** The fraction of the *end-diastolic volume* that is ejected during systole is called the *ejection fraction*. During diastole, the volume of each ventricle increases to about 110 to 120 ml. During systole, about 70 ml of this blood is ejected. The 40 to 50 ml of blood that remain in each ventricle is called the *end-systolic volume*.

104. **a** Listening with a stethoscope, the "lub" sound is associated with closure of the A-V valves at the beginning of systole, and the "dub" sound is associated with closure of the semilunar valves at the end of systole. Because the cardiac cycle is considered to start with the beginning of systole, the "lub" sound is called the *first heart sound,* and the "dub" sound is called the *second heart sound.*

105. **e** The pulse pressure, which is the difference between the systolic and diastolic pressures, is increased when the amount of blood that is ejected during systole increases or when the distensibility of the arterial tree decreases.

106. **a** Nearly 75% of the blood enters the ventricles during the first third of diastole, called the *period of rapid filling of the ventricles.* Atrial contraction during the last third of diastole accounts for only about 25% of the filling of the ventricles.

107. **d** When the left ventricular pressure rises above the diastolic pressure in the aorta (about 80 mmHg), the aortic valve opens, and blood is ejected from the ventricle.

108. **d** Under resting conditions, the cardiac muscle derives approximately 70% of its energy from the metabolism of fatty acids instead of carbohydrates. Anaerobic glycolysis is called upon during exercise for extra amounts of energy, but this can supply very little energy in relation to the large amounts of energy required by the heart.

109. **a** The strong compression of the ventricular muscle around the coronary blood vessels causes the coronary blood flow to fall to a low value during systole. During diastole, the ventricular muscle relaxes completely, allowing the blood to flow rapidly throughout diastole.

110. **e** During fetal life, the pressure in the pulmonary artery is higher than in the aorta, and the ductus arteriosus shunts blood from the pulmonary artery into the aorta. If the ductus does not close after birth, blood will be shunted from the aorta into the pulmonary artery throughout the entire cardiac cycle because the pressure in the aorta is always greater than the pressure in the pulmonary artery.

111. **e** The Frank-Starling law of the heart states that the more the heart is filled during diastole, the greater will be the amount of blood pumped into the aorta; that is, within physiological limits, the heart can pump all of the blood that comes to it without excessive damming of blood in the veins. The ability of stretched muscle to contract with greater force is characteristic of all striated muscles. Stretching the muscle is believed to increase interdigitation of the actin and myosin filaments and thus to facilitate a more forceful contraction.

112. **c** Resistance is equal to the pressure difference divided by the flow: $(60 - 20)/200 = 0.2$ mmHg/ml/min.

113. **c** The specific gravity of mercury is 13.6, which means that a column of mercury 10 mmHg high exerts the same pressure as a column of water 13.6 cm high. Because the specific gravity of blood is similar to that of water, a column of blood 68 cm high would exert a pressure of about 50 mmHg. Therefore, the pressure in the larger arteries of the hand is equal to the pressure at the level of the heart minus the distance (in mmHg) above the heart: $100 - 50 = 50$ mmHg.

114. **e** As the diameter of a vessel changes, the resistance of the vessel changes in inverse proportion to the fourth power of the diameter. Therefore, increasing the diameter of a vessel to twice the initial diameter would decrease the vessel resistance to one sixteenth of the initial resistance.

115. **d** The arterioles are often called the resistance vessels of the body because they account for about half the resistance of the entire systemic circulation. The arteriolar wall has a thick smooth muscle coat in relation to the size of the vessel, and it is innervated richly by the autonomic nervous system.

116. **a** Because the systemic veins contain about 60% of all the blood in the circulatory system, they are referred to collectively as the blood reservoir of the circulation. When the liver sinuses and venous plexus of the skin become constricted, they can each contribute several hundred milliliters of blood to the remainder of the circulation. The large abdominal veins can contribute about 300 ml, and the spleen can contribute about 150 ml. The heart and lungs are also important blood reservoirs.

117. **b** The pulmonary blood flow (cardiac output) can increase greatly without causing much increase in pulmonary arterial pressure because the pulmonary resistance decreases almost as much as the pulmonary flow increases. This decrease in resistance is caused by recruitment of previously closed pulmonary capillaries as well as distention of the capillaries.

118. **d** Angiotensin acts directly on the kidneys to decrease sodium and water excretion. In addition,

angiotensin stimulates aldosterone secretion, which also causes the kidneys to retain sodium and water. Although angiotensin is a powerful vasoconstrictor, constriction of peripheral blood vessels cannot cause *long-term* increases in arterial pressure unless the renal vessels are constricted as well.

119. **d** The renal–body fluid volume mechanism is slow to act, but it is a very powerful mechanism for regulating arterial pressure extremely accurately over long periods of time. The most rapid control of arterial pressure is achieved by the cardiovascular nervous reflexes.

120. **c** In left heart failure, large amounts of blood are pumped from the systemic circulation into the lungs, leading to pulmonary edema. The amount of blood transferred into the lungs is obviously dependent on the pumping capabilities of the right heart.

121. **a** Although all of the choices given can affect cardiac output, their influence on cardiac output is secondary to the metabolic needs of the tissues for blood.

122. **b** Low levels of oxygen in the myocardium cause the local tissues to release adenosine, which in turn acts to dilate the local blood vessels.

123. **a** Blood flow through the brain is controlled almost entirely by autoregulation, mainly in response to carbon dioxide released from the brain tissue.

124. **e** A simple example of a vicious cycle common to many types of shock is the following: decreased cardiac output causes decreased coronary blood flow and deterioration of the heart, which further decreases cardiac output, and so on. If the positive feedback cycle is allowed to continue, the patient will expire.

125. **a** Septic shock is often associated with a so-called hyperdynamic state in which the cardiac output is greatly increased and the peripheral vascular resistance is decreased. The hyperdynamic state may be an appropriate cardiovascular response to the high metabolic demands of sepsis.

126. **e** When the blood pressure falls below about 60 mmHg, the vasomotor center becomes ischemic, and the neurons within the vasomotor center become strongly excited, thereby exciting vasoconstrictor neurons of the sympathetic nervous system. The degree of sympathetic vasoconstriction is often so great that many of the peripheral blood vessels become totally or almost totally occluded in this "last-ditch effort" to maintain blood flow to the ischemic tissues of the brain by elevating blood pressure.

127. **d** In congestive heart failure, the right atrial pressure, and therefore the venous pressure, is elevated mainly because of the increased blood volume caused by the retention of fluid. The increase in right atrial pressure can maintain the cardiac output at a normal level during *resting* conditions despite continued weakness of the heart itself.

128. **c** Sympathetic stimulation of the peripheral arterioles causes the vessels to constrict, which increases their resistance and decreases the flow of blood. When the veins are stimulated by the sympathetic nervous system they become *less* compliant.

129. **c** Endurance training stimulates angiogenesis in skeletal muscle, causing a very significant increase in both the density of capillaries and the number of capillaries around each muscle fiber. Also, marathon runners often have a greater proportion of small, slow-twitch fibers in the muscles that is thought to have a genetic basis. The number of capillaries per unit mass of fibers is greater in the vicinity of slow muscle fibers when compared to the very large, fast-twitch fibers that are more abundant in the muscles of sprinters and weight lifters.

130. **b** Angiotensin is one of the most powerful vasoconstrictor substances in the body.

131. **b** The increase in blood volume caused by moderate fluid retention is beneficial in *mild* heart failure because it increases venous return to the heart, resulting in a normal cardiac output. In more severe cases of heart failure, the heart is already pumping at its maximum capacity and excess fluid retention no longer has a beneficial effect. Instead, very severe edema develops throughout the body.

132. **c** The increase in sympathetic activity that occurs during exercise causes vasoconstriction in many tissues throughout the body, but not in the active muscles or in the brain. The increase in blood pressure caused by the vasoconstriction contributes to the marked increase in blood flow to the muscles.

133. **e** The maximum breathing capacity is about 50% greater than the pulmonary ventilation during maximum exercise, whereas the cardiac output is increased to about 90% of its maximum value during maximum exercise. Therefore, the cardiovascular system is normally much more limiting on the maximum rate of oxygen consumption than is the respiratory system.

134. **c** Increasing the resistance to fluid filtration through the glomerular membranes will decrease the glomerular filtration rate and thereby cause the kidneys to retain salt and water, but these effects subside gradually over a period of days to weeks because the renal retention of sodium and water leads to increased arterial pressure. Once the pressure has risen fully, normal amounts of fluid are filtered by the kidneys because of the increased

pressure, and normal amounts of sodium and water are excreted.

135. **e** All of these diseases, as well as many other types of renal disease that reduce the ability of the kidneys to excrete sodium and water, usually lead to hypertension.

136. **a** The resistance to blood flow is *inversely* proportional to the fourth power of the vessel diameter.

137. **e** The precise mechanism of blood flow autoregulation has not been determined; however, several vasodilator substances, such as adenosine, carbon dioxide, potassium ions, and others, may be released in great enough amounts from the active skeletal muscle to cause dilation of the local arterioles.

138. **a** Sympathetic stimulation of the splanchnic vessels decreases the splanchnic blood flow, allowing more of the cardiac output to supply the skeletal muscles. Sympathetic stimulation of the skeletal muscle arterioles tends to decrease the muscle blood flow.

139. **c** The resistance to blood flow through the portal vasculature is increased in the cirrhotic liver, and this increases the portal venous pressure and thus the liver lymph flow. If the resistance increases slowly, large collateral vessels develop between the portal veins and esophageal vessels. When these collaterals protrude deeply into the lumen of the esophagus, they are called esophageal varicosities.

140. **b** The flows through the systemic and pulmonary circulations are nearly the same. Pulmonary blood volume is only about one tenth of total blood volume.

141. **a** Increased pressure in the carotid sinus activates the baroreceptor reflect, which in turn elicits mechanisms that tend to decrease blood pressure: vagal stimulation of the heart decreases heart rate, and decreased sympathetic stimulation of the entire cardiovascular system decreases both heart rate and contractility and produces widespread vasodilation.

142. **d** The ductus arteriosus is a right-to-left shunt in the fetus because the pulmonary arterial pressure is greater than the aortic pressure in the fetus. When the ductus arteriosus remains patent after birth, blood flows in the opposite direction because the aortic pressure is now greater than the pulmonary arterial pressure. Cyanosis does not occur unless the heart fails or the lungs become congested.

143. **b** When conduction through the A-V nodal tissues is slowed until the PR interval is 0.25 to 0.45 second, the action potentials are sometimes not strong enough to pass through the A-V node. Therefore, the atria beat at a faster rate than the ventricles.

144. **c** The capillaries have the greatest cross-sectional area and thus the slowest velocity of blood flow.

145. **e** Veins must have the lowest hydrostatic pressure so that blood can flow down a pressure gradient from the arteries to the veins.

146. **a** One might suspect that the large veins would have the lowest resistance, but they are usually partially collapsed, which increases their resistance above the arterial value.

147. **c** The total surface area of all the capillaries is many times greater than that of the other vessels.

148. **a** Surfactant is a surface active substance that decreases the surface tension of the alveolar fluid. Decreased surface tension causes increased pulmonary compliance, which decreases the work required to expand the lungs.

149. **d** Contraction of the external intercostals causes the ribs to rotate upward. This increases the volume of the thoracic cavity, causing the lungs to expand. The abdominal muscles and internal intercostals are muscles of expiration.

150. **b** Alveolar ventilation = respiration rate × (tidal volume – anatomic dead space volume). Therefore, alveolar ventilation = $10 \times (550 - 250) = 3,000$ ml/min.

151. **d** Much of the increase in respiration rate simply moves air back and forth in the anatomic dead space, and this does not contribute to alveolar ventilation, according to the equation given in Answer 150. A shorter snorkel would decrease the effective anatomic dead space and thus increase alveolar ventilation.

152. **b** The tidal volume can never be greater than the vital capacity, because the vital capacity is the maximum amount of air that can be expired after the deepest possible breath has been taken.

153. **e** Blood that perfuses nonventilated portions of the lungs cannot be oxygenated. This blood mixes with fully oxygenated blood from ventilated alveoli, decreasing the arterial Po_2 below the alveolar value. Although oxygen must diffuse down a partial pressure gradient from the alveoli into the blood, the capillary Po_2 becomes virtually identical to the alveolar Po_2 when the red blood cell is about one third of the way through the capillary.

154. **c** About 2% of the blood that enters the aorta has passed through the bronchial circulation, which is not exposed to the pulmonary air and thus has an oxygen tension similar to that of venous blood, about 40 mmHg. The bronchiolar blood mixes with the blood in the pulmonary veins, causing the oxygen tension to decrease from about 104 mmHg to about 95 mmHg.

155. **e** Even during rest, about 70% of the oxygen in the

arterial blood is removed as it passes through the coronary circulation, causing the coronary venous oxygen tension to be very low, about 20 mmHg. Mixed venous blood in the pulmonary artery has an oxygen tension of about 40 mmHg.

156. **d** At 66 feet (~20 meters) below sea level the pressure is three atmospheres, one atmosphere of pressure for each 33 feet (~10 meters) of water plus one atmosphere caused by the air above the water. Therefore, a 10-liter volume of air at 66 feet is equivalent to a 30-liter volume at sea level.

157. **b** Oxygen therapy is of little value in anemia because plenty of oxygen is already available in the alveoli and the hemoglobin in the blood has fully equilibrated with the alveolar oxygen. Instead, the problem in anemia is too little hemoglobin in the blood, which reduces the amount of oxygen that is carried in the blood. Nevertheless, oxygen therapy can cause small amounts of extra oxygen to be transported in the *dissolved* state even though the amount transported by the hemoglobin is hardly altered.

158. **a** About 70% of the carbon dioxide in the blood is carried in the form of bicarbonate ions. Dissolved carbon dioxide entering red blood cells reacts very rapidly with water because the red blood cells contain carbonic anhydrase, an enzyme that catalyzes the reaction between water and carbon dioxide to form carbonic acid. The carbonic acid then dissociates into hydrogen and bicarbonate ions.

159. **e** Carbon dioxide is transported in the blood as dissolved gas (10%), as bicarbonate (70%), and as carbamino compounds (20%). Carbamino compounds are formed by the combination of carbon dioxide with terminal amine groups of blood proteins. The most important protein for transporting carbon dioxide in the carbamino form is hemoglobin.

160. **a** Stretch receptors located in the walls of the bronchi and bronchioles throughout the lungs transmit signals through the vagi into the dorsal respiratory group of neurons when the lungs become overstretched. This activates an appropriate feedback response that inhibits the inspiratory center and thereby protects the lungs against overinflation.

161. **a** During resting conditions, arterial blood is almost fully saturated with oxygen. Therefore, it is not possible to increase significantly the arterial oxygen content by increasing alveolar ventilation.

162. **c** Hematocrit and hemoglobin concentration can vary widely without significantly affecting the arterial oxygen tension because oxygen diffuses along a partial pressure gradient from the alveoli into the blood until the gradient is virtually dissipated. This event is nearly independent of the oxygen-carrying capacity of the blood, as exemplified by the fact that arterial oxygen tension is usually normal during anemia and polycythemia. In contrast, hematocrit and hemoglobin concentrations have a great effect on arterial oxygen content.

163. **a** High-altitude hypoxia decreases the size of the skeletal muscle fibers, which facilitates acclimatization by decreasing the distances between the capillaries.

164. **b** If a diver has been beneath the sea long enough for large quantities of nitrogen to build up in the body, and then suddenly comes back to the surface of the sea, nitrogen bubbles can form in the body fluids. The most significant problems arise from bubbles that form in the nervous system, causing severe pain, paralysis, dizziness, and loss of consciousness. If the diver is brought to the surface slowly, that is, if decompression occurs slowly, decompression sickness can be avoided.

165. **d**

166. **c**

167. **b**

168. **e** The movement of sodium ions to the inside of the membrane causes the neuron to depolarize and therefore to be stimulated.

169. **d** These neurons are part of a pain control system, called an analgesia system.

170. **a** Stimulation of a single large neuron in the motor cortex might lead to stimulation of several thousand muscle fibers.

171. **c** In a reverberating circuit, the output of a neuronal circuit feeds back to reexcite the same circuit. This makes it possible for the circuit to discharge repetitively for a very long time.

172. **d** Pressure on the bottom of the feet causes the extensor muscles of the legs to tighten, helping to support the weight of the body. This reflex, called the positive supportive reflex, is believed to be integrated entirely in the spinal cord.

173. **c** The exteroceptive system, which transmits impulses from the skin, would sense the air pressure against the skin when one is running against the wind and cause the body to lean forward to oppose this force.

174. **c** Parkinson's disease results almost invariably from widespread destruction of areas in the substantia nigra that send dopamine-secreting nerve fibers to the caudate nucleus and putamen.

175. **a** Such an intention tremor is usually caused by failure of the cerebellum to dampen the motor movements. Damage to certain of the basal ganglia will also cause a tremor, but this tremor usually continues as long as the person is awake.

176. **c** Adrenergic stimulation causes the liver to release glucose, thereby *increasing* the blood glucose concentration.

177. **d** The cerebrospinal fluid is found in the cisterns around the brain, in the ventricles of the brain, and in the subarachnoid space around both the brain and the spinal cord. Because the brain and cerebrospinal fluid have approximately the same specific gravity, the brain simply floats in the fluid.

178. **b** The myelin sheaths of the myelinated neuron virtually eliminate ion flow through the neuronal membrane except at the juncture of two adjacent Schwann cells that make up the myelin sheaths. These breaks in myelination, called *nodes of Ranvier*, occur about every 1 to 3 mm along the length of an axon and allow the ions to move with ease between the extracellular fluid and the axon. Therefore, the depolarization process can occur only at the nodes, causing the action potential to jump relatively large distances from node to node. This mechanism increases the velocity of nerve transmission as much as 5-fold to 50-fold.

179. **d** Several structures of the limbic system, including the hypothalamus, are particularly concerned with the affective nature of sensory sensations, that is, whether the sensations are pleasant or unpleasant. Electrical stimulation of certain areas evokes pleasant sensations, whereas electrical stimulation of other areas causes pain, fear, defense or escape reactions, and other unpleasant sensations.

180. **a** Among other effects, sympathetic stimulation causes dilation of the pupils, increased heart rate, decreased peristalsis, and increased blood pressure.

181. **d** Each sympathetic pathway from the spinal cord comprises a preganglionic neuron and a postganglionic neuron. Postganglionic neurons can originate in one of sympathetic chain ganglia or in the prevertebral ganglion, and from there each neuron travels to a tissue, where it terminates. In contrast, the preganglionic neurons of the parasympathetic nervous system travel all the way to the target organ where they synapse with relatively short postganglionic neurons.

182. **b** The preganglionic neurons of the parasympathetic and nervous systems are cholinergic; that is, they release acetylcholine at the terminal synapse. The postganglionic neurons of the parasympathetic nervous system are all cholinergic. On the other hand, most of the postganglionic sympathetic neurons are adrenergic; that is, they release norepinephrine at the effector organ; notable exceptions include postganglionic cholinergic fibers to the sweat glands, piloerector muscles, and a few blood vessels.

183. **b** The typical motor neuron receives excitatory and inhibitory inputs from other neurons, approximately 80% to 95% of them on the dendrites and only 5% to 20% on the soma.

184. **c** When the body is too cold, heat production increases, piloerection occurs, and the blood vessels in the skin constrict.

185. **b** Long-term memory is believed to result from structural changes at the synapses that augment or attenuate signal conduction.

186. **d** A person with retrograde amnesia cannot recall memories from the past, even though the memories are still there. The degree of amnesia for recent events is likely to be much greater than for events of the distant past.

187. **d**

188. **d**

189. **b** The flexor reflex, also called the *withdrawal reflex*, is elicited most powerfully by stimulation of pain endings, which cause the limb to withdraw from the stimulus.

190. **d** The Golgi tendon apparatus is located at the juncture of the muscle and tendon. Several muscle fibers are connected in series with the tendon organ, and the organ is stimulated when the tension of these muscle fibers increases. Stimulation of the Golgi tendon apparatus produces reflex inhibition of muscle contraction and thereby prevents the muscle from developing too much tension.

191. **e** The muscle spindles, distributed throughout the belly of a muscle, send information to the central nervous system regarding muscle length and rate of change of muscle length. Stimulation of the muscle spindles causes the muscle to contract and thereby prevents it from being overstretched. The knee-jerk test is based on stimulation of the muscle spindles.

192. **c** The pacinian corpuscle is a rapidly adapting mechanoreceptor, located in the skin and deep fascial tissues, that is capable of detecting rapid movements of the tissues, such as vibrations.

193. **a** Meissner's corpuscles are found in nonhairy parts of the skin where touch sensations are highly developed, such as the lips and fingertips.

194. **e** Other modalities of sensation detected by free nerve endings are heavy pressure and probably warmth and cold.

195. **e** Visceral pain is usually caused by stimulation of pain endings over a wide area; for example, the organs of the abdomen are usually insensitive to a pin prick or even a sharp knife cut.

196. **a** The macula of the utricle is a receptor organ of the vestibular apparatus. Its function is independent of the hearing apparatus.

197. **c** Wernicke's area is a general interpretative area that has a critical role in the higher levels of brain

function commonly referred to as intelligence. When it is damaged in the left hemisphere of a right-handed person, the person may lose the ability to put together sensory information to determine the overall meaning. However, the person will still hear perfectly well and may even be able to read certain words.

198. **c** The fibers of the pyramidal tract begin at pyramidal cells in the primary motor cortex. They usually cross to the contralateral side at the juncture of the medulla and spinal cord, and most of them synapse with interneurons in the spinal cord gray matter.

199. **e**

200. **e**

201. **b** Orange has a wavelength closer to that of red light than to that of green light.

202. **d** When a loud sound is transmitted into the central nervous system, an attenuation reflex occurs after a latent period of 40 msec to 80 msec. The reflex involves the contraction of two muscles that pull the malleus and stapes toward each other, thereby causing the entire ossicular system to develop a high degree of rigidity. In turn, the ossicular conduction of low-frequency sounds to the cochlea can be reduced by as much as 30 to 40 decibels. Since loud sounds are usually low-frequency sounds, the attenuation reflex can protect the cochlea from damage caused by loud sounds when they develop slowly.

203. **b** Many naturally occurring plant poisons have a bitter taste, causing animals to reject them.

204. **a** The ciliary muscle encircles the lens and is attached to the lens by ligaments. When an object moves closer to the eye, the ciliary muscle contracts, which decreases the tension on the ligaments. The elastic lens can then change passively from a relatively flat shape to a round shape, allowing the image to be focused on the retina.

205. **b** Bright light decreases the quantity of rhodopsin in the rods by splitting it into retinal and scotopsin, which makes the rods less sensitive to light. Complete adaptation usually requires several minutes.

206. **a** Because the entire retina is likely to be involved in the reflex, discrete damage to the fovea would have little effect on the reflex.

207. **c** Because the cochlea is embedded in bone, vibrations in the bone can be transmitted directly to the cochlear fluid. For this reason, damage to the ossicles or tympanic membrane would not be detected from a bone conduction test.

208. **a** The fovea is located in the very center of the retina and has an area of only 0.4 mm. Cones provide greater visual acuity than rods primarily because the ratio of cones to optic nerve fibers is much greater than that of rods to optic nerve fibers.

209. **c** Swallowing is initiated voluntarily when the tongue forces a bolus of food upward and backward against the palate. Once the food is forced into the pharynx, the swallowing process becomes involuntary.

210. **a** The propulsive movement of the gastrointestinal tract result from smooth muscle contraction, and smooth muscle is not striated.

211. **e** Chyme is the semifluid material produced by gastric digestion of food. Gastrin promotes growth of the exocrine pancreas and mucosa of the colon, small intestine, and acid-secreting portion of the stomach. Therefore, gastrin is a gastrotrophic hormone secreted by the stomach.

212. **b** Gastrin, in high concentrations, can also cause the gallbladder to contract, but the effect may not have physiological relevance.

213. **a**

214. **b**

215. **d** Bile salts are formed in the hepatic cells from cholesterol, and in the process of secreting the bile salts about 1 to 2 g of cholesterol are also secreted each day. Under abnormal conditions, the cholesterol may precipitate, causing cholesterol gallstones to develop in the gallbladder. Some of the causes of gallstone formation include too much absorption of water or bile acids from bile, too much cholesterol in bile, and inflammation of gallbladder epithelium.

216. **b** The breakdown of complex foodstuffs, such as carbohydrates, fats, and proteins is accomplished by the same basic process of hydrolysis. The only difference is that different enzymes are required to promote the reactions for each type of food.

217. **d** Pancreatic secretion contains a large quantity of alpha-amylase, a digestive enzyme that hydrolyzes starches, glycogen, and most other carbohydrates to form disaccharides and a few trisaccharides.

218. **c** Pepsinogen is an inactive precursor of the proteolytic enzyme, pepsin. Following secretion from the peptic and mucous cells of the gastric glands, the pepsinogen comes into contact with hydrochloric acid and previously formed pepsin, which split the pepsinogen to form active pepsin.

219. **c**

220. **e** In addition to these functions, cholecystokinin also has trophic effects. It stimulates DNA synthesis and growth of the exocrine pancreas, but it has little or no trophic influence on the small intestine or stomach.

221: **b** Transporting hydrogen ions out of the gastric mucosa decreases the local hydrogen ion concentration, and this is believed to offer some protection against autodigestion of the stomach.

222. e Mucus is secreted by all segments of the gastrointestinal tract. Mucus is an excellent lubricant, and it protects the mucosa from the intestinal juices as well as from different types of food.

223. a Secretin is released by the presence of acid in the duodenum. Actions of secretin that function to decrease the amount of acid in the duodenum include inhibition of gastric acid secretion, inhibition of gastric emptying, and release of pancreatic bicarbonate. For these reasons, secretin has been nicknamed nature's antacid. Secretin also inhibits intestinal motility.

224. e

225. e Evaporation will occur as long as the relative humidity is below 100%. For each gram of water that evaporates from the body surface, 580 calories of heat are lost from the body.

226. d When more food energy is consumed than is utilized each day, the excess is stored as fat.

227. b Fat is transported from one part of the body to another almost entirely in the form of free fatty acids. On leaving the fat cells, the free fatty acids ionize strongly in the plasma and immediately combine with albumin. The concentration of free fatty acid in plasma under resting conditions is about 15 mg/dl, and there is only about 0.45 g of fatty acids in the entire circulatory system.

228. c The essential amino acids must be present in the diet, and not all dietary proteins contain all ten of the essential amino acids.

229. a When the hypothalamus becomes too cold, heat loss is decreased by constriction of skin blood vessels, and heat production is increased by shivering and by an epinephrine-induced increase in metabolic rate. These mechanisms help return the body temperature to the hypothalamic set-point temperature.

230. b During the course of febrile illness, pyrogens are released from degenerating tissues or secreted by toxic bacteria. These pyrogens increase the set-point temperature of the hypothalamus to a value greater than the normal body temperature. All of the mechanisms for raising body temperature— shivering, constriction of skin blood vessels, and so on—are then brought into play, and within a few hours the body temperature rises to the set-point temperature.

231. e When the hypothalamus becomes overheated, its temperature-regulating capabilities are greatly diminished, sweating may cease to occur, and the person may become poikilothermic. The rise in body temperature will perpetuate itself by increasing the metabolic rate. When the core temperature rises above 106° F to 108° F, the person is likely to develop heat stroke.

232. a Sucrose is a disaccharide that is digested in the small intestine to make a molecule of glucose and a molecule of fructose. Essentially all carbohydrates are absorbed from the gut as monosaccharides.

233. b Creatine phosphate (also called phosphocreatine) is the most abundant store of high-energy phosphate bonds in the cells. Although it cannot energize directly many of the intracellular reactions, it can transfer energy interchangeably with ATP; for example, the slightest decrease in ATP levels leads to rapid transfer of energy from creatine phosphate to replenish the ATP stores. When extra amounts of ATP become available, the stores of creatine phosphate are replenished. During anaerobic metabolism the stores of creatine phosphate are used up within a few minutes.

234. d The hypothalamic–hypophyseal venous portal system carries prolactin-inhibitory hormone from the hypothalamus to the anterior pituitary gland. In the absence of this hormone, prolactin secretion increases to about three times normal levels.

235. b Thyroxine decreases the plasma concentrations of triglycerides, cholesterol, and phospholipids, but increases the level of free fatty acids.

236. a Thyroid-stimulating hormone has no known effect on the synthesis of thyroxine-binding globulin.

237. c Cortisol suppresses inflammation in part by stabilizing lysosomal membranes.

238. e The brain and red blood cells are among the few tissues of the body that do not respond to insulin. Even so, the overall effect of insulin of keeping the blood glucose concentration constant has important implications for the nutrition of brain tissue.

239. e Growth hormone decreases carbohydrate metabolism.

240. c Glucagon helps correct hypoglycemia within minutes by increasing the rate of breakdown of glycogen by the liver. It acts more slowly to promote glyconeogenesis.

241. a The general model for the action of steroid hormones is the following: The steroid hormone enters the target cell, is transported to the nucleus with a receptor protein molecule, and finally interacts with one or more specific parts of the genome to initiate or increase synthesis of a specific protein. This mechanism is different from the action of most protein hormones, which rely on a second-messenger system, usually the cyclic AMP system, to mediate their intracellular effects.

242. c Addison's disease results from failure of the adrenal cortices to produce adrenocortical hormones. Loss of cortisol secretion makes it impos-

sible to maintain normal blood glucose concentration between meals because glucose cannot be synthesized in significant quantities by gluconeogenesis.

243. **e** Most individuals with hyperthyroidism have an enlarged thyroid gland with each cell secreting more than normal amounts of thyroid hormone; however, the plasma levels of thyroid-stimulating hormone (TSH) are found to be less than normal and often zero. Instead, thyroid-stimulating antibodies, designated as TSAb, that bind to the same membrane receptors as TSH are found in the plasma, and the high levels of thyroid hormone in turn suppress anterior pituitary formation of TSH.

244. **d** Glucagon increases blood glucose concentration, mainly by causing glycogenolysis and gluconeogenesis in the liver. Growth hormone increases blood glucose concentration by decreasing glucose utilization and uptake by the cells. Also, growth hormone increases the mobilization of fatty acids from adipose tissue and increases the use of fatty acids for energy.

245. **b**

246. **a** Insulin inhibits the action of hormone-sensitive lipase, an enzyme that causes hydrolysis of the triglycerides already stored in the fat cells.

247. **b** Lack of iodine in the diet prevents the production of both thyroxine and triiodothyronine but does not stop the formation of thyroglobulin. No hormone is thus available to inhibit secretion of TSH, allowing the anterior pituitary to secrete large quantities of TSH. The TSH causes the thyroid cells to secrete excessive amounts of thyroglobulin into the follicles, and the gland then grows larger and larger.

248. **a** Exophthalmos occurs in many individuals with hyperthyroidism, but the condition is not *caused* by the high levels of thyroxine in the plasma. Instead, exophthalmos is thought to result from an autoimmune process in which antibodies directed against the extraocular muscles cause the muscles to weaken and the eyeball to protrude.

249. **b** Though parathyroid hormone increases the absorption of both calcium and phosphate from bone, the extracellular phosphate concentration often actually decreases because parathyroid hormone increases the rate of excretion of phosphate by the kidneys.

250. **b** Vitamin D_3 *is* cholecalciferol. Vitamin D_3 is converted to 25-hydroxycholecalciferol in the liver and this, in turn, is converted in the kidney to the active form, 1,25-dihydroxycholecalciferol.

251. **d** Parathyroid hormone increases tubular reabsorption of calcium in the ascending limbs of the loops of Henle, distal tubules, and collecting ducts, and at the same time it decreases reabsorption of phosphate in the proximal tubules. Parathyroid hormone also enhances calcium and phosphate reabsorption from the intestines by increasing the formation of 1,25-dihydroxycholecalciferol from vitamin D in the kidneys, and increases absorption of calcium and phosphate from the bone by stimulating both the proliferation and activity of the osteoclasts.

252. **a**

253. **d** The decline in plasma phosphate concentration caused by infusion of parathyroid hormone is caused by its powerful effect on the kidney to decrease phosphate reabsorption, an effect that is usually great enough to override increased phosphate absorption from the bone and intestine.

254. **b** The collagen fibers of bone have great tensile strength, which means that they can bear great longitudinal stress without tearing apart.

255. **d** The major crystalline salt of the bone, hydroxyapatite, is composed mainly of calcium and phosphate. The great compressional strength of hydroxyapatite crystals, combined with the tensile strength of collagen fibers, provides a type of construction not unlike reinforced concrete, with the sand, mortar, and rock providing the compressional strength and the iron rods providing the tensile strength.

256. **d**

257. **b** Erection of the female clitoris and associated erectile tissues occurs in a similar manner.

258. **b**

259. **b** During a woman's reproductive life about 450 of the primordial follicles grow into vesicular follicles and ovulate, which corresponds to one ova per month for about 37 years.

260. **b** Hair develops in the pubic region and in the axillae after puberty, but androgens formed by the adrenal glands are mainly responsible for this.

261. **a** Progesterone promotes development of lobules and alveoli of the breasts; however, progesterone does not cause the alveoli to actually secrete milk.

262. **c** Only vasopressin (also called antidiuretic hormone) and oxytocin are secreted by the posterior pituitary.

263. **a** Growth hormone causes the liver to release several small proteins called somatomedins that function to increase the growth of bones and other peripheral tissues.

264. **b** Cortisol increases the rate of gluconeogenesis by the liver cells, and this helps increase the blood glucose concentration. Cortisol *activates* hormone-sensitive lipase.

265. **e** Mechanical stimulation of the nipple causes oxy-

tocin to be released into the general circulation, and the oxytocin in turn causes the myoepithelial cells of both breasts to contract and milk to be ejected. Appropriate auditory and visual sensations apparently cause oxytocin to be released from the posterior pituitary gland.

266. **a** Renin is released from the kidneys when they become ischemic, and it initiates a series of reactions that lead to the formation of angiotensin. Angiotensin strongly stimulates aldosterone secretion. Adrenocorticotropic hormone slightly increases aldosterone secretion.

267. **a** Diabetes mellitis is associated with decreased intracellular glucose concentration in those tissues that depend on insulin for the uptake of glucose; the brain and red blood cells are exceptions.

268. **a** The physiological effects of hypothyroidism are the same regardless of the cause. They include fatigue, extreme muscular weakness, decreased heart rate, decreased cardiac output, decreased metabolic rate, myxedema, decreased blood volume, sometimes increased body weight, constipation, decreased respiratory rate, and mental sluggishness.

269. **e** Stress of almost any type causes increased cortisol secretion.

270. **a** Contraction of the uterus is inhibited by progesterone and stimulated by estrogens.

271. **e** Loss of blood flow through the placenta increases the total peripheral resistance, and expansion of the lungs pulls open the pulmonary vessels, decreasing the pulmonary vascular resistance.

272. **c** In the developed fetus the right and left hearts pump in parallel rather than in series as in the adult. The left ventricle pumps only about 30% of the combined ventricular output.

273. **b** In vitamin D deficiency, extra amounts of parathyroid hormone are released, which maintains the plasma calcium concentration at a value only slightly lower than normal. However, plasma phosphate concentration falls to extremely low levels because the increased parathyroid activity increases the excretion of phosphates in the urine.

274. **e**

Rypins' Questions & Answers for Basic Sciences Review, Second Edition, edited by Edward D. Frohlich. J. B. Lippincott Company, Philadelphia © 1993.

C H A P T E R

4
Biochemistry

Robert Roskoski, Jr., M.D., Ph.D.

Brazda Professor and Head, Department of Biochemistry and Molecular Biology, Louisiana State University Medical Center

Directions. *Choose the best answer.*

1. Except for succinate dehydrogenase, the enzymes of the Krebs tricarboxylic acid cycle are found in the:
   (a) Outer mitochondrial membrane
   (b) Intermembranous space
   (c) Inner mitochondrial membrane
   (d) Mitochondrial matrix
   (e) Cristae

2. Which of the following substances is able to pass through biological membranes in the absence of a translocase, permease, or specific transport protein?
   (a) Glucose
   (b) ATP
   (c) Oxygen
   (d) Sodium
   (e) Hydrogen ion

3. Which of the following organelles contains enzymes that degrade proteins, complex carbohydrates, and lipids?
   (a) Lysosome
   (b) Peroxisome
   (c) Mitochondrion
   (d) Endoplasmic reticulum
   (e) Plasma membrane

4. The enzymes of glycolysis, gluconeogenesis, glycogenesis, glycogenolysis, and fatty acid synthesis *de novo,* are located in the:
   (a) Smooth endoplasmic reticulum
   (b) Nucleus

   (c) Peroxisome
   (d) Plasma membrane
   (e) Cytosol

5. Which of the following chemical bonds has a strength of about 100 kcal/mol?
   (a) Hydrophobic bond
   (b) Covalent bond
   (c) Hydrogen bond
   (d) Salt bridge
   (e) van der Waals bond

6. Which of the following substances contains the energy-rich phosphoamidate (P-N) bond?
   (a) ATP
   (b) Phosphoenolpyruvate
   (c) 1,3-bisphosphoglycerate
   (d) Creatine phosphate
   (e) Uridine diphosphate glucose

7. The amino acid _____ is not normally found in proteins.
   (a) Alanine
   (b) Cysteine
   (c) Glutamine
   (d) Ornithine
   (e) Phenylalanine

8. Which of the following amino acids contains an R group or side chain that normally bears a positive charge at pH 7?
   (a) Arginine
   (b) Asparagine
   (c) Glutamate
   (d) Proline
   (e) Tyrosine

9. The pK_a of the physiological phosphate buffer system is 6.8. If the concentration of $H_2PO_4^{-1}$ is 5.0 mM at pH 6.8, the concentration of HPO_4^{-2} is:
   (a) 0.5 mM
   (b) 1.0 mM
   (c) 5.0 mM
   (d) 6.8 mM
   (e) 50 mM

10. Following the oxygenation of hemoglobin, the α and β subunits move relative to one another. This describes a change in the _____ structure of the protein.
    (a) Covalent
    (b) Primary
    (c) Secondary
    (d) Tertiary
    (e) Quaternary

11. Which of the following enzymes catalyzes a hydrolysis reaction and is a hydrolase?
    (a) Glucose-6-phosphatase
    (b) Aldolase
    (c) Aminoacyl-tRNA synthetase
    (d) Glycogen phosphorylase
    (e) Hexokinase

12. Enzymes perform their catalytic function by:
    (a) Increasing the entropy of a reaction
    (b) Increasing the equilibrium constant
    (c) Increasing the total kinetic energy of reactants relative to products
    (d) Decreasing the standard free-energy change ($\Delta G°$) of a reaction
    (e) Decreasing the free energy of activation ($\Delta G^{\ddagger}$) of a reaction

13. Competitive inhibitors:
    (a) Increase the apparent K_m of the substrate in an enzyme-catalyzed reaction
    (b) Decrease the maximal velocity (V_{max}) of an enzyme-catalyzed reaction
    (c) Are irreversible
    (d) Decrease the equilibrium constant of a reaction
    (e) Bind covalently to the enzyme to alter its activity

14. When the plot of substrate concentration versus physiological effect is sigmoidal, this indicates that:
    (a) The process is exponential
    (b) The process exhibits positive cooperativity
    (c) The process has a negative free-energy change
    (d) The rate of the process approaches a minimum at high substrate concentration
    (e) The process is accompanied by a decrease in entropy

15. Which of the following substances contains an energy-rich or high-energy bond?
    (a) Creatine
    (b) Glucose-6-phosphate
    (c) Glycerol-3-phosphate
    (d) Phosphatidylcholine
    (e) Phosphoenolpyruvate

16. The conversion of glucose to pyruvate by the Embden-Meyerhof glycolytic pathway:
    (a) Occurs in a series of nine reversible steps
    (b) Is exergonic
    (c) Occurs in skeletal muscle but not erythrocytes
    (d) Occurs within the mitochondrion
    (e) Results in the formation of 38 moles of ATP per mole of glucose

17. Which of the following substances is the C4 epimer of glucose?
    (a) Sucrose
    (b) Mannose
    (c) Glucuronic acid
    (d) Galactose
    (e) Fructose

18. Which of the following is not a reducing sugar?
    (a) Glucose
    (b) Galactose
    (c) Lactose
    (d) Mannose
    (e) Sucrose

19. Which reaction in the Embden-Meyerhof glycolytic pathway is reversible?
    (a) Hexokinase
    (b) Phosphofructokinase
    (c) Phosphoglycerate kinase
    (d) Pyruvate kinase

20. The conversion of one mole of glucose to two moles of lactate is associated with:
    (a) The net formation of two moles of NADH
    (b) The net formation of two moles of ATP
    (c) An increase in free energy
    (d) The reduction of oxygen to form water
    (e) The utilization of GTP

21. The enzyme _____ is inhibited by fluoride.
    (a) Hexokinase
    (b) Triose phosphate isomerase
    (c) Glyceraldehyde-3-phosphate dehydrogenase
    (d) Enolase
    (e) Pyruvate kinase

22. Fructose-2,6-bisphosphate activates the liver enzyme _____ by an allosteric mechanism.
    (a) Hexokinase
    (b) Phosphofructokinase
    (c) Pyruvate kinase
    (d) Lactate dehydrogenase

(e) Fructose-1,6-bisphosphatase

23. Glucokinase:
    (a) Is inhibited by glucose-6-phosphate
    (b) Is found in muscle
    (c) Has a higher K_m for glucose than does hexokinase
    (d) Catalyzes the phosphorylation of galactose
    (e) Catalyzes a reversible reaction

24. The cofactor _____ is *not* associated with the pyruvate dehydrogenase reaction.
    (a) NAD^+
    (b) FAD
    (c) Coenzyme A
    (d) Biotin
    (e) Lipoic acid

25. Isocitrate dehydrogenase is:
    (a) Activated by NADH
    (b) Inhibited by NAD^+
    (c) Activated by ADP
    (d) Inhibited by AMP

26. The enzyme _____ participates in substrate-level phosphorylation.
    (a) Aconitase
    (b) Fumarase
    (c) Malate dehydrogenase
    (d) Succinate dehydrogenase
    (e) Succinate thiokinase

27. The irreversible step in the Krebs citric acid cycle that makes the cycle unidirectional is catalyzed by:
    (a) Aconitase
    (b) Alpha-ketoglutarate dehydrogenase
    (c) Succinate thiokinase
    (d) Succinate dehydrogenase
    (e) Fumarase

28. Carbon dioxide is a product of the enzyme-catalyzed reaction:
    (a) Aconitase
    (b) Alpha-ketoglutarate dehydrogenase
    (c) Succinate thiokinase
    (d) Succinate dehydrogenase
    (e) Malate dehydrogenase

29. The electron transport chain of oxidative phosphorylation is located in the:
    (a) Mitochondrial matrix
    (b) Inner mitochondrial membrane
    (c) Inner membranous space
    (d) Outer mitochondrial membrane
    (e) Endoplasmic reticulum

30. Which component of the electron transport chain reacts physiologically with oxygen?
    (a) NADH dehydrogenase
    (b) Coenzyme Q
    (c) Cytochrome b
    (d) Cytochrome c

(e) Cytochrome aa_3

31. _____ carries electrons from complex III to complex IV of the electron transport chain.
    (a) Coenzyme Q
    (b) Cytochrome b
    (c) Cytochrome c
    (d) Cytochrome aa_3
    (e) NADH

32. Which of the following is the initiating amino acid for protein biosynthesis?
    (a) Phenylalanine
    (b) Methionine
    (c) Cysteine
    (d) Tryptophan
    (e) Serine

33. Which of the following is *not* a component of the electron transport chain of oxidative phosphorylation?
    (a) Flavin mononucleotide (FMN)
    (b) Cytochrome b
    (c) Cytochrome c_1
    (d) Iron sulfur
    (e) Cytochrome P-450

34. Which of the following bases does not normally occur in DNA?
    (a) Guanosine
    (b) Cytosine
    (c) Adenine
    (d) Uracil
    (e) Thymine

35. The enzyme _____ catalyzes the phosphorolysis of the α-1,4-glycosidic bonds of glycogen.
    (a) Glycogen synthase
    (b) UDPG pyrophosphorylase
    (c) Glycogen phosphorylase
    (d) Debranching enzyme
    (e) Branching enzyme

36. The following enzyme is converted to a *less* active form following phosphorylation as catalyzed by cyclic AMP-dependent protein kinase (protein kinase A).
    (a) Glycogen synthase
    (b) UDPG pyrophosphorylase
    (c) Glycogen phosphorylase
    (d) Debranching enzyme
    (e) Branching enzyme

37. The enzyme _____ is activated following phosphorylation by cyclic AMP-dependent protein kinase (protein kinase A).
    (a) Glycogen synthase
    (b) Hexokinase
    (c) Phosphoglucomutase
    (d) Pyruvate dehydrogenase
    (e) Phosphorylase kinase

38. The enzyme _____ participates in both glycolysis and gluconeogenesis.
    (a) Pyruvate carboxylase
    (b) Phosphoenolpyruvate carboxykinase
    (c) Fructose-1,6-bisphosphatase
    (d) Glucose-6-phosphatase
    (e) Phosphohexose isomerase
39. 5'-AMP is an allosteric activator of the enzyme:
    (a) Glycogen synthase
    (b) Glycogen phosphorylase
    (c) Pyruvate carboxylase
    (d) Phosphoenolpyruvate carboxykinase
    (e) Glucose-6-phosphatase
40. The enzyme _____ functions in the oxidative
segment of the pentose phosphate pathway.
    (a) 6-phosphogluconate dehydrogenase
    (b) Glyceraldehyde-3-phosphate dehydrogenase
    (c) Fructose-1,6-bisphosphatase
    (d) Transaldolase
    (e) Transketolase
41. The main function of the pentose phosphate
pathway in humans is:
    (a) ATP production
    (b) NADH production
    (c) Carbon dioxide production
    (d) NADPH producttion
    (e) NAD^+ utilization
42. Which of the following substances is transported
across the inner mitochondrial membrane by a
specific translocase?
    (a) Malate
    (b) Oxaloacetate
    (c) NADH
    (d) Palmitoyl-CoA
    (e) NADPH
43. The action of acyl-CoA dehydrogenase in the β
oxidation of fatty acids requires:
    (a) Carnitine
    (b) FAD
    (c) Fumarate
    (d) NAD^+
    (e) Thiamine pyrophosphate
44. The oxidation of one mole of β-hydroxyl fatty
acyl-CoA to β-keto fatty acyl-CoA during the β
oxidation of fatty acids results in the production
of _____ mole(s) of ATP by oxidative
phosphorylation.
    (a) 0
    (b) 1
    (c) 2
    (d) 3
    (e) 12
45. Which of the following participates in fatty acid
biosynthesis but *not* in β oxidation of fatty acids?

    (a) NAD^+
    (b) The mitochondrion
    (c) Acetyl coenzyme A
    (d) Water
    (e) Acyl carrier protein (ACP)
46. Which of the following participates in *both* fatty
acid biosynthesis and β oxidation of fatty acids?
    (a) Malonyl coenzyme A
    (b) NADH
    (c) Acetyl coenzyme A
    (d) NAD^+
47. Which of the following compounds, is *not* a participant in the salvage pathway for the synthesis
of phosphatidylcholine?
    (a) ATP
    (b) S-adenosylmethionine
    (c) CDP-choline
    (d) Phosphatidic acid
    (e) CTP
48. Which of the following compounds, is *not* a participant in the pathway for the synthesis *de novo*
of sphingomyelin?
    (a) Palmitoyl coenzyme A
    (b) Serine
    (c) NADPH
    (d) NAD^+
    (e) CDP-choline
49. Ketone bodies are synthesized in the:
    (a) Liver
    (b) Spleen
    (c) Heart
    (d) Brain
    (e) Muscle
50. Ketone bodies react with _____ prior to their
degradation.
    (a) ATP
    (b) GTP
    (c) CTP
    (d) Palmitoyl coenzyme A
    (e) Succinyl coenzyme A

*Directions. Each group of questions consists of several
lettered headings followed by a list of numbered statements. For each numbered phrase, select the one lettered
heading that is most closely associated with each statement.*

Questions 51–52

    (a) NADH dehydrogenase
    (b) Coenzyme Q (ubiquinone)
    (c) Cytochrome b
    (d) Cytochrome c
    (e) Cytochrome aa₃

51. Accepts electrons from succinate dehydrogenase (complex II)
52. Directly inhibited by cyanide

Questions 53–55

(a) Enoyl ACP-reductase
(b) 3-ketoacyl-ACP synthase
(c) 3-ketoacyl-ACP reductase
(d) D-3-hydroxyacyl ACP-dehydratase
(e) Acetyl coenzyme A carboxylase

53. Reaction pulled forward by a decarboxylation
54. Rate-limiting reaction in fatty acid biosynthesis
55. Contains biotin

Questions 56–57

(a) Glucose-6-phosphatase
(b) Hypoxanthine guanine phosphoriboxyltransferase (HGPRT)
(c) Adenosine deaminase
(d) Hexosaminidase A
(e) Phenylalanine hydroxylase

56. Deficiency associated with von Gierke's disease
57. Deficiency associated with Lesch-Nyhan disease

Questions 58–59

(a) Albumin
(b) Chylomicrons
(c) VLDL
(d) LDL
(e) HDL

58. Transports triacylglycerol from liver to extra-hepatic tissues
59. Transports free fatty acids from adipose tissue to other tissues

Questions 60–62

(a) Citrate synthase
(b) Isocitrate dehydrogenase
(c) Alpha-ketoglutarate dehydrogenase
(d) Succinate thiokinase
(e) Succinate dehydrogenase

60. Activated by ADP
61. Catalyzes both a condensation reaction and hydrolysis reaction
62. Inhibited by malonate

Questions 63–65

(a) Ribosomal RNA
(b) Transfer RNA
(c) Messenger RNA
(d) 5S RNA
(e) DNA

63. Capped by 7-methylguanosine in humans
64. CCA at the 3' end
65. Contains a poly A tail in humans

Questions 66–68

(a) UDPG pyrophosphorylase
(b) Debranching enzyme
(c) Branching enzyme
(d) Glycogen phosphorylase
(e) Glycogen synthase

66. Activated by glucose-6-phosphate
67. Contains pyridoxal phosphate
68. Rate-limiting reaction in glycogen biosynthesis

Questions 69–71

(a) Acyl carrier protein (ACP)
(b) Biotin
(c) NADPH
(d) Beta ketothiolase
(e) Carnitine

69. Contains pantetheine
70. Prosthetic group for ATP-dependent acetyl coenzyme A carboxylation
71. Participates directly in ketone body formation

Questions 72–74

(a) Lipoate
(b) Thiamine pyrophosphate
(c) Vitamin B_{12}
(d) Biotin
(e) Pyridoxal phosphate

72. Cofactor of alanine amino transferase (glutamate-pyruvate transaminase)
73. Required for the conversion of methylmalonyl coenzyme A to succinyl coenzyme A
74. Cofactor for the decarboxylation of glutamate to γ-aminobutyric acid (GABA)

Questions 75–76

(a) Acetoacetyl coenzyme A
(b) Oxaloacetate
(c) Alpha-ketoglutarate
(d) Succinyl coenzyme A
(e) Pyruvate

75. Breakdown product of serine
76. Breakdown product of leucine

Questions 77–79

(a) DNA polymerase α
(b) DNA polymerase β
(c) DNA polymerase γ
(d) DNA polymerase δ
(e) DNA polymerase ϵ

77. Catalyzes mitochondrial DNA elongation reactions
78. DNA repair
79. Synthesis of the leading DNA strand in eukaryotes

Questions 80–81

(a) Transcription unit
(b) Terminator
(c) Enhancer
(d) Monocistronic
(e) Promoter

80. Increases frequency of transcription
81. RNA polymerase binding site

Questions 82–83

(a) <4 kcal/g
(b) 4 kcal/g
(c) 7 kcal/g
(d) 9 kcal/g
(e) 12 kcal/g

82. Metabolic energy derived from cholesterol oxidation in humans
83. Metabolic energy derived from carbohydrate metabolism in humans

Questions 84–86

(a) Kwashiorkor
(b) Marasmus
(c) Pernicious anemia
(d) Beri beri
(e) Pellagra

84. Produced in children by adequate calorie but deficient protein intake
85. Niacin deficiency
86. Impaired transketolase activity

Questions 87–89

(a) Glycine
(b) Aspartate
(c) Lysine
(d) Threonine
(e) Leucine

87. Lacks an asymmetrical carbon atom
88. R group is positively charged at physiological pH
89. R group is hydrophobic

Questions 90–92

(a) Serine
(b) Phenylalanine
(c) Proline
(d) Cysteine
(e) Glutamate

90. Essential dietary constituent in humans
91. Participates in the formation of interchain covalent bonds in insulin
92. R group contains a hydroxyl group

Directions: *For each of the following questions answer:*

(a) if only 1,2, and 3 are correct
(b) if only 1 and 3 are correct
(c) if only 2 and 4 are correct
(d) if only 4 is correct
(e) if all are correct

93. Which of the following may play a role in determining the conformation of a protein?
    1. Ionic bonds (salt bridges)
    2. Hydrogen bonds
    3. Hydrophobic bonds
    4. Disulfide bond formation
94. GTP is a substrate for which of the following?
    1. Phosphoenolpyruvate (PEP) carboxykinase
    2. RNA polymerase
    3. Succinate thiokinase
    4. Cyclic GMP-dependent protein kinase
95. Which of the following inhibit liver phosphofructokinase by an allosteric mechanism?

1. Fructose-2,6-bisphosphate
2. Citrate
3. AMP
4. ATP

96. Cholesterol contains:
   1. 27 carbon atoms
   2. An aromatic A ring
   3. A hydroxyl group on C4
   4. An aldehyde at C19

97. Hexokinase catalyzes the phosphorylation of:
   1. Glucose
   2. Fructose
   3. Mannose
   4. Galactose

98. The debranching enzyme of glycogen metabolism:
   1. Mediates a phosphorolysis reaction
   2. Catalyzes a transglycosylation reaction
   3. Mediates cleavage of an α-1,4-glucosyl bond
   4. Catalyzes the hydrolysis of an α-1,6-glucosyl bond

99. Which of the following is used to prepare DNA clones corresponding to RNA?
   1. Plasmids
   2. Reverse transcriptase
   3. Restriction endonucleases
   4. Dideoxyadenosine triphosphate

100. Helicase:
   1. Is required to initiate RNA transcription
   2. Requires ATP for activity
   3. Combines Okazaki fragments
   4. Catalyzes an early step in replication

101. Enzymes:
   1. Are protein catalysts
   2. Increase the equilibrium constant of a reaction
   3. Decrease the free energy of activation of a reaction
   4. Increase the standard free-energy change of a reaction

102. Which of the following enzymes catalyze irreversible reactions?
   1. Fructose-1,6-bisphosphatase
   2. Glyceraldehyde-3-phosphate dehydrogenase
   3. Glucose-6-phosphatase
   4. Enolase

103. The enzyme _____ utilizes NADP$^+$ or NADPH.
   1. Glucose-6-phosphate dehydrogenase
   2. Glutathione reductase
   3. 6-phosphogluconate dehydrogenase
   4. Succinate dehydrogenase

104. The hydrolysis of pyrophosphate serves to pull which of the following reactions forward?
   1. DNA polymerase
   2. Fatty acyl coenzyme A synthetase
   3. RNA polymerase
   4. Aminoacyl-tRNA synthetase

105. Phosphatidate is an intermediate in the biosynthesis of:
   1. Phosphatidylcholine
   2. Triacylglycerol
   3. Phosphatidylethanolamine
   4. Sphingomyelin

106. The enzyme _____ participates in the synthesis of ketone bodies.
   1. Beta ketothiolase
   2. Hydroxymethylglutaryl coenzyme A synthase
   3. Hydroxymethylglutaryl coenzyme A lyase
   4. Hydroxymethylglutaryl coenzyme A reductase

107. Which of the following amino acids are both glycogenic and ketogenic?
   1. Serine
   2. Isoleucine
   3. Histidine
   4. Phenylalanine

108. Which of the following amino acids is metabolized in humans in reactions involving tetrahydrofolate derivatives?
   1. Glycine
   2. Histidine
   3. Serine
   4. Tyrosine

109. Transfer RNAs:
   1. End with a . . . CCA at the 3' end
   2. Are synthesized in eukaryotes in reactions catalyzed by RNA polymerase II
   3. Base pair with the codon of mRNA in an antiparallel fashion
   4. Are directly required for the termination reactions of ribosome-dependent protein biosynthesis

110. Maple syrup urine disease is associated with a defect in the metabolism of:
   1. Valine
   2. Leucine
   3. Isoleucine
   4. Proline

111. The amino acid essential in adult humans is:
   1. Tryptophan
   2. Tyrosine
   3. Lysine
   4. Serine

112. _____ serves as a precursor of heme.
   1. Succinyl coenzyme A
   2. Ferrous iron
   3. Glycine
   4. N^5,N^{10}-methylenetetrahydrofolate

Directions: Each set of lettered headings below is followed by a list of numbered statements. For each statement answer:

A if the term is associated with (a) *only*
B if the term is associated with (b) *only*
C if the term is associated with *both* (a) *and* (b)
D if the item is associated with *neither* (a) *nor* (b)

Questions 113–114

(a) Trypsin
(b) Chymotrypsin
(c) Both
(d) Neither

113. Zinc cofactor
114. Hydrolyzes proteins on the carboxyl terminal side of lysine and arginine

Questions 115–116

(a) Transaldolase
(b) Transketolase
(c) Both
(d) Neither

115. Catalyzes the interconversion of ribose-5-phosphate and xylulose-5-phosphate to sedoheptulose-7-phosphate and glyceraldehyde-3-phosphate
116. Catalyzes an irreversible reaction

Questions 117–118

(a) RNA synthesis
(b) DNA synthesis
(c) Both
(d) Neither

117. Pyrophosphate is a product of the elongation reaction.
118. Okazaki fragments

Questions 119–121

(a) Glycolysis
(b) Glyconeogenesis from pyruvate
(c) Both
(d) Neither

119. Requires GTP
120. Occurs in the cytosol
121. NADPH required

Questions 122–124

(a) Fatty acid synthesis
(b) Beta oxidation of fatty acids
(c) Both
(d) Neither

122. Associated with acetyl coenzyme A
123. Associated with malonyl coenzyme A
124. NAD^+ required

Questions 125–127

(a) Glycogenolysis
(b) Glycogenesis
(c) Both
(d) Neither

125. Activated by epinephrine
126. Activated by insulin
127. Occurs in liver and muscle

Questions 128–129

(a) Cholesterol biosynthesis
(b) Ketone body synthesis
(c) Both
(d) Neither

128. Mevalonate is an intermediate.
129. Phosphoribosylpyrophosphate energy donor

Questions 130–132

(a) Purine biosynthesis
(b) Pyrimidine biosynthesis
(c) Both
(d) Neither

130. Aspartate is required as a reactant.
131. Phosphoribosylpyrophosphate is required.
132. Glycine is a direct precursor.

Questions 133–134

(a) ATP
(b) GTP
(c) Both
(d) Neither

133. Required for protein biosynthesis
134. Required for the stimulation of adenylate cyclase in response to epinephrine

Questions 135–137

(a) Dietary fat
(b) Dietary carbohydrate
(c) Both
(d) Neither

135. Bile acids required for digestion
136. Metabolites oxidized in the Krebs citric acid cycle
137. Transported in chylomicrons

Directions. *Each group of questions consists of several lettered headings followed by a list of numbered statements. For each numbered phrase, select the one lettered heading that is most closely associated with each statement.*

Questions 138–140

(a) Phosphofructokinase
(b) Acetyl coenzyme A carboxylase
(c) Aspartate transcarbamoylase
(d) Hydroxymethylglutaryl coenzyme A reductase
(e) Carbamoyl phosphate synthetase II

138. Rate-limiting enzyme for cholesterol biosynthesis
139. Rate-limiting enzyme for pyrimidine biosynthesis in humans
140. Activated by citrate

Questions 141–142

(a) Glycogen synthase
(b) Hormone sensitive lipase
(c) Glycogen phosphorylase
(d) Heparin-sensitive lipase
(e) Pyruvate dehydrogenase

141. Activity increased following direct phosphorylation catalyzed by cyclic AMP-dependent protein kinase
142. Activity decreased following direct phosphorylation catalyzed by a mitochondrial protein kinase

Questions 143–145

(a) Argininemia
(b) Maple syrup urine disease
(c) Alkaptonuria
(d) Hyperammonemia
(e) Phenylketonuria

143. Phenylalanine hydroxylase deficiency

144. Branched-chain keto acid dehydrogenase deficiency
145. Homogentisate oxidase deficiency

Questions 146–148

(a) Streptomycin
(b) Tetracycline
(c) Chloramphenicol
(d) Puromycin
(e) Cycloheximide

146. Produces mistakes in bacterial translation (misreading of the genetic code)
147. Inhibits bacterial ribosomal peptidyltransferase activity
148. Causes premature chain termination during protein synthesis in prokaryotes and eukaryotes

Questions 149–151

(a) Tyrosine hydroxylase
(b) Aromatic amino acid decarboxylase
(c) Dopamine β-hydroxylase
(d) Phenylethanolamine N-methyltransferase
(e) Monoamine oxidase

149. Pyridoxal phosphate as cofactor
150. Uses ascorbate as reductant
151. Uses tetrahydrobiopterin as reductant

Questions 152–154

(a) Lipoate
(b) Pantothenate
(c) Riboflavin
(d) Niacin
(e) Thiamine pyrophosphate

152. Coenzyme forms an α-hydroxyethyl adduct with pyruvate.
153. Coenzyme forms the prosthetic group of NADH dehydrogenase (complex I) of the electron transport chain.
154. Coenzyme participates in hydride ion $(H:^-)$ transfer reactions.

Directions. *Choose the best answer.*

155. Tay-Sachs disease is associated with an enzyme defect in the _____.
    (a) Mitochondrion
    (b) Cytosol
    (c) Nucleus

(d) Peroxisome

(e) Lysosome

156. Which of the following compounds is an end-product in the degradation of cholesterol?

(a) Mevalonate

(b) Farnesyl pyrophosphate

(c) Lanosterol

(d) Bile acid

(e) Squalene

157. Two carbon equivalents are exported from the mitochondrion for fatty acid biosynthesis as:

(a) Acetate

(b) Malate

(c) Oxaloacetate

(d) Aspartate

(e) Citrate

158. The lipoprotein responsible for the majority of cholesterol transport to the liver from extra-hepatic tissues is:

(a) Chylomicrons

(b) VLDL

(c) LDL

(d) HDL

(e) Albumin

159. Which of the following amino acids is glycogenic only?

(a) Aspartate

(b) Isoleucine

(c) Leucine

(d) Lysine

(e) Tyrosine

160. Which of the following amino acids is ketogenic only?

(a) Asparagine

(b) Glutamate

(c) Isoleucine

(d) Leucine

(e) Serine

161. The predominant amino group acceptor in mammalian intermediary metabolism is:

(a) Cystathionine

(b) Alpha-ketoglutarate

(c) Alpha-ketoisocaproate

(d) Alpha-ketoadipate

(e) Argininosuccinate

162. Carbamoyl phosphate synthetase I (the enzyme that participates in the biosynthesis of urea):

(a) Occurs in the cytosol

(b) Is inhibited by N-acetylglutamate

(c) Requires GTP as the energy donor

(d) Utilizes ammonia as nitrogen donor

(e) Occurs in all nucleated cells of the body

163. Hydrolysis of the amino acid _____ yields urea.

(a) Ornithine

(b) Argininosuccinate

(c) Aspartate

(d) Citrulline

(e) Arginine

164. Transamination involving the amino acid _____ directly yields an intermediate of the citric acid cycle.

(a) Alanine

(b) Aspartate

(c) Glutamine

(d) Methionine

(e) Tyrosine

165. The amino acid _____ is the major donor of one-carbon fragments to tetrahydrofolate.

(a) Alanine

(b) Aspartate

(c) Glutamate

(d) Serine

(e) Tyrosine

166. Tetrahydrobiopterin is required for the metabolism of _____.

(a) Isoleucine

(b) Methionine

(c) Phenylalanine

(d) Serine

(e) Valine

167. The metabolism of which of the following amino acids leads to the production of small amounts of nicotinic acid in humans?

(a) Cysteine

(b) Methionine

(c) Serine

(d) Tryptophan

(e) Valine

168. A metabolite of which of the following amino acids is a substrate for branched-chain keto acid dehydrogenase?

(a) Arginine

(b) Lysine

(c) Methionine

(d) Proline

(e) Valine

169. The amino acid _____ is essential in adult humans.

(a) Cysteine

(b) Proline

(c) Serine

(d) Threonine

(e) Tyrosine

170. _____ biosynthesis is catalyzed by an enzyme that converts ATP to ADP and P_i.

(a) Glutamine

(b) Asparagine

(c) Tyrosine

(d) Glycine

(e) Serine

171. The initiating codon for protein biosynthesis is:
(a) UUU
(b) AUG
(c) UGA
(d) UAA
(e) UAG

172. The biosynthesis of _____ is associated with the splitting of ATP to both P_i and PP_i.
(a) Glutamine
(b) Asparagine
(c) Serine
(d) Cystathionine
(e) S-adenosylmethionine

173. The transfer of the methyl group from N^5-methyl-tetrahydrofolate to homocysteine requires:
(a) Pyridoxal phosphate
(b) Thiamine pyrophosphate
(c) Nicotinic acid
(d) Vitamin B_{12}
(e) Lipoic acid

174. *Unlike* the pathway for purine biosynthesis:
(a) Aspartate is not required for pyrimidine biosynthesis.
(b) Pyrimidine biosynthesis occurs in the cytosol.
(c) The ribose group is added to the pyrimidine base *after* its synthesis.
(d) One of the carbon atoms of the pyrimidine ring is derived from carbon dioxide.
(e) One of the nitrogens of the pyrimidine ring is derived from methenyl-tetrahydrofolate.

175. The reactants for the thymidylate synthase reaction include:
(a) dUMP
(b) dTMP
(c) dAMP
(d) dGMP
(e) dCMP

176. The products of the thymidylate synthase reaction include thymidylate and:
(a) Tetrahydrofolate
(b) Dihydrofolate
(c) S-adenosylhomocysteine
(d) Oxidized thioredoxin
(e) N^5,N^{10}-methylene tetrahydrofolate

177. Which of the following serves as a substrate for the ribonucleotide reductase reaction in the biosynthesis of deoxynucleotides?
(a) UMP
(b) AMP
(c) TTP
(d) ATP
(e) UDP

178. Which of the following is complementary to guanosine in the Watson-Crick sense?
(a) Guanosine
(b) Adenine
(c) Uracil
(d) Cytosine
(e) Thymine

179. The molar percentage of G in human DNA is 30%. The molar percentage of A is:
(a) 10%
(b) 20%
(c) 30%
(d) 40%
(e) 50%

180. The haploid human genome contained within 23 chromosomes consists of about _____ nucleotide base pairs.
(a) 3.5×10^5
(b) 3.5×10^7
(c) 3.5×10^9
(d) 3.5×10^{11}
(e) 3.5×10^{13}

181. The chief enzyme responsible for replication of the lagging DNA strand in humans is
(a) DNA polymerase α
(b) DNA polymerase β
(c) DNA polymerase γ
(d) DNA polymerase δ
(e) DNA polymerase ϵ

182. The editing or proofreading function of DNA polymerases refers to their:
(a) 5' to 3' exonuclease activity
(b) 3' to 5' exonuclease activity
(c) RNAse activity
(d) Topoisomerase activity
(e) DNA ligase activity

183. The energy donor in the human DNA ligase reaction is:
(a) UTP
(b) NAD^+
(c) GTP
(d) ATP
(e) CTP

184. DNA polymerase requires each of the following for its activity *except*:
(a) A template
(b) A primer
(c) A free 3'-hydroxyl group
(d) An incoming deoxynucleoside triphosphate
(e) NAD^+ as an energy donor

185. The two high-energy bonds of ATP are expended during the formation of:
(a) Aminoacyl-tRNA
(b) Glucose-6-phosphate
(c) Glutamine from glutamate
(d) Malonyl coenzyme A from acetyl coenzyme A and carbon dioxide

(e) Choline phosphate from choline

186. The protein required for the proper initiation of *E. coli* RNA polymerase is the _____ subunit.
    (a) α (alpha)
    (b) β (beta)
    (c) β' (beta prime)
    (d) γ (gamma)
    (e) σ (sigma)

187. The enzyme _____ is required for the transcription of eukaryotic heterogeneous nuclear RNA (the mRNA precursor).
    (a) RNA polymerase γ
    (b) RNA polymerase I
    (c) RNA polymerase II
    (d) RNA polymerase III
    (e) polynucleotide phosphorylase

188. The chief site of ribosomal RNA biosynthesis is:
    (a) The mitochondrion
    (b) Cytosol
    (c) Golgi
    (d) Nucleosome
    (e) Nucleolus

189. Which of the following substances inhibits the initiation of RNA biosynthesis in bacteria?
    (a) Methotrexate
    (b) Actinomycin D
    (c) Rifamycin
    (d) Streptomycin
    (e) Chloramphenicol

190. The genetic code is:
    (a) Overlapping
    (b) Nondegenerate
    (c) Different in *E. coli* and humans
    (d) A triplet
    (e) Ambiguous

191. DNA ligase joins:
    (a) Parallel and antiparallel strands
    (b) Processed Okazaki fragments
    (c) Primer and template strands
    (d) Major and minor grooves

192. The formation of aminoacyl-tRNA corresponding to each of the 20 genetically encoded amino acids:
    (a) Requires one generic amino acid tRNA ligase enzyme
    (b) Requires one generic tRNA for all 20 of the amino acids
    (c) Requires GTP as the universal energy donor of protein synthesis
    (d) Requires a 2'- or 3'-hydroxyl group at the 3'-end of the tRNA
    (e) Involves the attachment of the amino acid to the anticodon loop

193. Which of the following eukaryotic elongation fac-

tors of protein synthesis binds GTP and aminoacyl-tRNA?
    (a) eIF1
    (b) eIF3
    (c) EF1
    (d) EF2
    (e) eRF

194. Chain elongation during fatty acid biosynthesis by the fatty acid synthase complex is:
    (a) From the methyl to the carboxyl terminus
    (b) From the carboxyl to the methyl terminus
    (c) Central to peripheral
    (d) Dispersed
    (e) Semiconservative

195. Chain elongation during protein biosynthesis is:
    (a) Carboxyl to the amino terminus
    (b) Amino to the carboxyl terminus
    (c) Dispersed
    (d) Central to peripheral
    (e) Palindromic

196. The synthesis of the peptide bond per se is mediated by
    (a) EF1
    (b) EF2
    (c) GTP
    (d) The ribosome
    (e) Aminoacyl-tRNA synthetase

197. Which of the following compounds is required for the formation of N-linked glycoprotein biosynthesis?
    (a) Heme
    (b) Ubiquinol
    (c) Dolichol
    (d) Beta carotene
    (e) Farnesyl pyrophosphate

198. _____ is an example of a DNA palindrome:
    (a) AAAA
    (b) GAATTC
    (c) ATTA
    (d) GCCG
    (e) AUGGUA

199. Restriction fragment length polymorphisms (RFLPs) are observed on:
    (a) Northern blots
    (b) Western blots
    (c) Southern blots
    (d) Eastern blots
    (e) C$_o$t curves

200. Which of the following enzymes catalyzes RNA-dependent DNA synthesis and is used in preparing complementary DNA (cDNA)?
    (a) DNA polymerase
    (b) RNA polymerase
    (c) Polynucleotide phosphorylase

(d) Reverse transcriptase

(e) Polynucleotide kinase

201. Myasthenia gravis is due to the adventitious production of antibodies against:

(a) Acetylcholine

(b) Choline acetyltransferase

(c) Acetylcholinesterase

(d) The muscarinic cholinergic receptor

(e) The nicotinic cholinergic receptor

202. The chief excitatory transmitter in the human brain is:

(a) Dopamine

(b) Serotonin

(c) Glutamate

(d) Gamma-aminobutyric acid (GABA)

(e) Norepinephrine

203. Dopamine is synthesized in two steps from:

(a) Tyrosine

(b) Tryptophan

(c) Choline

(d) Acetyl-CoA

(e) Arachidonic acid

204. Cardiac glycosides inhibit directly:

(a) Aromatic amino acid decarboxylase

(b) Tryptophan hydroxylase

(c) Tyrosine hydroxylase

(d) Dopamine β-hydroxylase

(e) Sodium–potassium ATPase

205. Hormones that alter gene transcription by interacting with receptors located in the nucleus include each of the following *except:*

(a) Testosterone

(b) Triiodothyronine

(c) Cholecalciferol

(d) ACTH (adrenocorticotrophic hormone)

(e) Estradiol

206. Action of the enzyme _____ liberates diacylglycerol and inositol-1,4,5-trisphosphate from phosphatidylinositol-4,5-bisphosphate.

(a) Phospholipase A_1

(b) Phospholipase A_2

(c) Phospholipase C

(d) Phospholipase D

(e) Lecithin cholesterol acyltransferase

207. The protein kinase activity of _____ phosphorylates tyrosine residues in acceptor proteins.

(a) The insulin receptor

(b) Cyclic AMP-dependent protein kinase

(c) Cyclic GMP-dependent protein kinase

(d) Protein kinase C

(e) Calcium/calmodulin protein kinase II

208. Which of the following enzymes is a serine protease that digests fibrin clots?

(a) Factor XIII

(b) Plasmin

(c) Gamma-carboxylglutamate

(d) Heparin

(e) Warfarin

209. The plasma volume of a 60-kg human is about _____ liters.

(a) 3

(b) 9

(c) 12

(d) 30

(e) 42

210. The caloric equivalent of 1 kg (2.2 lb) of triacylglycerol is _____ kilocalories (Calories).

(a) 4

(b) 9

(c) 7,000

(d) 9,000

(e) 12,000

211. Acyl carrier protein contains:

(a) Pantothenate

(b) Riboflavin

(c) Lipoate

(d) Vitamin B_{12}

(e) Niacin

212. The reducing substrate for the enzyme-catalyzed reaction _____ is deficient in scurvy.

(a) Tyrosine hydroxylase

(b) Phenylalanine hydroxylase

(c) Tryptophan hydroxylase

(d) Prolyl hydroxylase

(e) Cytochrome P-450

213. The protein _____ is located in the thick filament.

(a) Troponin I

(b) Troponin C

(c) Tropomyosin

(d) Actin

(e) Myosin

214. The protein _____ sterically blocks the interaction of myosin and actin.

(a) Creatine phosphokinase

(b) Sodium–potassium ATPase

(c) Troponin C

(d) Tropomyosin

(e) Calmodulin

215. Procollagen contains but mature collagen lacks:

(a) Proline

(b) Glycine

(c) Cysteine

(d) Tryptophan

(e) Alanine

216. Classical hemophilia is due to a deficiency of factor:

(a) III

(b) IV
(c) VI
(d) VIII
(e) IX

217. Factor III, or thromboplastin of the blood-clotting scheme:
    (a) Directly activates prothrombin
    (b) Activates the intrinsic pathway
    (c) Activates the extrinsic pathway
    (d) Directly activates the common pathway
    (e) Is a serine protease

218. Fibrinopeptides are derived from Factor:
    (a) I
    (b) III
    (c) IV

(d) IX
(e) XIII

219. Gamma-carboxylglutamate participates in complex formation with:
    (a) Sodium
    (b) EDTA
    (c) Citrate
    (d) Calcium
    (e) Potassium

220. _____ is the rate-limiting enzyme in prostaglandin biosynthesis.
    (a) Endoperoxidase
    (b) Cyclo-oxygenase
    (c) Lipoxygenase
    (d) Phospholipase C
    (e) Phospholipase A$_2$

1. **d** The enzymes of the Krebs cycle are soluble and occur within the mitochondrial matrix. Succinate dehydrogenase is embedded within the inner mitochondrial membrane, where it can transfer its electrons to other components (coenzyme Q) of the electron transport chain, also found in the inner mitochondrial membrane. The outer mitochondrial membrane is permeable to all low-molecular-weight molecules and even small proteins. In contrast, the inner mitochondrial membrane is impermeable to low-molecular-weight molecules except for those transported by protein translocases.

2. **c** Oxygen, carbon dioxide, urea, and a few small uncharged molecules are able to diffuse through biological membranes. ATP, sodium, and hydrogen ion are charged and do not readily diffuse through biological membranes. Glucose is polar and is too large to pass through a membrane by simple diffusion.

3. **a** Lysosomes contain cathepsins (proteases with an acid pH optimum), DNAses, RNases, and hexosaminidases and other carbohydrate digestive enzymes. Lysosomes function as the wastebasket of the cell. Peroxisomes contain catalase and peroxidase. The mitochondrion is the powerhouse of the cell and contains the electron transport chain, the Krebs cycle enzymes, and the enzymes of β oxidation of fatty acids. Most ATP synthesis occurs in the mitochondrion. The endoplasmic reticulum is the site of complex lipid biosynthesis and the cytochrome P-450 system. The plasma membrane contains the sodium–potassium ATPase, many permeases that mediate the transport of molecules into the cell, and many hormone receptors such as the insulin receptor.

4. **e** Cytosol. The cytosol contains the enzymes of glycolysis, gluconeogenesis, glycogenesis, glycogenolysis, fatty acid synthesis, the pentose phosphate pathway, steroid biosynthesis, and purine and pyrimidine biosynthesis.

5. **b** Covalent bonds are strong (100 kcal/mole). In contrast, hydrophobic bonds, hydrogen bonds, salt bridges, and van der Waals bonds are considerably weaker (0.5–5 kcal/mole).

6. **d** Creatine phosphate contains an energy rich P—N linkage. ATP contains two energy-rich acid anhydride bonds. UDPG contains an energy-rich acid anhydride bond and an energy-rich glycosidic bond. 1,3-Bisphosphoglycerate contains an energy-rich acid anhydride bond at C1 and an energy-poor phosphate ester at C3. Phosphoenolpyruvate contains a very high-energy phosphate bond attached to C2.

7. **d** Ornithine is a five-carbon amino acid that occurs in the Krebs urea cycle along with citrulline. Neither of these two amino acids is incorporated into proteins by ribosome-dependent protein synthesis. Alanine, cysteine, glutamine, and phenylalanine are among the genetically encoded amino acids that occur in proteins.

8. **a** Two amino acids (lysine and arginine) are positively charged at physiological pH. Two amino acids (glutamate and aspartate) are negatively charged at pH 7. Asparagine, proline, and tyrosine have polar R groups that are uncharged at physiological pH.

9. **c** 5.0 mM. The pK is the pH at which the acidic ($H_2PO_4^{-1}$) and basic (HPO_4^{-2}) components of a buffer are present at equal concentration.

10. **e** The interaction of protein subunits represents the quaternary structure. The primary structure is the amino acid sequence. The secondary structure refers to hydrogen bonding found in α helices and β sheets. The tertiary structure represents the overall three-dimensional structure.

11. **a** Glucose-6-phosphatase, which catalyzes the hydrolysis of glucose-6-phosphate to form glucose and inorganic phosphate, is an example of a hydrolase. Aldolase is a lyase. Aminoacyl-tRNA synthetase is a ligase. Phosphorylase and hexokinase are transferases.

12. **e** Catalysts accelerate reactions by decreasing the free energy of activation. Catalysts and enzymes do not alter the equilibrium constant or the kinetic energy of the substrates. Enzymes or catalysts do not alter the thermodynamics (standard free-energy change or entropy) of the net reaction.

13. **a** Competitive inhibitors are reversible and increase the apparent K_m. Competitive inhibitors have no effect on the V_{max} of a reaction. Competitive inhibitors do not alter the equilibrium constant and they do not bind covalently with the enzyme.

14. **b** A sigmoidal curve is the *sine qua non* for positive cooperativity.

15. **e** Phosphoenolpyruvate contains an exceptionally energy-rich bond with a standard free-energy of hydrolysis of –15 kcal per mole. The phosphate ester bonds of glucose-6-phosphate and glycerol-3-phosphate have a standard free energy of hydrolysis of about –3 kcal per mole.

16. **b** The glycolytic pathway, and essentially all

metabolic pathways, are exergonic and proceed with the liberation of free energy. Glycolysis occurs in muscle, erythrocytes, and virtually all living cells in humans. The enzymes and metabolites of the pathway are in the cytosol. The net production of ATP is two.

17. **d** Galactose is the C4 epimer of glucose and mannose is the C2 epimer. Sucrose is a disaccharide made of glucose and fructose, and fructose is a ketohexose. Glucuronic acid contains a carboxyl group at C6 and occurs in proteoglycans and other complex carbohydrates.

18. **e** Sucrose is a disaccharide made up of glucose and fructose covalently bonded through their respective hemiacetal and hemiketal bonds, thereby eliminating the reducing properties of the compound. Lactose is milk sugar composed of glucose and galactose. The C1 of the glucosyl residue in lactose is free. The C1 is able to undergo mutarotation and is able to reduce alkaline copper solutions.

19. **c** Of the four kinase reactions in the Embden-Meyerhof glycolytic pathway, only phosphoglycerate kinase catalyzes a reversible reaction. The 1-phosphate is bonded to 3-phosphoglycerate via an energy-rich, mixed-acid anhydride. 1,3-Bisphosphoglycerate reacts reversibly with ADP to form ATP and 3-phosphoglycerate.

20. **b** Two moles of ATP are required for priming reactions in glycolysis (one for hexokinase and the second for phosphofructokinase). Two moles of ATP are formed from each mole of glucose in the phosphoglycerate kinase reaction and the pyruvate kinase reaction. The overall yield is $-2 + 2 + 2 = 2$ net ATP formed. 2 NADH are formed and 2 NAD^+ are regenerated as glucose in converted into two moles of lactate.

21. **d** Inhibition of enolase by fluoride was important in elucidating the glucolytic pathway. Millimolar concentrations of fluoride are required, and this concentration is unlikely to be obtained in the physiological situation. Glyceraldehyde-3-phosphate dehydrogenase is inhibited by iodoacetate. This was important in elucidating the role of ATP in muscle contraction.

22. **b** Fructose-2,6-bisphosphate activates liver phosphofructokinase and is the most important physiological regulator of the Embden-Meyerhof glycolytic pathway in this organ. Fructose-2,6-bisphosphate also inhibits hepatic fructose-1,6-bisphosphatase. Liver pyruvate kinase is inhibited following phosphorylation by cyclic AMP-dependent protein kinase.

23. **c** Glucokinase has a higher K_m for glucose than does hexokinase (glucokinase requires a higher concentration of glucose to reach $V_{max}/2$). Hexokinase, but not glucokinase, is saturated by glucose at concentrations that appear postprandially in the hepatic portal vein. Glucokinase is found in liver and is not inhibited by glucose-6-phosphate (a product of the reaction) as is hexokinase. Galactose phosphorylation is catalyzed specifically by galactokinase. The conversion of ATP and glucose to products is physiologically irreversible and is accompanied by the loss of one high-energy bond.

24. **d** NAD^+, FAD, coenzyme A, lipoic acid, and FAD are the five cofactors of the pyruvate, α-ketoglutarate, and branched-chain keto acid dehydrogenases. Biotin is a cofactor for ATP-dependent carboxylation reactions.

25. **c** Activation of isocitrate dehydrogenase by ADP is the most important regulatory process in the Krebs cycle. The presence of ADP indicates that ATP levels are submaximal and serves as a signal to increase Krebs cycle activity.

26. **e** Substrate-level phosphorylation represents the formation of a high-energy bond in the absence of an electron transport chain. This occurs in the succinate thiokinase reaction (succinyl-CoA + GDP + P_i → succinate + GTP + CoA). The high-energy bond of GTP is equivalent of that of ATP.

27. **b** The α-ketoglutarate dehydrogenase reaction is irreversible and makes the Krebs cycle function in a unidirectional fashion. The citrate synthase reaction is an irreversible reaction leading into the Krebs cycle. The other Krebs cycle reactions are reversible.

28. **b** Carbon dioxide is given off in two steps of the Krebs cycle in reactions catalyzed by α-ketoglutarate dehydrogenase and isocitrate dehydrogenase.

29. **b** The electron transport chain and the ATP synthase of oxidative phosphorylation are located in the inner mitochondrial membrane. Succinate dehydrogenase, which donates electrons to the electron transport chain, is also located there. The electron transport chain associated with the cytochrome P-450 system is located in the endoplasmic reticulum.

30. **e** Cytochrome aa_3, or cytochrome oxidase, reacts with oxygen to form metabolic water. This cytochrome contains heme iron and also two moles of copper. Cytochrome aa_3 corresponds to site 3 of oxidative phosphorylation. Electron transport through site 3 is inhibited by cyanide, azide, and carbon monoxide. The other components of the electron transport chain may form reactive and adventitious intermediates (superoxide, hydrogen peroxide) with oxygen.

31. **c** Cytochrome c is a low-molecular-weight, soluble protein that carries electrons from complex III to

complex IV. The other cytochromes are associated with the inner mitochondrial membrane. Coenzyme Q is a mobile, lipid-soluble electron transporter that carries electrons from NADH dehydrogenase (complex I) and succinate dehydrogenase (complex II) to complex III.

32. **b** Methionine is the initiating amino acid for protein synthesis in prokaryotes and eukaryotes. The initiating codon is AUG. In prokaryotes, N-formylmethionine tRNA^i participates in the initiation process, where i refers to initiation. The formyl group eliminates the positive charge from methionine and the absence of a charge is crucial in allowing N-formylmet-tRNA^i to be placed in the P site of the bacterial ribosome. In eukaryotes, methionine is not formylated. IF2 (prokaryotes) or eIF2 (eukaryotes) is the initiation factor (IF) that specifically recognizes methionine covalently linked to the initiator tRNA. These initiation factors form a ternary complex consisting of the initiation factor, GTP, and methionine-tRNA^i or fmet-tRNA^i. The elongation factors, which recognize met-tRNA^{met}, do not recognize met-tRNA^i.

33. **e** Cytochrome P-450 participates in oxidation-reduction reactions (*e.g.,* steroid hormone hydroxylation reactions) involving the endoplasmic reticulum. FMN and iron sulfur are found in complex I of the electron transport chain.

34. **d** Uracil is a component of RNA and does not normally occur in DNA. The spontaneous hydrolysis of cytosine in DNA yields uracil. Uracil is recognized by repair enzymes as abnormal, and uracil in DNA is replaced by repair enzymes. Cytosine, adenine, guanosine, and thymine occur in DNA.

35. **c** Phosphorylase catalyzes the cleavage of α-1,4-glycosidic bonds by phosphate (phosphorolysis). Glycogen synthase catalyzes the synthesis of the α-1,4-glycosidic bonds. UDPG pyrophosphorylase catalyzes the formation of UDPG from glucose-1-phosphate and UTP. Branching enzyme catalyzes the formation of α-1,6-glycosidic branches, and debranching enzyme catalyzes the hydrolysis of α-1,6-glycosidic bonds.

36. **a** Glycogen synthase is inactivated following phosphorylation by cyclic AMP-dependent protein kinase. Glycogen phosphorylase is not phosphorylated directly by cyclic AMP-dependent protein kinase but is phosphorylated by phosphorylase kinase. The phosphorylation of phosphorylase by its kinase results in activation.

37. **e** Phosphorylase kinase is activated following phosphorylation by cyclic AMP-dependent protein kinase. Phosphorylase kinase, in turn, catalyzes the phosphorylation and activation of phosphorylase. Pyruvate dehydrogenase is not a physiological substrate for cyclic AMP-dependent protein kinase. Pyruvate dehydrogenase kinase mediates the inactivation of pyruvate dehydrogenase.

38. **e** Phosphohexose isomerase catalyzes the reversible interconversion of glucose-6-phosphate and fructose-6-phosphate. Pyruvate carboxylase, phosphoenolpyruvate carboxykinase, fructose-1,6-bisphosphatase, and glucose-6-phosphatase participate in gluconeogenesis.

39. **b** 5'-AMP serves as a signal that ATP levels are submaximal. 5'-AMP stimulates glycogenolysis by activating phosphorylase. 5'-AMP inhibits gluconeogenesis by inhibiting fructose-1,6-bisphosphatase.

40. **a** Glucose-6-phosphate dehydrogenase, lactonase, and 6-phosphogluconate dehydrogenase are the three enzymes that make up the oxidative portion of the pentose phosphate pathway. Transaldolase and transketolase occur in the nonoxidative portion of the pentose phosphate pathway. Fructose-1,6-bisphosphatase occurs in the gluconeogenic pathway and glyceraldehyde-3-phosphate dehydrogenase is a reversible enzyme that particpates in both glycolysis and gluconeogenesis.

41. **d** The primary function of the pentose phosphate pathway is to generate NADPH for reductive biosynthesis, especially lipid and steroid biosynthesis. A secondary function is to provide five-carbon sugars for nucleotides. Carbon dioxide is produced in the oxidative portion of the pentose phosphate pathway, but this is not the main function of the pathway. ATP is not derived from the reactions of the pathway directly or indirectly.

42. **a** Malate is transported across the inner mitochondrial membrane in exchange for α-ketoglutarate. Oxaloacetate, NADH, NADPH, coenzyme A, and acyl coenzyme A per se are not transported across the inner mitochondrial membrane.

43. **b** The first step in the β oxidation of fatty acids within the mitochondrion is catalyzed by acyl-CoA dehydrogenase; this enzyme contains FAD. Acyl-CoA dehydrogenase is found in the inner mitochondrial membrane, and this dehydrogenase passes its electrons to coenzyme Q. Two moles of ATP will result from oxidative phosphorylation as a result of this process.

44. **d** NAD$^+$ is associated with the second oxidation of the β oxidation scheme involving β-hydroxyl acyl-CoA. The resulting NADH passes its electrons to the electron transport chain with an ATP yield of 3.

45. **e** Acyl carrier protein serves as a swinging arm in transporting acyl derivatives from active site to active site of the fatty acid synthase complex. NAD$^+$ and the mitochondrion participate in fatty acid

oxidation. Acetyl coenzyme A and water participate in both fatty acid synthesis and oxidation.

46. **c** Acetyl coenzyme A serves as the primer for fatty acid biosynthesis and is also generated during β oxidation of fatty acids. NADH and NAD^+ participate in β oxidation only. Malonyl coenzyme A participates in fatty acid biosynthesis only.

47. **b** S-adenosylmethionine is a methyl donor that converts phosphatidylethanolamine to phosphatidylcholine in the *de novo* pathway of phosphatidylcholine biosynthesis. ATP, CTP, CDP-choline, and phosphatic acid are *bona fide* intermediates in the salvage pathway of phosphatidylcholine biosynthesis.

48. **d** Palmitoyl-CoA, serine, NADPH, and CDP-choline are participants in the pathway for sphingomyelin biosynthesis, but NAD^+ is not a participant. NAD^+ is generally associated with catabolic reactions and not biosynthetic reactions.

49. **a** Only liver mitochondria contain the enzymes for ketone body biosynthesis including HMG-CoA lyase.

50. **e** Succinyl-CoA reacts with acetoacetate to form acetoacetyl-CoA and succinate. Liver lacks the enzyme that mediates the conversion of acetoacetate to acetoacetyl-CoA, but this transferase is present in most extrahepatic tissues. Acetoacetyl-CoA is cleaved by thiolase to form two moles of acetyl-CoA that are oxidized by the Krebs cycle.

51. **b** Coenzyme Q is a mobile, lipid soluble component of the electron transport chain. Coenzyme Q accepts electrons from succinate dehydrogenase (bypassing site 1) and passes electrons distally. Two moles of ATP result from the oxidation of each mole of succinate to fumarate and the functioning of the electron transport chain and ATP synthase.

52. **e** Cyanide, azide, and carbon dioxide are site 3 (cytochrome aa_3 or cytochrome oxidase) electron transport inhibitors.

53. **b** 3-Ketoacyl-ACP synthase catalyzes a reaction between malonyl-ACP and an acyl thioester primer; the products include an acyl-acetyl-ACP and carbon dioxide. The decarboxylation reaction is exergonic and promotes the condensation reaction.

54. **e** Acetyl coenzyme A carboxylase is the rate-limiting reaction in fatty acid biosynthesis. Citrate is an allosteric activator of the enzyme and mediates the formation of more active enzyme aggregates from less active monomeric enzyme. Fatty acyl coenzyme A is an inhibitor of acetyl coenzyme A carboxylase.

55. **e** Acetyl-CoA carboxylase, pyruvate carboxylase, and propionyl-CoA carboxylase all contain biotin, which participates in ATP-dependent carboxylation reaction.

56. **a** Type I glycogen storage disease (von Gierke's disease) is due to a deficiency of glucose-6-phosphatase.

57. **b** Hypoxanthine guanine phosphoribosyltransferase (HGPRT) is deficient in Lesch-Nyhan disease. This disorder is associated with hyperuricemia. Lesch-Nyhan disease and its severity provided the first indication of the importance of the salvage pathway of purines in humans. Adenosine deaminase is associated with immunodeficiency. Hexosaminidase A is deficient in Tay-Sachs disease, which is a lysosomal disorder. Phenylalanine hydroxylase deficiency results in phenylketonuria. Phenylalanine hydroxylase is found in liver and is responsible for the first step in the catabolism of phenylalanine.

58. **c** VLDL is synthesized in liver and is responsible for the transport of triacylglycerol from the liver to extrahepatic tissue.

59. **a** Hormone-sensitive lipase in adipose tissue catalyzes the hydrolysis of triacylglycerol to fatty acids and glycerol. The free fatty acids are transported as a complex with albumin. Chylomicrons transport dietary lipid from the gut to liver and other tissues. HDL ("good cholesterol") transports cholesterol from extrahepatic tissues to the liver. LDL ("bad cholesterol") transports cholesterol from the liver to extrahepatic tissues.

60. **b** Isocitrate dehydrogenase is the main regulatory enzyme of the Krebs cycle. When ATP concentrations are submaximal, ADP concentrations increase and activate Krebs cycle activity.

61. **a** Citrate synthase catalyzes the condensation of acetyl-CoA and oxaloacetate. The enzyme also catalyzes the release of CoA from the adduct by an exergonic hydrolysis reaction. The hydrolysis reaction provides the free energy that makes the overall citrate synthase reaction physiologically irreversible.

62. **e** Succinate dehydrogenase is inhibited competitively by malonate. This observation was important in the elucidation of the Krebs cycle. The electron acceptor of succinate dehydrogenase is FAD. FAD donates its electrons eventually to coenzyme Q. Site 1 of the electron transport chain is bypassed, and two ATP molecules will result per mole of succinate oxidized. The reductant for isocitrate dehydrogenase and α-ketoglutarate dehydrogenase is NAD^+.

63. **c** mRNA is synthesized from hnRNA (heterogeneous nuclear RNA) by several processing reactions. Processing includes capping the 5' end with 7-methylguanosine, adding up to 200 A residues to the 3' end by polyadenylation, and excising introns by splicing reactions.

64. b All transfer RNAs end with CCA at the 3' end. The amino acid forms a covalent high-energy bond with the A residue at the 3' end. A single enzyme exists for replacing all three nucleotides at the 3' end of tRNA in the event that they are removed.

65. c As noted in question 63, hnRNA is processed to form mRNA. A part of this processing (posttranscriptional modification) involves the addition of the poly A tail. ATP is the nucleotide donor. The enzyme that performs the addition reactions operates without a template. The poly A tail appears to increase the stability of mRNA. These modifications of mRNA occur only in eukaryotes. Histone is the only protein whose message lacks the poly A tail.

66. e Glycogen synthase is activated by glucose-6-phosphate. This is an example of a feed-forward activation mechanism. The D-form or phosphorylated glycogen synthase is *d*ependent upon glucose-6-phosphate for full activity. The I-form or unphosphorylated form is *i*ndependent of glucose-6-phosphate for full activity.

67. d Glycogen phosphorylase contains pyridoxal phosphate linked to an enzymic lysine via a Schiff base. This cofactor plays a structural role in the protein. Reduction of the Schiff base does not inhibit the function of the pyridoxal derivative in phosphorylase. This is a unique aspect of the biochemistry of pyridoxal phosphate and glycogen phosphorylase.

68. e Glycogen synthase is the rate-limiting reaction in the pathway for glycogenesis. Phosphorylase is the rate-limiting enzyme for glycogenolysis. The straight chain portion of glycogen is made up of α-1,4-glycosidic bonds. The branch points are made up of α-1,6-glycosidic bonds. Branching enzyme transfers several glucosyl residues en bloc with the concomitant formation of an α-1,6-glycosidic bond during glycogenesis. Debranching enzyme catalyzes the hydrolytic cleavage of glucose from the α-1,6-branch points during glycogenolysis.

69. a Pantothenic acid is the vitamin that serves as a precursor to coenzyme A and acyl carrier protein. The *pan* of *pantothenic acid* refers to the ubiquitous distribution of this factor in nature (as the *pan* of *pandemic* refers to a worldwide epidemic). Deficiency of pantothenic acid per se rarely, if ever, occurs as an isolated entity. Deficiency might occur during prolonged starvation in which multiple vitamin deficiencies are manifest.

70. b Biotin is a cofactor for many ATP-dependent carboxylation reactions. Following activation in an ATP-dependent process (yielding ADP and P_i), activated carbon dioxide forms an intermediate with biotin. The activated carbon dioxide is next trans-

ferred to the acceptor to form the carboxylated product.

71. d The first step in ketone body formation (which occurs exclusively in liver) involves the condensation of two molecules of acetyl-CoA to form acetoacetyl-CoA and coenzyme A. This conversion is catalyzed by β ketothiolase. This reaction goes in the direction opposite to that which occurs during the β oxidation of fatty acids. Acetoacetyl-CoA reacts with a third molecule of acetyl-CoA to form hydroxymethylglutaryl-CoA. A lyase then mediates the conversion of HMG-CoA to acetoacetate and coenzyme A. Acetoacetate and its reduction product (β-hydroxybutyrate) are transported from liver to extrahepatic tissues for oxidative metabolism.

72. e Pyridoxal phosphate (vitamin B_6) is a universal cofactor for transamination reactions. Pyridoxal phosphate also participates in other reactions involving amino acid derivatives. These include several decarboxylation and dehydration reactions.

73. c Vitamin B_{12} catalyzes the conversion of methylmalonyl coenzyme A to succinyl coenzyme A in a mutase reaction. This reaction is important in the degradation of odd-numbered-carbon-chain fatty acids, branched-chain amino acids (valine and isoleucine), and threonine. Vitamin B_{12} also mediates a reaction between methyl-tetrahydrofolate and homocysteine to produce methionine.

74. e One of the decarboxylation reactions mediated by pyridoxal phosphate involves the formation of γ-aminobutyric acid (GABA) from glutamate. GABA is an inhibitory neurotransmitter in the mammalian central nervous system and is present in millimolar concentrations. Glutamate is an excitatory neurotransmitter in the mammalian CNS and is also present in millimolar concentrations. Different neurons release GABA or glutamate. Thiamine pyrophosphate is the coenzyme for many oxidative decarboxylation reactions (involving NAD^+) and for transaldolase.

75. e Serine is a three-carbon amino acid that is converted to the three-carbon pyruvate.

76. a Leucine is a six-carbon amino acid that is entirely ketogenic. Leucine is metabolized to acetoacetyl coenzyme A and acetyl coenzyme A.

77. c DNA polymerase γ is required for mitochondrial DNA replication.

78. b DNA polymerase β is involved in repair synthesis and removal of the DNA-RNA primers of Okazaki fragments. The role of DNA polymerase ϵ in repair synthesis is an open question.

79. d DNA polymerase δ mediates the synthesis of the leading DNA strand in eukaryotes. DNA polymerase δ requires PCNA (proliferating cell nuclear antigen) for activity. PCNA is also called cyclin, denoting an

important role in traversing the cell cycle. DNA polymerase α is the enzyme that catalyzes the synthesis of the lagging strand.

80. **c** Enhancers are DNA elements that increase the frequency of transcription. Enhancers may be several thousand bases removed from the gene. Silencers are DNA regulatory elements that decrease the rate of transcription.

81. **e** RNA polymerase binds to the promoter. The transcription unit extends from the promoter (5'-end) to the terminator (3'-end) of a gene. DNAs corresponding to a single polypeptide are monocistronic. Nearly all eukaryotic genes are monocistronic. A polycistronic gene is transcribed to produce an mRNA corresponding to two or more proteins. Each protein of the polycistronic message is translated independently. Many bacterial genes are polycistronic.

82. **a** Humans lack the ability to degrade the four-membered ring of cholesterol. Only the side chain of cholesterol can be metabolized to carbon dioxide and water. The energy yield of cholesterol is much less than 4 kcal per gram. Bile acids are the chief metabolites of cholesterol in humans. A few hundred milligrams per day are eliminated in the feces.

83. **b** The caloric equivalent of carbohydrate and protein is about 4 kcal per gram. The caloric value of lipid (excluding cholesterol) is about 9 kcal per gram. The caloric yield of ethanol is about 7 kcal per gram.

84. **a** Kwashiorkor occurs in children and is related to deficient protein intake, but adequate caloric intake. Marasmus in children results from a deficiency of both caloric and protein intake.

85. **e** Niacin deficiency is associated with pellagra. Niacin occurs in NAD^+ and $NADP^+$ and thus participates in many oxidation-reduction reactions.

86. **d** The cofactor of transketolase is thiamine pyrophosphate, and beri beri is the disorder associated with thiamine deficiency. Thiamine is also the cofactor for several oxidative decarboxylation reactions such as those mediated by pyruvate dehydrogenase and α-ketoglutarate dehydrogenase. Vitamin B_{12} deficiency is pernicious anemia.

87. **a** The only genetically encoded amino acid lacking an asymmetric carbon atom (a carbon atom with four different substituents) is glycine.

88. **c** Two amino acids have R groups that are positively charged at pH 7: lysine and arginine. The R group of histidine is an imidazole group with a pK of about 7. Histidine bears a partial positive charge at pH 7 (some imidazoles are charged, and others are uncharged; hence the term *partial positive charge*).

89. **e** The R group of leucine is a hydrophobic hydrocarbon side chain. Aspartate is negatively charged at physiological pH. Threonine contains a polar hydroxyl group.

90. **b** Phenylalanine cannot be synthesized by humans and is therefore an essential amino acid. Phenylalanine is converted into tyrosine in the liver by a reaction catalyzed by phenylalanine hydroxylase. Dietary tyrosine decreases the dietary requirement for phenylalanine in a process called sparing. In addition to phenylalanine, the essential amino acids include valine, threonine, tryptophan, isoleucine, methionine, histidine, arginine, leucine, and lysine. Histidine and arginine may be essential only in growing humans. (PVT TIM HALL is an acronym for the essential amino acids.)

91. **d** Cysteine participates in the formation of interchain disulfide bonds linking together the A and B chains of insulin. Two cysteines also form an intrachain disulfide bond in the A chain. The acid-catalyzed hydrolysis of such proteins yields cystine (two cysteine residues linked by a disulfide bond).

92. **a** Three genetically encoded amino acids contain a hydroxyl group: serine, threonine, and tyrosine. Each of these hydroxyl groups serve as a phosphate acceptor in reactions catalyzed by protein kinases.

93. **e** Ionic bonds, hydrogen bonds, hydrophobic bonds, and disulfide bonds are important in determining the overall conformation of a protein.

94. **a** GTP is a substrate of PEP carboxykinase that plays a role in hepatic gluconeogenesis. Four ribonucleoside triphosphates (ATP, GTP, UTP, and CTP) are substrates for the RNA polymerase reaction. GTP is also a substrate for the succinate thiokinase reaction. The substrate for cyclic GMP-dependent protein kinase is ATP.

95. **c** Citrate (present during extensive lipolysis and fatty acid oxidation) and ATP inhibit phosphofructokinase (PFK), glycolysis, and ATP production. Fructose-2,6-bisphosphate and AMP are activators of hepatic PFK.

96. **b** Cholesterol contains 27 carbon atoms, four rings, and a hydroxyl group at C4. Estradiol, not cholesterol, has an aromatic A ring. Aldosterone, not cholesterol, has an aldehyde at C19.

97. **a** Hexokinase catalyzes the phosphorylation of several hexoses but not galactose. Galactokinase is the only enzyme that catalyzes the phosphorylation of galactose.

98. **c** Debrancher catalyzes the transfer of several glycosyl residues from an α-1,6-branch point to form a new α-1,4 bond. The debrancher then catalyzes the

hydrolytic removal of the remaining glucosyl group bound in α-1,6 linkage.

99. **a** Reverse transcriptase is used to synthesize DNA and RNA. The resulting complementary DNA (target) is inserted into plasmid DNA (vehicle) for propagation and cloning. Oftentimes the target is inserted into specific restriction endonuclease sites at palindromic sequences. Dideoxynucleoside triphosphate is an inhibitor of DNA polymerase and is used in DNA sequencing procedures.

100. **c** Helicase is an ATP-dependent enzyme that opens the replication fork of DNA ahead of the growing DNA. DNA ligase is the enzyme that combines Okazaki fragments during lagging strand biosynthesis.

101. **b** Enzymes are protein catalysts that decrease the free energy of activation of a reaction. Enzymes do not alter the equilibrium constant nor do they alter the free-energy change for the overall reaction.

102. **b** Fructose-1,6-bisphosphatase and glucose-6-phosphatase catalyze hydrolysis reactions. Essentially all hydrolysis reactions are irreversible. Glyceraldehyde-3-phosphate dehydrogenase and enolase catalyze reversible reactions.

103. **a** Glucose-6-phosphate dehydrogenase, glutathione reductase, and 6-phosphogluconate dehydrogenase are specific for the $NADP^+$ system. Glutamate dehydrogenase utilizes either NAD^+ or $NADP^+$. Succinate dehydrogenase contains FAD as its cofactor.

104. **e** DNA polymerase, RNA polymerase, amino acid-tRNA synthetase, and fatty acyl coenzyme A synthetase catalyze reactions that are pulled forward by pyrophosphate hydrolysis.

105. **a** Phosphatidylcholine, triacylglycerol, and phosphatidylethanolamine are synthesized from phosphatidate. Sphingomyelin is not a glycerol derivative and is not synthesized from phosphatidate.

106. **a** Beta ketothiolase, hydroxymethylglutaryl coenzyme A synthase, and hydroxymethylglutaryl coenzyme A lyase constitute the machinery for acetoacetate production. HMG-CoA reductase is the rate-limiting enzyme in the pathway for cholesterol biosynthesis.

107. **c** Isoleucine and phenylalanine are both glycogenic and ketogenic. Serine and histidine are glycogenic only.

108. **a** Glycine and serine yield N^5,N^{10}-methylenetetrahydrofolate. Histidine yields N^{10}-formiminotetrahydrofolate. Tyrosine metabolism does not involve tetrahydrofolate.

109. **b** Transfer RNAs end with a CCA at the 3' end. The anticodon of tRNA interacts with the codon of mRNA. All base pairing in biology is antiparallel in

nature. RNA polymerase III in eukaryotes, not RNA polymerase II, mediates the synthesis of tRNAs. The release factors and a termination codon (UAA, UAG, UGA) are required for polypeptide chain termination independent of any tRNAs.

110. **a** The three branched-chain amino acids (valine, leucine, and isoleucine) are metabolized by branched-chain keto acid dehydrogenase. Proline is converted to glutamate during its metabolism. A deficiency of the branched-chain keto acid dehydrogenase is associated with maple syrup urine disease.

111. **b** Tryptophan and lysine are the two amino acids listed that are essential. Tyrosine can be synthesized in humans from phenylalanine. Serine can be synthesized from dihydroxyacetone phosphate.

112. **a** Succinyl coenzyme A, ferrous ion, and glycine account for all of the atoms present in heme.

113. **D** Trypsin and chymotrypsin are simple proteins and contain no organic or metal cofactors. Carboxypeptidase from pancreas contains zinc as an essential cofactor. Carboxypeptidase, an exopeptidase, catalyzes the hydrolysis of amino acids from the carboxyl terminal end.

114. **A** Trypsin catalyzes the hydrolysis of the interior of proteins (endopeptidase activity) on the carboxyl terminal side of arginine and lysine (basic amino acids). Chymotrypsin catalyzes the hydrolysis on the carboxyl terminal side of hydrophobic amino acids (valine, leucine, isoleucine, and the three aromatic amino acids—phenylalanine, tyrosine, and tryptophan).

115. **B** Transketolase catalyzes the transfer of two-carbon fragments. The active site of transketolase contains thiamine pyrophosphate. Transaldolase catalyzes the transfer of three-carbon fragments. The active site of transaldolase (and aldolase) contains lysine.

116. **C** Both transaldolase and transketolase catalyze reversible reactions.

117. **C** Pyrophosphate is liberated from the reactant triphosphates in both DNA and RNA biosynthesis. Subsequent pyrophosphate hydrolysis catalyzed by pyrophosphatase pulls the reaction of DNA and RNA synthesis forward.

118. **B** The lagging strand of DNA is synthesized discontinuously as Okazaki fragments. RNA is synthesized continuously.

119. **B** The phosphoenolpyruvate carboxykinase reaction of the gluconeogenic pathway requires GTP. The products of this reaction include phosphoenolpyruvate, carbon dioxide, and GDP. None of the reactions of glycolysis requires GTP.

120. **C** Both glycolysis and gluconeogenesis occur in

the cytosol. The conversion of pyruvate to ox-aloacetate, however, occurs in the mitochondrion.

121. **D** NADPH is not required directly for glycolysis or gluconeogenesis. NAD^+ is required for glycolysis and NADH is required for gluconeogenesis. Both compounds participate in the glyceraldehyde-3-phosphate dehydrogenase reaction.

122. **C** Acetyl coenzyme A is the product of the β oxidation of fatty acids. Acetyl coenzyme A is the primer for fatty acid biosynthesis. Moreover, acetyl coenzyme A is the precursor for malonyl coenzyme A which, in turn, provides all of the carbon atoms of the fatty acid chain except for the two carbon atoms most distant from the carboxyl end.

123. **A** Malonyl coenzyme A is used only for fatty acid biosynthesis and not for fatty acid oxidation.

124. **B** NAD^+ is required for fatty acid oxidation. NAD^+ is not required for fatty acid synthesis.

125. **A** Epinephrine activates glycogenolysis. This process is initiated by a membrane-associated β-adrenergic receptor and a G protein that activates adenylate cyclase. Cyclic AMP-dependent protein kinase catalyzes the phosphorylation of phosphorylase kinase. Phosphorylase kinase, in turn, mediates the phosphorylation of phosphorylase b to form phosphorylase a. Phosphorylase a is the more active enzyme. Phosphorylase a catalyzes the degradation of glycogen (glycogenolysis).

126. **B** Insulin promotes the storage of carbohydrate as glycogen. The insulin receptor has protein tyrosine kinase activity. The molecular details concerning insulin's activation of glycogenesis are unknown.

127. **C** The highest concentration of glycogen occurs in the liver. Since muscle makes up about half of the lean body mass, most of the body's store of glycogen occurs in muscle. Glycogen metabolism is thus important in both liver and muscle.

128. **A** The six-carbon mevalonate is a precursor of cholesterol. Mevalonate is not on the pathway for ketone body formation. Cholesterol is synthesized in the cytosol of all nucleated cells. Ketone bodies are synthesized in liver mitochondria and oxidized in the mitochondria of extrahepatic cells.

129. **D** The pyrophosphates, which occur in dimethylallyl pyrophosphate, isopentenyl pyrophosphate, geranyl pyrophosphate, and farnesyl pyrophosphate, are derived from ATP by two sequential kinase reactions. PRPP is not a reactant in cholesterol biosynthesis.

130. **C** Aspartate contributes four atoms to the pyrimidine ring (three carbons and a nitrogen) and aspartate contributes one nitrogen to the purine ring (N1).

131. **C** Purines are synthesized on ribose phosphate derived from phosphoribosylpyrophosphate (PRPP).

Pyrimidines are first synthesized and ribose phosphate is added afterward. PRPP is also the donor in pyrimidine biosynthesis.

132. **A** Glycine contributes C4, C5, and N7 of the purine ring. Aspartate and carbamoyl phosphate contribute all of the atoms that constitute the pyrimidine ring.

133. **C** ATP is required for the formation of aminoacyl-tRNA. GTP is required to implant aminoacyl-tRNA in the P site of the ribosome. GTP is also required for the translocation reaction following peptide bond formation. Translocation is necessary for moving peptidyl-tRNA from the P site to the A site in parallel with translocating mRNA relative to the ribosome.

134. **B** G proteins serve as intermediaries in the activation or inhibition of adenylate cyclase. G proteins consist of a trimer of $\alpha\beta\gamma$ subunits. After the receptor binds hormone, the complex interacts with the G protein. The α subunit exchanges GTP for bound GDP and becomes activated following its dissociation from the $\beta\gamma$ subunit dimer. The activated G protein then stimulates adenylate cyclase. The α subunit possesses intrinsic GTPase activity. The α-GTP complex is inactivated by hydrolysis of GTP and α-GDP recombines with the $\beta\gamma$ subunits to form an inactive trimer.

135. **A** Ingested fat must be emulsified prior to digestion by lipases and prior to absorption. Bile acids, which are detergent molecules synthesized from cholesterol, are the chief agents used for emulsification. Fat-soluble vitamins (A, D, E, and K) dissolved in dietary lipid are absorbed concomitantly.

136. **C** Carbohydrates, fats, and amino acids are degraded by the Krebs citric acid cycle. The Krebs cycle represents the final common pathway of intermediary metabolism.

137. **A** Ingested triacylglycerol is partially digested, absorbed by the gut, and reconverted into triacylglycerol. Dietary fat is transported from the gut by chylomicrons in the lymphatic system.

138. **d** HMG-CoA reductase is the committed step in cholesterol biosynthesis and this is the rate-limiting reaction.

139. **e** Carbamoyl phosphate synthetase II is the rate-limiting step in pyrimidine biosynthesis in humans. Carbamoyl phosphate synthetase I is involved in urea biosynthesis. The main regulatory step in pyrimidine biosynthesis in *E. coli* is aspartate transcarbamoylase.

140. **b** Citrate converts less active acetyl coenzyme A carboxylase monomers into more active enzyme aggregates. Phosphofructokinase is allosterically inhibited by citrate. Phosphofructokinase is the rate-limiting and controlling step in glycolysis.

141. **b** Hormone-sensitive lipase in adipose tissue is activated by the cyclic AMP second-messenger system. Glycogen phosphorylase is activated indirectly by cyclic AMP-dependent protein kinase. Phosphorylase kinase must first be activated by cyclic AMP-dependent protein kinase. The activated form of phosphorylase kinase then phosphorylates and activates glycogen phosphorylase.

142. **e** Pyruvate dehydrogenase is phosphorylated and inhibited by its protein kinase (pyruvate dehydrogenase kinase). Pyruvate dehydrogenase kinase is not related to the cyclic AMP second-messenger system, and pyruvate dehydrogenase kinase is located in the mitochondrion. Glycogen synthase is a substrate for cyclic AMP-dependent protein kinase. Following phosphorylation, glycogen synthase is less active.

143. **e** Phenylalanine hydroxylase deficiency and phenylketonuria is the most common inborn error of metabolism in caucasians.

144. **b** Maple syrup urine disease is named because of the odor of the urine resulting from a deficiency of branched-chain keto acid dehydrogenase, the enzyme that catabolizes valine, leucine, and isoleucine.

145. **c** Alkaptonuria is due to a deficiency of homogentisate oxidase. Tyrosine metabolites are excreted in urine and form dark-colored products following reaction with dissolved oxygen.

146. **a** Streptomycin produces mistakes in bacterial translation (*e.g.*, incorporation of leucine in response to a phenylalanine codon). Streptomycin also inhibits the initiation of bacterial protein synthesis.

147. **c** Chloramphenicol inhibits bacterial peptidyltransferase activity. The toxicity of chloramphenicol in humans is postulated to be due to inhibition of the mitochondrial protein synthesis machinery at the peptidyltransferase step. Mitochondrial ribosomes differ from those in the cytosol, and mitochondrial ribosomes resemble those of bacteria in many properties.

148. **d** Puromycin is a phenylalanine-tRNA analogue that results in premature chain termination of the nascent polypeptide chain in both prokaryotic and eukaryotic systems. Tetracycline inhibits the attachment of aminoacyl-tRNA to ribosomes of prokaryotes. Cycloheximide inhibits eukaryotic ribosomal peptidyltransferase activity. Cycloheximide and puromycin are not used in human therapeutics.

149. **b** Aromatic amino acid decarboxylase and many other decarboxylases (*e.g.*, glutamate decarboxylase) use pyridoxal phosphate (vitamin B_6) as cofactor.

150. **c** Dopamine β-hydroxylase uses dopamine, oxygen, and ascorbate as substrates. Products include norepinephrine, water, and an oxidized form of ascorbate.

151. **a** Tyrosine hydroxylase, phenylalanine hydroxylase, and tryptophan hydroxylase are three known human enzymes that use tetrahydrobiopterin as substrate. All three enzymes contain iron.

152. **e** Thiamine pyrophosphate of E1 of pyruvate dehydrogenase forms an α-hydroxyethyl adduct with pyruvate.

153. **c** FMN (flavin mononucleotide) forms a portion of NADH dehydrogenase of the mitochondrial electron transport chain.

154. **d** Niacin forms a portion of NAD^+ and $NADP^+$. Both of these substances participate in hydride ($H:^-$) transfer reactions. Pantothenate forms a portion of coenzyme A and acyl carrier protein. Lipoate participates in oxidation-reduction reactions which generate acyl-thioesters in the pyruvate dehydrogenase and α-ketoglutarate dehydrogenase reactions.

155. **e** Tay-Sachs, Niemann-Pick, and Gaucher disease are sphingolipidoses resulting from a deficiency of a lysosomal hydrolytic enzyme.

156. **d** As noted in question 82, cholesterol is not degraded to carbon dioxide and water. Quantitatively, the most important derivative and chief excreted form of cholesterol are bile acids. Mevalonate, farnesyl pyrophosphate, lanosterol, and squalene are biosynthetic intermediates of cholesterol biosynthesis.

157. **e** Pyruvate is converted to acetyl-CoA in the mitochondrion, and the acetyl group is a two-carbon metabolite. Acetyl-CoA condenses with citrate and citrate is exported from the mitochondrion. Citrate is converted into acetyl-CoA and oxaloacetate in an ATP-dependent citrate cleavage or lyase reaction. Acetyl-CoA serves as a precursor for malonyl-CoA used by the fatty acid synthase multienzyme complex.

158. **d** HDL transports cholesterol to the liver from extrahepatic tissues. VLDL transports triacylglycerol (triglyceride) from the liver to extrahepatic tissues. LDL transports cholesterol from the liver to extrahepatic tissues. Chylomicrons transport dietary lipid from the intestine. Albumin transports free fatty acids from adipose tissue to other tissues.

159. **a** Aspartate is converted to oxaloacetate, which is glycogenic. Leucine is ketogenic only. Isoleucine, lysine, and tyrosine are both glycogenic and ketogenic. In whole animal experiments lysine is metabolized to both glucose and ketone bodies. The reactions responsible for the conversion of lysine to carbohydrate in humans is unknown.

160. **d** Leucine is converted into acetyl coenzyme A and acetoacetyl coenzyme A and is entirely ketogenic. Isoleucine, lysine, phenylalanine, tyrosine, and tryptophan are both glycogenic and ketogenic. The other amino acids listed are glycogenic only. The majority of the 20 genetically encoded amino acids are glycogenic.

161. **b** Alpha-ketoglutarate plays a pivotal role in amino acid metabolism in humans. Alpha-ketoglutarate accepts amino groups by various transamination reactions. Alpha-ketoglutarate also undergoes reductive amination as catalyzed by glutamate dehydrogenase to form glutamate.

162. **d** Carbamoyl phosphate synthetase I utilizes ammonia as nitrogen donor. Carbamoyl phosphate synthetase II, in the pathway for pyrimidine biosynthesis, utilizes glutamine as nitrogen donor. Synthetase I occurs in the mitochondrion, is activated by N-acetylglutamate, utilizes ATP as energy donor, and is found in liver and kidney.

163. **e** The last step in the urea cycle involves the hydrolysis of arginine to produce urea and ornithine. Other intermediates in the urea cycle include argininosuccinate and citrulline. Aspartate is the precursor of one of the two nitrogens found in urea.

164. **b** Transamination of aspartate yields oxaloacetate, an intermediate in the Krebs cycle, in a single step. Transamination of glutamate yields α-ketoglutarate, an intermediate in the Krebs cycle, in a single step. Transamination of alanine yields pyruvate (not in the Krebs cycle). Glutamine is hydrolyzed to glutamate and the resulting glutamate can be transaminated to form α-ketoglutarate (two steps). Methionine and tyrosine are metabolized to Krebs cycle intermediates (glucogenic) in several steps. Tyrosine is also converted into acetoacetate (ketogenic).

165. **d** Serine reacts with tetrahydrofolate to form N^5,N^{10}-methylenetetrahydrofolate, water, and glycine. Serine is the major source of one-carbon fragments in mammalian metabolism. Glycine also reacts with tetrahydrofolate to form N^5,N^{10}-methylenetetrahydrofolate, ammonia, and carbon dioxide. Glycine is a minor source of one-carbon fragments.

166. **c** Tetrahydrobiopterin is a reducing cosubstrate for three aromatic amino acid hydroxylases (phenylalanine, tyrosine, and tryptophan). Phenylalanine hydroxylase (deficient in phenylketonuria) is a catabolic enzyme. The two other amino acid hydroxylases are on the biosynthetic pathway for catecholamines (tyrosine hydroxylase) and serotonin (tryptophan hydroxylase).

167. **d** Tryptophan is the only amino acid that is metabolized to form a vitamin in humans. The amount of nicotinic acid formed, however, is minor, and niacin is an essential human dietary constituent.

168. **e** Valine is the only branched-chain amino acid listed in this question. Two other branched-chain amino acids that are metabolized by the branched-chain keto acid dehydrogenase include leucine and isoleucine.

169. **d** As noted in question 90, threonine is the only essential amino acid listed here. Threonine was the last genetically encoded amino acid to be discovered (1934).

170. **a** Glutamine synthetase catalyzes a reaction between glutamate, ammonia, and ATP to form glutamine, ADP, and P_i. Asparagine synthetase catalyzes a reaction between aspartate, glutamine, and ATP and the products include asparagine, glutamate, AMP, and PP_i.

171. **b** AUG in the initiating codon in prokaryotes and eukaryotes. AUG also codes for internal methionines. The AUG near the 5' end of mRNA is used for initiation. The AUG is not at the 5' end and may be a hundred nucleotides from the end. Methionine (and tryptophan) have a single codon. Methionine and tryptophan are rare amino acids in proteins. UUU was the first codon discovered when it was found that polyuridylic acid leads to the ribosome-dependent synthesis of polyphenylalanine. UAA, UAG, and UGA are the termination codons and do not correspond to any tRNAs or amino acids.

172. **e** The biosynthesis of S-adenosylmethionine involves an unusual reaction between ATP, methionine, and water. The products include S-adenosylmethionine, P_i, and PP_i.

173. **d** The transfer of the methyl group from methyltetrahydrofolate to homocysteine requires vitamin B_{12}. The other reaction in humans that requires vitamin B_{12} is the conversion of D-methylmalonyl-CoA to succinyl-CoA as catalyzed by a mutase. The reduction of methylene-tetrahydrofolate to methyl-tetrahydrofolate is irreversible. In pernicious anemia, methyl-tetrahydrofolate accumulates and cannot be metabolized due to a deficiency of vitamin B_{12}. This is the "methyl trap" hypothesis.

174. **c** Purines are synthesized on ribose phosphate. In pyrimidines, ribose phosphate is added after the formation of the pyrimidine ring. Both purine and pyrimidine synthesis occur in the cytosol. Aspartate is required for both purine and pyrimidine biosynthesis. Carbon dioxide is incorporated into both purine and pyrimidine rings. Nitrogen in the pyrimidine ring is derived from aspartate and from carbamoyl phosphate.

175. **a** Deoxyuridylate (dUMP) is the acceptor of the methyl group from methylenetetrahydrofolate.

The product is thymidylate (5-methyldeoxyuridylate).

176. **b** N^5,N^{10}-methylenetetrahydrofolate is the methyl donor in the thymidylate synthase reaction. The methylene group must be reduced to the methyl state, and the reducing equivalents are derived from the donor itself; dihydrofolate is therefore the product. Thymidylate synthase is inhibited by a metabolite of 5-fluorouracil. The conversion of dihydrofolate to tetrahydrofolate is inhibited by methotrexate.

177. **e** Substrates for human ribonucleotide reductase are purine and pyrimidine nucleoside *diphosphates*. UDP is converted into dUDP. dUDP is converted to dUTP and hydrolyzed to dUMP; the latter is a substrate for thymidylate synthase (question 175).

178. **d** GC, AT, and AU represent Watson-Crick complementary base pairs.

179. **b** A + T + G + C = 100%. A = T; G = C. G = 30%, then C = 30%. A + T = 100 − 60 = 40%, A = T = 20%.

180. **c** The human haploid genome consists of 3.5×10^9 base pairs. The one-letter sequence of the human genome corresponds to the equivalent of 13 sets of the entire *Encyclopedia Britannica*.

181. **a** DNA polymerase α is the enzyme responsible for synthesis of the lagging DNA strand. DNA polymerase β is responsible for repair synthesis, and polymerase γ is responsible for replication of the mitochondrial genome. Polymerase δ is responsible for leading strand biosynthesis, and the role of polymerase ϵ in replication has not been determined. Similarly, the role of DNA polymerase II in the replication of *E. coli* has not been determined.

182. **b** 3' to 5' exonuclease activity removes the last deoxynucleotide incorporated into the growing primer strand. If a noncomplementary base is added to the primer, the mismatched base is removed by proofreading activity. 5' to 3' exonuclease is used for the removal of oligonucleotide primers and for repair synthesis. Topoisomerase activity adjusts the extent of supercoiling. DNA ligase removes the nick between a free 3'-hydroxy group and a 5'-phosphate group.

183. **d** ATP adenylates the free 5' phosphate present at the DNA nick; this adenylation results in the formation of an energy-rich acid anhydride bond. The activated 5'-phosphate reacts with the free 3'-hydroxyl group to form a phosphodiester bond. AMP is displaced. NAD^+ is the adenylate donor in the *E. coli* DNA ligase reaction.

184. **e** NAD^+ is the energy donor in the *E. coli* DNA ligase reaction and is not required for DNA polymerase activity. Template, primer, a free 3'-hydroxyl, and an incoming deoxynucleoside triphosphate are required for DNA polymerase activity.

185. **a** Amino acid activation as aminoacyl-tRNA and fatty acid activation as acyl coenzyme A involves the conversion of ATP to AMP and PP_i. PP_i is degraded by hydrolysis catalyzed by ubiquitous pyrophosphatase enzymes to $2 P_i$. Two high-energy bonds are expended for the synthesis of aminoacyl-tRNA from the amino acid and tRNA.

186. **e** The σ subunit is required for proper initiation of transcription in *E. coli*. The holoenzyme core is made up of $\alpha_2\beta\beta'$ subunits. The ρ (rho) factor mediates RNA chain termination for many (not all) RNA molecules.

187. **c** RNA polymerase II is responsible for mRNA biosynthesis in eukaryotes. RNA polymerase I is required for ribosomal RNA synthesis in the nucleolus. RNA polymerase III is responsible for the biosynthesis of tRNA and other small RNA molecules. Polynucleotide phosphorylase catalyzes the degradation of RNA in prokaryotes. In the reverse direction, polynucleotide phosphorylase catalyzes template-independent RNA synthesis from nucleoside diphosphates (and not triphosphates).

188. **e** rRNA synthesis occurs in the nucleolus.

189. **c** Rifamycin, used in the treatment of human tuberculosis, inhibits the initiation but not elongation reactions of prokaryotic RNA biosynthesis. Methotrexate inhibits dihydrofolate reductase. Actinomycin D inhibits RNA elongation reactions both in bacteria and humans. Streptomycin and chloramphenicol inhibit bacterial protein synthesis.

190. **d** The genetic code consists of 4^3, or 64, triplet codons. All but three of the codons represent 1 of the 20 genetically encoded amino acids. The code is nonoverlapping, nonambiguous, and nearly universal (the mitochondrial genetic code is somewhat different than that of bacteria and of cytosolic ribosome-dependent protein synthesis).

191. **b** Okazaki fragments are stretches of DNA from 100 to 1,000 deoxynucleotides long associated with the biosynthesis of the lagging strand. 5' to 3' exonuclease removes RNA primers. Repair polymerase fills in the gaps, and DNA ligase seals the nicks.

192. **d** The amino acid is covalently linked to the 2' or 3' hydroxyl group of an adenine at the 3'-end of tRNA. All tRNAs end with a . . . CCA sequence. The anticodon loop is the portion of the tRNA which interacts with the mRNA codon. There is one amino acid-tRNA synthetase for each of the 20 amino acids used in protein biosynthesis. There are at least two tRNAs for those amino acids with more than three

codons. ATP furnishes the chemical energy for the amino acid-tRNA synthetase reaction.

193. **c** EF1 forms a ternary complex with GTP and aminoacyl-tRNA. EF2 binds GTP and mediates the translocation reaction of the ribosome relative to mRNA. eIF1 and eIF3 are eukaryotic initiation factors that do not bind aminoacyl tRNA. eIF2 binds GTP and the initiator met-tRNA^i. eRF is a eukaryotic release factor. eRF does not bind aminoacyl-tRNA.

194. **a** The elongation reactions of fatty acid biosynthesis occur from the methyl to the carboxyl end.

195. **b** The elongation reactions of protein biosynthesis occur from the amino to the carboxyl terminus.

196. **b** Peptidyl transferase activity, which catalyzes the biosynthesis of peptide bonds, is an integral activity of the ribosome. The precise components of the ribosome that catalyze this reaction are unknown.

197. **c** Dolichol phosphate and dolichol diphosphate carry sugars in glycosidic linkage that are intermediates in N-linked glycoprotein synthesis.

198. **b** GAATTC. The Watson-Crick complement of this structure is 3'CTTAAG 5'. In the 5' to 3' direction, this corresponds to GAATTC.

199. **c** Restriction fragment length polymorphisms are obtained from DNAs that differ in the location of restriction enzyme sites because of differences in the sequence of the bases. Following digestion with restriction enzymes, the resulting DNAs are electrophoresed and the resulting fragments are resolved by length. In Southern blots (named after the originator), DNA is electrophoresed. In northern blots, RNA is run on the electrophoretic gels. In western blots, protein is electrophoresed and usually identified immunochemically. C$_o$t curves refer to the kinetics of nucleic acid hybridization.

200. **d** Reverse transcriptase catalyzes RNA-dependent DNA biosynthesis, using RNA as a template. Complementary DNA is DNA complementary to RNA. DNA polymerase catalyzes DNA-dependent DNA synthesis. Polynucleotide kinase catalyzes the addition of phosphate from ATP to a polynucleotide chain. Polynucleotide phosphorylase, which occurs in prokaryotes, catalyzes the phosphorolytic breakdown of RNA into nucleoside diphosphates.

201. **e** Antibodies produced against the nicotinic receptor are responsible for myasthenia gravis. The nicotinic receptor occurs at the neuromuscular junction and is activated to produce muscle contraction. Receptor-antibody interactions interfere with neurotransmission and result in weakness.

202. **c** As noted in question 74, glutamate is the chief excitatory neurotransmitter in mammalian brain. Dopamine, serotonin, GABA, and norepinephrine are also postulated to function as neurotransmitters in brain. GABA is the chief inhibitor neurotransmitter. The other agents may have both excitatory and inhibitor effects, depending on the location in the brain.

203. **a** Tyrosine is converted to DOPA in the first step and to dopamine in the second step. Tryptophan is converted to serotonin in a two-step reaction sequence. Choline and acetyl-CoA are converted into acetylcholine in a one-step reaction. Arachidonic acid is a precursor of the prostaglandins, thromboxanes, prostacyclins, and leukotrienes.

204. **e** Cardiac glycosides are specific in their inhibition of sodium–potassium ATPase.

205. **d** ACTH is a water-soluble hormone that acts at cell-surface receptors on target cells to activate adenylate cyclase via a G protein. Testosterone, triiodothyronine, and estradiol enter the cell and interact with intracellular receptors, which function in the nucleus to alter gene transcription. In some cases transcription of target genes is increased, and in other cases transcription is decreased.

206. **e** Phospholipase C mediates the hydrolysis of phosphatidylinositol-4,5-bisphosphate to yield diacylglycerol and inositol-1,4,5-trisphosphate. Phospholipase A$_2$ catalyzes the hydrolytic removal of the acyl group attached to C2 to form a lysophosphatidyl derivative and a free fatty acid. The fatty acid that is linked to C2 is often arachidonate. Arachidonate is converted into active or regulatory eicosanoids such as prostaglandin or thromboxane.

207. **a** The insulin receptor is made up of two extracellular polypeptides and two intracellular polypeptides. Following the interaction of insulin with the extracellular domain, protein-tyrosine kinase activity of the intracellular domain is activated. The identity of the tyrosine phosphate acceptors is unknown. Cyclic AMP-dependent protein kinase, cyclic GMP-dependent protein kinase, protein kinase C, and calcium/calmodulin-dependent protein kinase are seryl/threonyl protein kinases.

208. **b** Plasmin is a serine protease that digests clots during the healing process. Plasmin is derived from plasminogen. Tissue plasminogen activator (TPA) is a serum protein that promotes plasmin formation from plasminogen.

209. **a** The plasma volume is about 5% of the lean body mass (0.05 × 60 = 3.0 liters).

210. **d** The caloric value of fat is about 9 kcal per gram or 9,000 kcal per kilogram.

211. **a** Acyl carrier protein contains a portion of coenzyme A. Pantothenic acid represents the vitamin portion of coenzyme A and acyl carrier protein.

212. **d** Scurvy is due to a dietary deficiency of ascorbate or vitamin C. Ascorbate is the reducing substance that maintains the iron of prolyl hydroxylase in the

ferrous state. Ascorbate plays a similar role in the lysyl hydroxylase reaction. Both of these enzymes catalyze posttranslational modifications of collagen. This explains some of the symptomatology of scurvy related to connective tissue pathology.

213. **e** Myosin is the predominant thick filament protein. Myosin contains the ATPase activity of the myofibril responsible for transducing chemical to mechanical energy.

214. **d** Tropomyosin is located between myosin and actin and prevents their interaction in noncontracting muscle.

215. **c** Procollagen fibers contain cysteine residues, which form intramolecular disulfide bonds. These interchain disulfide links are removed with peptides during the conversion of procollagen to collagen.

216. **d** Classical hemophilia (hemophilia A) is due to a deficiency of Factor VIII. Christmas disease (hemophilia B) resembles classical hemophilia clinically, but Christmas disease (named after a patient) is due to a deficiency of Factor IX.

217. **c** Factor III activates the extrinsic pathway. Factor III is also known as thromboplastin or tissue factor.

218. **a** Fibrinogen (Factor I) is the most abundant of the blood-clotting constituents in plasma. Following proteolysis, which is catalyzed by Factor II (thrombin), fibrinopeptides are cleaved from fibrinogen, and the resulting fibrin aggregates to form a loose clot. Under the aegis of Factor XIII, the fibrin undergoes cross-linking reactions to form a firm clot.

219. **d** Calcium (Factor IV) is an essential component of the blood clotting cascade. EDTA and citrate are calcium chelators that inhibit blood clotting.

220. **e** The hydrolytic removal of arachidonic acid from phospholipids, which is catalyzed by phospholipase A_2, is the rate-limiting reaction for ecosanoid biosynthesis.

Rypins' Questions & Answers for Basic Sciences Review, Second Edition, edited by Edward D. Frohlich. J. B. Lippincott Company, Philadelphia © 1993.

C H A P T E R

5

General Microbiology and Immunology

Ronald B. Luftig, Ph.D.

Professor and Head, Department of Microbiology, Immunology, and Parasitology, Louisiana State University Medical Center

MULTIPLE-CHOICE QUESTIONS

The following multiple-choice questions have been drawn in part from the computerized national *Microbiology and Immunology Test Item Bank* through a previous arrangement with the Association of Medical School Microbiology Chairmen (AMSMC).

Section A

Directions. Each of the following questions or incomplete statements is followed by suggested answers or completions. Choose the one best answer.

1. Which of the following stages in the life cycle of malaria is infective to mosquitoes?
   (a) Schizont
   (b) Merozoite
   (c) Ring stage
   (d) Gametocyte
   (e) Sporozoite

2. A skin biopsy taken from the lesion of an individual with mucocutaneous leishmaniasis is most likely to show:
   (a) Flagellated promastigotes in polymorphonuclear neutrophils
   (b) Schizonts
   (c) Amastigotes undergoing binary fission
   (d) Eosinophilic granuloma formation
   (e) Extensive tissue necrosis with only rare protozoal forms

3. The important pathogenic event that is responsible for the symptoms of malarial infections in humans is:
   (a) Infection of erythrocytes with subsequent rupture (hemolysis)
   (b) Acute malarial hepatitis
   (c) Invasion and replacement of bone marrow with resultant anemia
   (d) Increased stickiness of infected erythrocytes and subsequent thrombosis

4. Which of the following diseases is caused by a metazoan parasite (helminth)?
   (a) Giardiasis
   (b) Filariasis
   (c) Trichomoniasis
   (d) Leishmaniasis
   (e) Trypanosomiasis

5. Pathogenicity of group A beta hemolytic streptococci seems best correlated with which of the following?
   (a) Polysaccharide production
   (b) M protein
   (c) Streptokinase production
   (d) Erythrogenic toxin production
   (e) None of the above

6. With respect to "nonspecific" defense, leukotriene B4, an arachidonate metabolite, is most closely associated with which of the following?
   (a) Increased ciliary activity
   (b) PMN chemotaxis
   (c) Degranulation in phagolysosomes
   (d) PMN killing mechanism

(e) Maintaining tissue integrity

7. The complement protein that enhances the binding of antigen–antibody complexes to polymorphonuclear leukocytes (PMN) and macrophages is:
   (a) C1
   (b) C3a
   (c) C3b
   (d) 5b, 6, 7 complex
   (e) C8

8. Congenital toxoplasmosis is suspected in a newborn infant. A positive result on which of the following indirect immunofluorescent antibody techniques performed on cord blood would confirm *in utero* infection?
   (a) IgG
   (b) IgM
   (c) IgA
   (d) IgE

9. *Accolé* forms (in which a parasite appears to be on the cell surface) and multiple infected red blood cells are associated with infection by:
   (a) *P. vivax*
   (b) *P. malariae*
   (c) *P. falciparum*
   (d) *P. ovale*

10. Which of the following chemotherapeutic agents is most commonly used in the treatment of infections with *Trichomonas vaginalis?*
    (a) Metronidazole
    (b) Diiodohydroxyquin
    (c) Tetracycline
    (d) Chloroquine phosphate
    (e) Amphotericin B

11. The host that harbors the adult, or sexually mature, parasite is called the:
    (a) Reservoir host
    (b) Intermediate host
    (c) Final (definitive) host
    (d) Commensal host
    (e) Symbiotic host

12. A middle-aged woman fond of eating raw sausage presents with fever, urticaria, tender muscles, and a high eosinophil count. Which of the following investigations is most likely to give the fastest and most conclusive result?
    (a) Muscle biopsy
    (b) Stool examination for ova and parasites
    (c) Blood test for antibodies to *Echinococcus, Taenia solium, T. saginatum,* and *Toxoplasma gondii*
    (d) Examination of stained blood smear

13. Liver abscess is a complication of:
    (a) Infectious hepatitis
    (b) Infectious mononucleosis

(c) Gastroenteritis of infants
(d) Amebiasis
(e) *Giardia lamblia* infection

14. Which of the following is the most sensitive serologic technique for diagnosing acute or congenital toxoplasmosis?
    (a) Indirect fluorescent antibody test for IgG antibodies
    (b) Indirect fluorescent antibody test for IgM antibodies
    (c) Indirect hemagglutination test
    (d) Sabin-Feldman dye test

15. The drug of choice in treating tapeworm infections is:
    (a) Metronidazole
    (b) Quinacrine
    (c) Chloroquine
    (d) Niclosamide

16. Septate hyphae, 3 μm to 4 μm in diameter, are seen in lung tissue stained with hematoxylin and eosin. On the basis of this finding, you would most likely identify the fungus present in the sample as:
    (a) Rhizopus
    (b) Aspergillus
    (c) Mucor
    (d) *Blastomyces dermatitidis*
    (e) *Histoplasma capsulatum*

17. The agent that causes actinomycosis in humans is:
    (a) Part of the normal human oral flora
    (b) A soil organism
    (c) Associated with dead and decaying matter that has been fertilized by bird droppings
    (d) Found in bird fecal matter

18. The term *coenocytic* refers to:
    (a) True hyphae with cross walls or septa
    (b) True hyphae without cross walls or septa
    (c) Pseudohyphae without cross walls or septa
    (d) A type of thallospore
    (e) None of the above

19. In fungi, conidia are:
    (a) Sexual spores
    (b) Undifferentiated bits of hyphae
    (c) Asexual spores
    (d) Discharged from gills of mushrooms
    (e) The yeastlike phase of dimorphic fungi

20. Tests for capsular polysaccharide in clinical specimens of body fluids are used for diagnosis of which of the following infections?
    (a) *Cryptococcus neoformans*
    (b) *Histoplasma capsulatum*
    (c) *Paracoccidioides brasiliensis*
    (d) *Coccidioides immitis*
    (e) *Candida albicans*

21. Which of the following is most important in host defense against fungal infection?
    (a) Antibody neutralization of toxin
    (b) Lysis of fungi by complement
    (c) Phagocytosis and intracellular killing
    (d) Antibody-dependent cell-mediated cytolysis
    (e) Release of vasoactive amines from mast cells

22. The virion-associated "transcriptase" of rabies virus is:
    (a) A DNA-dependent DNA polymerase
    (b) A DNA-dependent RNA polymerase
    (c) An RNA-dependent RNA polymerase
    (d) An RNA-dependent DNA polymerase
    (e) None of the above

23. Which of the following components in the serum is most diagnostic of a past hepatitis B virus infection from which an individual has acquired immunity to subsequent hepatitis B virus infections?
    (a) HBsAg
    (b) HBcAg
    (c) HBeAg
    (d) Anti-HBsAg
    (e) Anti-HBcAg

24. The matrix (M) protein in orthomyxovirus maturation:
    (a) Acts as an attachment receptor
    (b) Regulates the synthesis of viral nucleic acid
    (c) Serves as a recognition site for the nucleocapsid at the plasma membrane
    (d) Regulates the posttranslational processing of viral mRNA
    (e) Initiates transcription of the parental genome

25. An icosahedral capsid:
    (a) Is in most cases fitted under an envelope that is also icosahedral
    (b) Consists of protomers, each of which in turn consists of several, usually 5 or 6, capsomers
    (c) Has 20 edges
    (d) Has 20 faces
    (e) Has 20 corners

26. The rabies vaccine currently recommended for use in humans is:
    (a) Human diploid fibroblast vaccine
    (b) Duck embryo vaccine (DEV)
    (c) Live attenuated tissue culture vaccine
    (d) Pasteur modified virus vaccine
    (e) All of the above

27. RNA tumor viruses may integrate their genomes into cellular DNA by means of which of the following?
    (a) RNA-dependent RNA-polymerase
    (b) RNA-dependent DNA-polymerase
    (c) DNA-dependent RNA-polymerase
    (d) DNA-dependent DNA-polymerase
    (e) Thymidine kinase

28. Reye's syndrome of children (encephalopathy and fatty degeneration of the liver) is most frequently associated epidemiologically with which of the following?
    (a) Hepatitis A virus
    (b) Influenza B virus
    (c) Coronavirus
    (d) Arthropod-borne viruses
    (e) Retroviruses

29. Which of the following events would *preclude* transformation of a cell by an oncogenic DNA virus?
    (a) Transcription of any viral early gene
    (b) Translation of any viral early mRNA
    (c) Transcription of any viral late gene
    (d) Translation of any viral late mRNA
    (e) Lytic release of progeny virus

30. Delivery by cesarean section is advised if the mother:
    (a) Has serum IgG specific for HSV2
    (b) Presents with gingivostomatitis
    (c) Has serum IgM specific for HSV2
    (d) Both a and b
    (e) a, b, and c

31. Which list correctly arranges the viruses in order of increasing size?
    (a) Poxvirus, rhabdovirus, parvovirus
    (b) Papovavirus, adenovirus, poxvirus
    (c) Orthomyxovirus, herpesvirus, togavirus
    (d) Picornavirus, rhabdovirus, parvovirus
    (e) Rhabdovirus, poxvirus, picornavirus

32. From which of the following viruses could an attenuated viral strain be prepared by genetic reassortment to be incorporated into a vaccine for human use?
    (a) Vaccinia virus
    (b) Herpes simplex virus
    (c) Rubeola virus
    (d) Influenza A virus
    (e) Rabies virus

33. The diagnosis of congenital rubella can be made by:
    (a) Detection of serum IgM antibody in the newborn
    (b) Isolation of rubella virus from the placenta
    (c) Detection of serum IgG antibody after the age of 3 months
    (d) Isolation of rubella virus from the fetus
    (e) All of the above

34. A primary viral isolate from a suspected case of poliomyelitis was inoculated into VERO cells, and a dramatic cytopathic effect (CPE) was noted within 24 hours. The isolate was confirmed as

poliovirus by neutralization with polyvalent anti-body to poliovirus types I, II, III; however, monospecific antibody to each type failed to block CPE. This finding suggests that the isolate contained which of the following?
(a) Recombinant type I and type II viruses
(b) Virus that shares a few antigenic determinants with poliovirus
(c) Mixture of polio and another type of picorna-virus
(d) Hybrid virus of type I and type II poliovirus
(e) Mixture of two types of poliovirus

35. What is the single most important factor differentiating viruses from *Chlamydia?*
(a) Obligate intracellular parasitism
(b) A complex life cycle
(c) Energy parasitism
(d) The presence of a single type of nucleic acid in one and not the other

36. Bence Jones proteins, which are often found in the urine of patients with multiple myeloma, are:
(a) Mu chains
(b) Gamma chains
(c) Kappa or lambda chains
(d) Albumin
(e) Fibrinogen split products

37. A secretory piece is attached to IgA:
(a) In epithelial cells
(b) In plasma cells
(c) By enzymes in mucous secretions
(d) By T cells
(e) By macrophages

38. Lysis of bacteria by specific antibody:
(a) Requires the presence *only* of late complement components (C5–C9)
(b) Requires both early and late complement components
(c) Is seen most frequently with gram-positive organisms containing highly antigenic capsular polysaccharide
(d) Is seen more frequently with bacilli than with cocci
(e) Is mediated by specific proteases secreted by phagocytic cells

39. Which of the following is associated with a deficiency of the third component of complement, C3?
(a) Pyogenic infections
(b) Systemic lupus erythematosus
(c) Xeroderma pigmentosum
(d) Poststreptococcal glomerulonephritis
(e) Immune complex diseases

40. Immune response (Ir) genes:
(a) Are linked to the X chromosome
(b) Control V-region amino acid sequence variability in immunoglobulins
(c) Are linked to the histocompatibility gene complex
(d) Control common region allotypes of immunoglobulins
(e) Are found in all animals, from sponges to humans

41. Parental incompatibility with respect to major ABO groups protects the fetus from hemolytic disease of the newborn (which might arise from concomitant Rh incompatibility) because:
(a) Maternal antibodies to fetal Rh antigens are IgM
(b) Antibodies to Rh antigens cannot cross the placenta
(c) Maternal antibodies clear the circulation of fetal erythrocytes before sensitization can occur
(d) Maternal antibodies, although they get to the fetus, will cause only minimal agglutination and not lysis, since fetal levels of complement are low
(e) Fetal agglutinins will suppress the maternal response to erythrocyte antigens

42. The mechanism by which antihistaminic compounds relieve allergic conditions involves:
(a) Acceleration of the excretion of histamine
(b) Neutralization of the effects of histamine
(c) Chemical combination with and inactivation of histamine
(d) Competition with histamine for attachment to cell receptors
(e) Activation of histamine oxidase

43. In order to prevent hemolytic disease in a newborn with an A-positive mother and an O-negative father, you would:
(a) Administer RhoGAM to the mother after the birth of her first child
(b) Administer RhoGAM to each of her subsequent children
(c) Administer RhoGAM to the mother after her first A-positive daughter
(d) Administer RhoGAM to her first O-negative child
(e) Do nothing—there is no danger to any of her children

44. In serum sickness due to administration of horse antivenom, which of the following is to be expected?
(a) Decrease of serum C4 but not of C3
(b) Decrease of serum C3 but not of C4
(c) Decrease of both serum C3 and C4

(d) Decrease of neither serum C3 nor C4
(e) Decrease of serum C2 but not of C5

45. T_H cells:
(a) Proliferate in response to free antigens
(b) Bear CD4 and CD8 cell surface markers
(c) Help convert CTL precursors into active killer cells
(d) Are restricted in their response to exogenous antigen by the requirement that they coordinately recognize HLA-A, B, or C molecules
(e) Are easily differentiated from T_{DTH} cells

46. Cell-mediated immunity is especially important for recovery from infections caused by bacteria that are:
(a) Encapsulated
(b) Facultative anaerobes
(c) Facultative intracellular pathogens
(d) Cell-wall deficient
(e) Gram-negative

47. A child with leukemia has blast cells that react with the monoclonal antibody to CD4, but not with monoclonal antibody to CD8. Their cell lineage is most likely:
(a) A bursa-equivalent cell line
(b) From a phagocytic cell
(c) Suppressor T cells
(d) Helper T cells
(e) None of the above

48. Which of the following bacterial substances binds to the Fc portion of immunoglobulin molecules?
(a) Endotoxin
(b) Coagulase
(c) Lipoteichoic acid
(d) M Protein
(e) Protein A

49. Haemophilus influenzae:
(a) Is hemolytic
(b) Contains X and V factors in the capsule
(c) Is a gram-positive pleomorphic bacillus
(d) Produces an immunogenic antiphagocytic capsule
(e) Produces neurotoxins

50. What component(s) of the pneumococcus is(are) purified and used in the manufacture of pneumococcal vaccine?
(a) Mucopeptides from the cell wall
(b) Capsular polysaccharide
(c) C-substance
(d) M protein

51. DNA is extracted from smooth type I cells and injected into a mouse along with living rough cells obtained from smooth type III cells. If mutation and selection rather than transformation occur, the mouse should die of a pneumo-

coccal infection produced by which of the following?
(a) Smooth type I cells
(b) Smooth type III cells
(c) Rough cells derived from smooth type I cells
(d) Rough cells derived from smooth type III cells
(e) None of the above

52. A positive test for cold agglutinins in a patient with pneumonia is presumptive evidence of infection with:
(a) Streptococcus pneumoniae
(b) Mycoplasma pneumoniae
(c) Klebsiella pneumoniae
(d) Influenza virus
(e) Adenovirus

53. The antiphagocytic property of the group A streptococcus is associated with which of the following?
(a) Hyaluronidase
(b) Streptolysin S
(c) M protein
(d) C carbohydrate
(e) Mucopeptide

54. A rising titer of antistreptolysin O indicates:
(a) Acute rheumatic fever
(b) Hemorrhagic glomerulonephritis
(c) A recent streptococcal infection
(d) Scarlet fever
(e) None of the above

55. Instruments used in diagnostic bacteriology include the gas–liquid chromatograph, which provides information on a culture's:
(a) Generation of hydrogen sulfide and methane
(b) pH in carbohydrate media
(c) Production of organic acid metabolic end-products
(d) Production of microbial antigens
(e) Production of pigments

56. Which of the following bacteria can in certain cases be found inside a human red blood cell?
(a) Bartonella bacilliformis
(b) Streptobacillus moniliformis
(c) Listeria monocytogenes
(d) Erysipelothrix rhusiopathiae
(e) None of the above

57. Mycoplasma pneumoniae can be differentiated from other species of human mycoplasma and from L forms of bacteria by:
(a) Its susceptibility to tetracycline
(b) Its ability to pass through bacterial filters
(c) The ability of its colonies to adsorb sheep red blood cells

(d) Its inability to revert to a bacterial form
(e) Its growth requirement for sterols

58. The total number of viable bacteria present in a broth culture is determined most accurately by:
   (a) Photometric measurement of turbidity
   (b) Direct microscopic count
   (c) Colony counts made by the agar pour plate method
   (d) Agglutination with specific antiserum
   (e) Analysis of total bacterial nitrogen

59. Which of the following is a unique aspect of cariogenic strains of *Streptococcus mutans* that sets them apart from other oral acidogenic microbes?
   (a) Four equivalents of acid formed per mole of glucose
   (b) Extracellular polysaccharide made from glucose
   (c) Formation of levans from fructose
   (d) Formation of glucans from sucrose
   (e) Secretion of proteolytic enzymes

60. Which of the following is the correct sequence of steps in performing a Gram stain?
   (a) Safranin stain, decolorization, crystal violet stain, iodine solution
   (b) Crystal violet stain, decolorization, safranin stain, iodine solution
   (c) Safranin stain, iodine solution, decolorization, crystal violet stain
   (d) Crystal violet stain, iodine solution, decolorization, safranin stain

61. Pasteurization is a process in which liquids are:
   (a) Heated to 62° C to kill vegetative bacteria
   (b) Heated to 100° C to kill vegetative bacteria and spores
   (c) Heated to 120° C to kill vegetative bacteria and spores
   (d) Filtered to remove vegetative bacteria and spores
   (e) Filtered to remove vegetative bacteria and spores and then heated to 120° C to inactivate viruses

62. A live attenuated bacterium is used as a vaccine for protection against which one of the following diseases?
   (a) Botulism
   (b) Pertussis
   (c) Tuberculosis
   (d) Tetanus
   (e) Meningococcal meningitis

63. Abnormal neutrophil function is most often associated with recurrent infections caused by which of the following?
   (a) *Mycobacterium tuberculosis*
   (b) *Staphylococcus aureus*

(c) *Legionella pneumophila*
(d) *Streptococcus pneumoniae*
(e) *Streptococcus pyogenes*

64. Which of the following statements concerning the glyoxylate shunt is true?
   (a) The glyoxylate shunt results in the net synthesis of 1 mole of glyoxylic acid from 2 moles of acetyl-CoA.
   (b) The glyoxylate shunt bypasses the conversion of citrate to isocitrate.
   (c) The glyoxylate shunt requires all of the enzymes of the tricarboxylic acid cycle.
   (d) The two key enzymes of the glyoxylate shunt are isocitrate lyase and malate synthetase.

65. Sulfanilamide and related sulfonamides:
   (a) Are bactericidal
   (b) Inhibit the enzyme dihydrofolate reductase
   (c) Prevent the transport of folic acid into bacterial cells
   (d) May fail to inhibit susceptible bacteria if necrotic tissue is present
   (e) Are selectively toxic to bacteria because they can enter bacterial cells but cannot enter mammalian cells

66. Which of the following is the prevalent bacterial species in the colon of an adult?
   (a) A facultative anaerobe
   (b) A microaerophilic bacterium
   (c) An obligate anaerobe
   (d) An aerotolerant bacterium
   (e) An obligate aerobe

67. Antibiotic-associated colitis has been linked to a toxin produced by which one of the following organisms?
   (a) *Clostridium perfringens*
   (b) *Bacteroides fragilis*
   (c) *Bacteroides corrodens*
   (d) *Clostridium difficile*
   (e) *Campylobacter fetus*

68. The most reliable method for diagnosis of primary syphilis is the:
   (a) VDRL test
   (b) FTA-ABS test
   (c) Microhemagglutinin test
   (d) Darkfield examination of chancre material
   (e) *Treponema pallidum* immobilization test

69. Which of the following protozoan infections is normally transmitted sexually (venereally)?
   (a) *Giardia lamblia*
   (b) *Entamoeba histolytica*
   (c) *Trichomonas vaginalis*
   (d) *Entamoeba gingivalis*
   (e) *Balantidium coli*

70. Which of the following types of cells are *not* infected by HIV-1?

(a) CD4+ T cells (T_H)
(b) CD8+ T cells ($T_{c/s}$)
(c) Peripheral blood monocytes
(d) Lung macrophages

71. Which of the following pertains to HPV (human papilloma virus):
(a) Plantar warts can become malignant if exposed to too much sunlight.
(b) *Epidermodysplasia verruciformis* (EV) lesions can become malignant.
(c) Cervical cancer is associated to a high degree with anogenital warts present in patients with condylomas (HPV types 6, 11).
(d) Keratinocytes that are terminally differentiated serve as a culture system for growing HPV.

72. The hepatitis virus or agent with similarities to plant viroids is:
(a) Hepatitis A
(b) Hepatitis B
(c) Hepatitis C
(d) Hepatitis E
(e) Delta Agent

73. The following best describes the antiviral action of AZT or ddI:
(a) Induces an oligonucleotide polymerase and protein kinase that interferes with the translation of viral mRNA
(b) Specific inhibitor of HIV-1 reverse transcriptase
(c) Prevents the uncoating of influenza A viruses
(d) An unusual base is responsible for its activity.

Section B

In each of the following series of questions, each statement is followed by four possible answers. For each question answer:

(a) if only 1, 2, and 3 are correct
(b) if only 1 and 3 are correct
(c) if only 2 and 4 are correct
(d) if only 4 is correct
(e) if all the answers are correct

74. Which of the following statements regarding the acquired immune deficiency syndrome (AIDS) are true?
1. The number of new cases reported has leveled off, thereby reducing the public health concern.
2. An individual is at significantly increased risk of contracting AIDS when giving blood as a donor.

3. The human T-cell leukemia viruses (HTLV-I or -II) have been proved to be related to the virus causing AIDS.
4. Individuals with AIDS have lymphopenia with a marked deficiency of T-helper cells.

75. Endospores are usually:
1. Readily stained by the Gram staining procedure
2. Produced by very young cells (less than 24 hours old)
3. Killed by heating to 62° C for 30 minutes (pasteurization)
4. Produced when the nutrient supply becomes limiting

76. Enzymatic digestion with papain of an immunoglobulin molecule will produce:
1. Fd fragments
2. Two Fab fragments
3. An F(ab)2 fragment
4. An Fc fragment

77. Which of the following are non–spore-forming anaerobic bacteria that assume major significance in disease processes?
1. *Bacteroides fragilis*
2. *Fusobacterium nucleatum*
3. *Peptostreptococcus anaerobius*
4. *Actinomyces israelii*

78. Combination antimicrobial chemotherapy is indicated for which of the following clinical conditions?
1. Enterococcal endocarditis
2. Pulmonary tuberculosis
3. Cryptococcal meningitis
4. *Haemophilus influenzae* pneumonia

79. Growth on a cell-free artificial solid medium is possible for:
1. *Ureaplasma urealyticum*
2. *Mycoplasma pneumoniae*
3. An L form of *Proteus vulgaris*
4. *Chlamydia*

80. Characteristics of the alpha toxin of *Clostridium perfringens* include which of the following?
1. Liberation of phosphoryl choline from lecithin
2. Liberation of free fatty acid from lecithin
3. Hemolysis
4. Paralysis of muscles of humans and animals

81. Enterococci:
1. Are members of group D streptococci
2. Are normal flora in the gastrointestinal tract
3. Are a significant cause of bacterial endocarditis
4. Are exquisitely sensitive to penicillin G

82. The antibacterial activity of beta-lactam antibiotics:

1. Is bactericidal under all circumstances
2. Results in the formation of a covalent linkage between the drug and the enzyme catalyzing transpeptidation
3. Is independent of bacterial autolytic activity
4. Occurs at a step in peptidoglycan synthesis following translocation of polyisoprenoid alcohol phosphate-linked intermediates to a site external to the plasma membrane

83. Which of the following serve(s) to distinguish between aerobic respiration and anaerobic respiration?
1. Only aerobic respiration results in the net oxidation of substrates.
2. The terminal electron acceptors in aerobic respiration are organic compounds.
3. Production of ATP by substrate-level phosphorylation occurs only during anaerobic respiration.
4. In anaerobic respiration an inorganic molecule other than O_2 serves as the terminal electron acceptor.

84. The Weil-Felix reaction:
1. Is a skin test used in the diagnosis of chlamydial infections
2. Involves the agglutination of certain strains of *Proteus* by serum antibodies
3. Distinguishes group A from group B togaviruses
4. Is useful in the diagnosis of rickettsial infections

85. Which of the following factors dispose to the development of toxic shock syndrome?
1. Vaginal colonization with *Staphylococcus aureus*
2. Presence of polyester material that binds Mg
3. Individual susceptibility to the involved toxin
4. Pharyngeal colonization with group A *Streptococcus*

86. Which of the following organisms produce(s) toxin(s) that act in organs and tissues distant from the site of colonization?
1. *Vibrio cholerae*
2. *Salmonella typhi*
3. *Escherichia coli*
4. *Corynebacterium diphtheriae*

87. Which of the following statements about diphtheria are true?
1. Immunity to diphtheria depends on circulating antitoxin.
2. Humans are the only hosts for the organism.
3. Toxin is produced only by strains lysogenic for bacteriophages carrying the tox gene.
4. Fragment A of the toxin is responsible for attachment to host cells.

88. Extracellular products of *Streptococcus pyogenes* include which of the following?
1. Streptokinase
2. Glucosyl transferase
3. Streptolysin O
4. C carbohydrate

89. Virulence of enteropathogenic *E. coli* as the causative agent in diarrhea is dependent on the:
1. Expression of serotype 0111 : B4 or 0127 : B8
2. Expression of colonization factor antigen
3. Depression of the concentration of iron in the intestine
4. Elaboration of an enterotoxin

90. Fibroblast interferon:
1. Inhibits translation of viral mRNA
2. Induces a host cell gene to effect its antiviral activity
3. Generally exhibits specificity for animal species in which it was induced
4. Is inhibitory only for the family of viruses that induced it

91. Which of the following diseases are primary zoonoses that are only occasionally the source of human infection?
1. Brucellosis
2. Leptospirosis
3. Anthrax
4. Diphtheria

92. Which of the following statements about rheumatic fever are correct?
1. It results from an immune response to a group A streptococcal infection.
2. Elevation in the ASO titer is a useful diagnostic criterion.
3. Subsequent infections with group A streptococci predispose the host to recurrent disease.
4. Treatment involves the use of penicillin G.

93. Which of the following products function as adherence factors for the colonization of mucous membranes?
1. Lipoteichoic acid of *Streptococcus pyogenes*
2. Capsular polysaccharide of *Streptococcus pneumoniae*
3. Pili of *Neisseria gonorrhoeae*
4. Lipid A of *Escherichia coli*

94. Which of the following statements about serologic tests for syphilis is are true?
1. The FTA-ABS (fluorescent treponemal antibody-absorbed) test is positive in almost all patients with secondary, latent, or tertiary syphilis.
2. The VDRL (Venereal Disease Research Laboratory) test detects antibodies that react with the nontreponemal antigen cardiolipin.

3. The FTA-ABS (fluorescent treponemal antibody-aborbed) test can be used to determine whether a positive VDRL test represents treponemal infection or a biologic false-positive reaction.
4. The TPI (*Treponema pallidum* immobilization) test is an indirect fluorescent antibody test for antitreponemal antigen in serum.

95. For which of the following organisms does opsonic antibody play a major role in acquired immunity to infection?
1. *Neisseria meningitidis*, group A
2. *Vibrio cholerae*
3. *Haemophilus influenzae*, type b
4. *Corynebacterium diphtheriae*

96. Which of the following organisms is/are associated with manifestations of "immune complex" disease?
1. *Plasmodium malariae*
2. *Streptococcus pyogenes*, group A
3. Hepatitis B virus
4. *Haemophilus influenzae*, type B

97. A cell containing an entire integrated SV-40 genome would likely be induced to start synthesizing infectious virus particles by:
1. Treatment with mutagenic chemicals
2. Infection with a cytocidal (cell-killing) virus
3. Fusion with another cell type permissive for SV-40 replication
4. Treatment with antiviral antibody

98. Which of the following statement(s) about viroids are true?
1. They are conventional viruses of very small size.
2. They have lipid envelopes.
3. They are not associated with human disease.
4. They are infectious nucleic acids.

99. Which of the following viruses possess(es) DNA, a capsid with icosahedral symmetry, and no lipid envelope?
1. Herpesvirus
2. Adenovirus
3. Poxvirus
4. Papovavirus

100. The hemagglutinin (HA) of influenza virus:
1. Induces antibodies that correlate with host resistance
2. Possesses cross-reactive A, B, and C antigens
3. Is responsible for attachment of the virus to susceptible cells
4. Must be cleaved into HA-1 and HA-2 before virus can be released from cells

101. Which of the following is/are known to exist in only one major antigenic type?
1. Measles
2. Rubella
3. Mumps
4. Adenovirus

102. All C-type retrovirus particles:
1. Have a centrally located core
2. Contain reverse transcriptase
3. Replicate via a DNA intermediate
4. Contain a lipid envelope

103. Which of the following induce(s) nuclear inclusions in infected cells?
1. Cytomegalovirus
2. Adenovirus
3. Papovaviruses
4. Smallpox virus

104. Which of the following statements is/are true of all paramyxoviruses?
1. They contain a single-stranded RNA genome of negative polarity.
2. Envelopes are derived from the host cells' plasma membrane.
3. They have a cytoplasmic site of replication.
4. They enter the body by the respiratory route.

105. The heterophile antibody that appears in the serum during infectious mononucleosis:
1. Is detected by agglutination of formalinized horse erythrocytes
2. Is removed from the serum by absorption with guinea pig kidney tissue
3. Is removed from the serum by absorption with bovine red blood cells
4. Persists in persons who have been infected with Epstein-Barr virus

106. Susceptible cultured cells infected with which of the following viruses would exhibit hemadsorption with the appropriate erythrocytes?
1. Sindbis virus
2. Rabies virus
3. Measles virus
4. Respiratory syncytial virus

107. Polyoma virus will:
1. Transform "nonpermissive" cells in culture
2. Replicate and cause a lytic infection in "permissive" cells in culture
3. Cause lytic infections with a much lower multiplicity of infection/cell as compared with that required for transformation
4. Replicate in transformed cells with the continued release of infectious virus during an extended period of time

108. Members of the herpetoviridae:
1. Are a leading cause of corneal blindness
2. Cause vesicular eruptions limited to the posterior portion of the oral cavity (tonsillar pillars, tonsils, pharynx)

3. Cause congenital infections of the fetus that may lead to mental retardation
4. Cause epidemic pleurodynia

109. In which of the following is the genome double-stranded nucleic acid?
    1. Orthomyxoviruses
    2. Poxviruses
    3. Parvoviruses
    4. Reoviruses

110. A segmented RNA genome is characteristic of which of the following?
    1. Arenaviruses
    2. Reoviruses
    3. Bunyaviruses
    4. Orthomyxoviruses

111. Which of the following contain(s) an RNA-dependent DNA polymerase as a structural component of the virion?
    1. Adenoviruses
    2. Orthomyxoviruses
    3. Rhabdoviruses
    4. RNA tumor viruses

112. Which of the following viral proteins are involved in viral attachment to host cells?
    1. Paramyxovirus nucleocapsid antigen
    2. Adenovirus fiber antigen
    3. Vaccinia virus DNA polymerases
    4. Influenza virus hemagglutinins

113. Immunoglobulin produced by a particular B cell and its progeny:
    1. Has antibody specificity encoded in the B-cell genome
    2. May switch from one idiotype to another during B-cell differentiation
    3. May switch from one isotype to another during B-cell differentiation
    4. Has antibody specificity induced by interaction with antigen

114. Which of the following vaccine(s) should *not* be given to an immunodeficient patient?
    1. Influenza vaccine
    2. Rubella vaccine
    3. Pneumococcal vaccine
    4. Trivalent oral polio vaccine

115. A quantitative precipitin test was performed using type 3 pneumococcal polysaccharide (S3) as antigen and rabbit antiserum against S3 as the source of antibody (anti-S3). Which of the following statements concerning this test are true?
    1. At any point on the precipitin curve, most or all of the protein in the precipitate will be immunoglobulin.
    2. The ratio of antibody to antigen in the pre-cipitate will be highest in the tubes that contain the smallest amount of antigen.
    3. In the equivalence zone the precipitate will contain essentially all of the S3 and anti-S3; no free S3 or anti-S3 will remain in the supernatant.
    4. In the zone of antigen excess some anti-S3 will remain in the supernatant as soluble complexes with S3.

116. Which of the following determinants are considered important in predicting the success of kidney transplants?
    1. The T-cell determinants that react with CD 3, 4, and 8 antibodies
    2. The HLA antigens
    3. The allotypic determinants on immuno-globulins
    4. The ABO antigens on red blood cells

117. Which of the following statements about anti-malarial drugs is/are correct?
    1. A standard course of treatment with chloro-quine will prevent relapses of vivax malaria.
    2. The 4-aminoquinolines are no longer useful for malaria prophylaxis.
    3. Primaquine is the antimalarial drug of choice for persons with glucose-6-phosphate de-hydrogenase deficiency.
    4. Pyrimethamine or trimethoprim, in combination with a sulfonamide, has been used successfully to treat chloroquine-resistant falciparum malaria.

118. Which of the following statements regarding poststreptococcal glomerulonephritis is/are correct?
    1. It represents an immune-complex disease.
    2. Treatment involves penicillin to suppress the immune response.
    3. Proteinuria, hematuria, and depressed serum complement levels are characteristic.
    4. Prevention is accomplished by active immunization using cell wall antigens.

119. Possible sources of "second signals" to a B cell bound by specific antigen include:
    1. EB virus
    2. Endotoxin
    3. Antigen-specific T cells
    4. Plasma cells

120. Mononuclear cells that are capable of suppressing immune responses include:
    1. Monocytes
    2. Polymorphonuclear leukocytes (PMN)
    3. CD-8 positive lymphocytes
    4. CD-13 positive lymphocytes

121. Interleukin-1 (IL-1):

1. Is the product of both lymphocytes and macrophages
2. Is the sole signal required for proliferation of T lymphocytes
3. Is an example of an antigen-specific factor
4. Induces the maturation of IL-2-producing lymphocytes

122. Complex, class II loci gene products:
1. Are designated HLA-D in humans
2. Are found as surface determinants on activated T lymphocytes
3. Stimulate T cells in mixed lymphocyte reactions
4. Elicit blocking antibodies during the course of renal allograft rejection

123. Which of the following parameters are increased in association with neutrophil phagocytosis?
1. Production of lactate
2. Oxygen consumption
3. Hydrogen peroxide formation
4. Rate of PMN cell division

124. Bacterial endospores are characterized by:
1. A low level of metabolic activity
2. An accumulation of dipicolinic acid
3. Many surface layers, one of which is peptidoglycan and another of which is keratin-like
4. Greater resistance to heat, drying, and radiation than vegetative cells

125. The NBT (nitro blue tetrazolium) reduction assay is used to:
1. Evaluate granulocyte function
2. Evaluate T-cell function
3. Determine whether polymorphonuclear leukocytes can produce superoxide
4. Stain B lymphocytes

126. Interleukin-2 (IL-2) is an important molecule in immune responses. Which of the following functions does it carry out?
1. Binds to and "presents" antigen
2. Helps generate cytotoxic T cells
3. Kills virus-infected cells
4. Is required for replication of helper T cells

127. *Pneumocystis carinii:*
1. Can be detected in a lung biopsy by the methenamine silver stain
2. Causes an exudative pneumonia with large numbers of plasma cells
3. Is a high-risk infectious agent for leukemic children under chemotherapy
4. Is best treated with amphotericin B

128. Cryptosporidiosis:
1. Is a zoonosis
2. Is self-limiting in immunocompetent persons
3. May be chronic and severe in immunosuppressed persons
4. Does not require an intermediate host

129. Pneumocystis:
1. Is a common cause of infection but usually causes disease only when immunity is impaired
2. Is usually diagnosed by serologic testing
3. Is best diagnosed by the finding of cysts in biopsy material
4. Is readily cultured for diagnosis

130. Which of the following stages of the *Plasmodium* cycle occur in humans?
1. Exoerythrocytic multiplication in liver parenchymal cells
2. Schizogony and formation of merozoites
3. Erythrocytic cyclic reinfection with merozoites
4. Sporogony and ookinete maturation to sporozoites and oocysts

131. Which of the following statements about host defenses against fungal infections is/are correct?
1. Antibody is not protective.
2. Leukocytes can kill fungi.
3. Mild illness can confer protection against future infections.
4. Interferon released from lymphocytes slows fungal metabolism.

132. Amphotericin B is:
1. Fungicidal
2. Dermotoxic
3. Administered parenterally
4. Effective against *Mycobacteria*

133. Asexual spores of fungi are:
1. Arthrospores
2. Chlamydospores
3. Blastospores
4. Ascospores

134. Which of the following characteristics distinguish(es) fungi from bacteria?
1. The presence of intracellular double-stranded DNA
2. The presence of ribosomes
3. The capacity to produce extracellular enzymes
4. The presence of mitochondria

135. *Coccidioides immitis* is identified in tissues on the basis of which of the following?
1. Budding yeast cells with pseudohyphae
2. Yeastlike forms with very large capsules
3. Arthrospores
4. Endosporulating spherules

136. The phenomenon of genetic reassortment:
1. Can occur during reovirus replication

2. Involves the crossing over of genes within an RNA segment
3. Can occur during influenza virus replication
4. Can occur only with RNA viruses of plus polarity

137. Interferon:
    1. Is species specific
    2. Reacts directly with virus particles to inactivate them
    3. Reacts with cells, and the affected cells then become resistant to a number of different viruses
    4. Is constitutively produced at high levels in cells but requires an inducer for activity

138. Bunyaviruses and arenaviruses share which of the following properties?
    1. Have segmented RNA genomes
    2. Contain ribosomes
    3. Can cause hemorrhagic fever
    4. Are transmitted by insect vectors

139. Which of the following is/are characteristics of both virulent and temperate bacteriophages?
    1. Always contain RNA as the genetic material
    2. Kill the host bacterium following productive (lytic) infection
    3. Integrate phage DNA into the host genome as part of normal lytic infection
    4. Life cycle includes both extracellular virion production and vegetative intracellular growth

140. Which of the following mechanisms may be involved in desensitization to an allergen?
    1. Enhanced production of circulating IgG, which binds the allergen before its adsorption to mast cells
    2. Enhanced production of IgG, which displaces the IgE on mast cells
    3. Enhanced production of T-suppressor cells
    4. Enhanced production of antihistamines

141. Activation of lymphocytes in type IV hypersensitivity (DTH) may result in the release of:
    1. Opsonins
    2. Interleukins
    3. Anaphylatoxins
    4. Mitogenic factor

142. Pre–B cells are characterized by:
    1. Monomeric IgM on the surface of the cells
    2. A large cytoplasm-to-nucleus ratio
    3. The presence of IgD in the cytoplasm
    4. The presence of monomeric IgM in the cytoplasm

143. Which of the following statements about the initiation of the classical complement cascade are correct?
    1. Two molecules of IgG are required to activate it.

2. A subunit of C1 attaches to the C(H2) subregion of the heavy chain.
3. The interaction of antigen and one molecule of IgM is sufficient to initiate it.
4. C3b interacts with factor B.at the cell membrane.

144. Phosphodiesterase inhibitors:
    1. Increase mast cell cyclic AMP levels
    2. Have an effect on mast cell degranulation analogous to stimulators of adenylate cyclase
    3. Include theophylline
    4. May enhance recovery from an asthmatic attack

145. IgA has which of the following properties?
    1. It neutralizes certain viruses.
    2. It fixes complement via the classical pathway.
    3. It is found in plasma cells located in the lamina propria of the gut.
    4. It occurs primarily as a polymer in both secretions and serum.

146. Soluble antigen–antibody complexes in the blood:
    1. May be trapped against the vessel basement membrane if they are greater than 19 S in size
    2. Activate complement via the classical pathway
    3. May be deposited in the kidney
    4. Initiate type IV (DTH) reactions

147. Capsules are involved with pathogenicity in which of the following?
    1. *Klebsiella pneumoniae*
    2. *Cryptococcus neoformans*
    3. *Neisseria meningitidis*
    4. *Bacillus anthracis*

148. Erythrogenic toxin:
    1. Is produced by lysogenic strains of *Streptococcus pyogenes*
    2. Occurs in three immunologically distinct forms
    3. Is responsible for the scarlatinal rash of scarlet fever
    4. Stimulates the production of antibodies that will prevent infection with group A streptococci

149. *Clostridium perfringens:*
    1. Is found in the genital tract of some healthy women
    2. Is found in the intestinal tract of some healthy humans
    3. Is a frequent cause of so-called food poisoning
    4. Produces a toxin that degrades lecithin

150. *Chlamydia trachomatis:*
    1. Is an obligate intracellular parasite
    2. Is a common cause of sexually transmitted disease

3. Is a common cause of eye infections
4. May be transmitted from infected animals to human beings

151. *Streptococcus pyogenes* with type 12 M protein:
1. Fails to adhere to host pharyngeal epithelium
2. Induces immune responses but not protective immunity
3. Adheres to epithelium but fails to induce an inflammatory response
4. Induces immune responses that may lead to acute glomerulonephritis in 10% to 15% of infections

152. Clinically important R-factor–mediated mechanisms of acquired antibiotic resistance include which of the following?
1. For penicillins (beta-lactam antibiotics): decreased accumulation because of decreased active transport across the cytoplasmic membrane
2. For aminoglycosides: inactivation by enzymatic modification
3. For tetracyclines: inactivation by enzymatic modification
4. For penicillins (beta-lactam antibiotics): decreased outer membrane permeability (in gram-negative bacteria) usually associated with periplasmic lactamase production

153. Infection by group B streptococci:
1. Can be followed by rheumatic fever
2. Frequently occurs in persons debilitated by underlying systemic disease
3. Can be prevented by vaccine directed against the capsule
4. Occurs in neonates

154. Antitoxic antibodies are not found in the serum of patients recovering from which of the following?
1. Diphtheria
2. Botulism
3. Cholera
4. Streptococcal pneumonia

155. *Legionella pneumophila:*
1. Is a small, gram-negative rod
2. Is transmitted from person to person
3. Grows best at 35° C in 50% CO_2
4. Grows on MacConkey's agar

156. BCG vaccine:
1. Raises antibodies that can passively transfer resistance to tuberculosis in guinea pigs
2. Is an acid-fast, non–spore-forming, aerobic bacillus
3. Is a formalin-killed bacterial suspension
4. Evokes delayed sensitivity against PPD (purified protein derivative)

Section C

Directions. *Preceding each group of numbered terms or statements is a diagram or a lettered set of possible answers. Match each numbered item with the correct answer. Answers may be used more than once in each group.*

The following diagram represents the amount of antigen present as a function of time after IV injection of antigen.

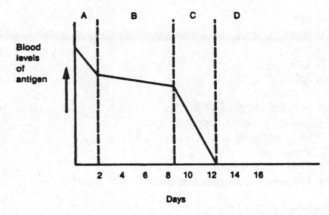

Questions 157–160

157. Indicates time of immune elimination
158. Indicates time of equilibrium with extravascular tissue
159. Indicates time when free antibody may be detected
160. Indicates time when soluble (*i.e.,* small) immune complexes may be formed in "serum sickness"–type hypersensitivity

Questions 161–165

(a) *Leishmania tropica*
(b) *Trypanosoma cruzi*
(c) *Leishmania donovani*
(d) *Trypanosoma gambiense*
(e) *Leishmania brasiliensis*

161. African sleeping sickness
162. Kala azar
163. Chagas' disease
164. Tropical ulcer
165. Mucocutaneous leishmaniasis

Quesions 166–167

(a) Macrophages, polymorphonuclear leukocytes (PMN)
(b) K cells and macrophages

(c) T lymphocytes
(d) B lymphocytes
(e) Thymocytes

166. Kill virus-infected cells through antibody-dependent cell-mediated cytolysis (ADCC)
167. Upon specific recognition of viral antigens, kill cells by attaching to virus-induced surface antigens

Questions 168–173

(a) IgA
(b) IgM
(c) IgE
(d) IgG
(e) IgD

168. Longest serum half-life
169. Lowest serum concentration
170. Best agglutinin
171. Pentamer
172. Highest sedimentation coefficient
173. Highest serum concentration

Questions 174–177

(a) B cells
(b) T cells
(c) Both B and T cells
(d) Neither B nor T cells

174. Stem cells arise in bone marrow
175. Possess antigen-specific receptors
176. Usually express IgG on their surface
177. Responsible for affinity maturation

Questions 178–183

(a) *Chlamydia trachomatis*
(b) Rubella virus
(c) Both
(d) Neither

178. Intracellular parasite
179. DNA genome
180. Segmented RNA genome
181. Surface infection
182. Vector transmitted
183. Hemagglutinin

Questions 184–191

(a) *Plasmodium vivax*
(b) *Plasmodium malariae*
(c) *Plasmodium falciparum*

(d) *Plasmodium ovale*

184. Visceral microinfarcts
185. Quartan fever pattern
186. Malignant form of the disease
187. Sausage-shaped gametocytes
188. Most common worldwide
189. Cerebral "ring" hemorrhages
190. Prefers old erythrocytes
191. Prefers reticulocytes

Questions 192–199

(a) Bancroftian filariasis
(b) Dracontiasis
(c) Onchocerciasis
(d) Chagas' disease

192. Megaesophagus
193. Blindness
194. Skin ulcers
195. Subcutaneous nodules
196. Cardiac failure
197. Hydrocele
198. Lymphangitis
199. Romana's sign

Questions 200–205

(a) Paramyxoviruses
(b) Retroviruses
(c) Reoviruses
(d) Picornaviruses
(e) Orthomyxoviruses

200. Contain double-stranded RNA, which is in segments
201. Purified naked RNA is infectious if inserted in cells; do not carry a polymerase for production of mRNA
202. Contain single-stranded RNA, which is in eight segments and is antimessenger
203. Carry an RNA-dependent DNA polymerase (reverse transcriptase) in the virion
204. Nucleic acid is in one long, single-stranded molecule that is antimessenger; virion carries a polymerase that produces multiple mRNAs
205. In their multiplication, produce DNA, which is integrated into the cell genome

Questions 206–210

(a) Echovirus
(b) Influenza virus
(c) Cytomegalovirus

(d) Rabies virus
(e) Hepatitis B virus

206. Segmented genome
207. Intranuclear inclusion body
208. Intracytoplasmic inclusion bodies
209. Aseptic meningitis
210. Very resistant to inactivation by physical and chemical agents

Questions 211–215

(a) Hepatitis B virus
(b) Adenovirus
(c) Both
(d) Neither

211. DNA genome
212. Oncogenic potential
213. Replication in cell culture
214. Dane particle
215. Hemagglutinin on viral surface

Questions 216–219

(a) Adenovirus, type 1
(b) Rous sarcoma virus
(c) Marek's disease virus
(d) Mammary carcinoma virus
(e) Papilloma virus

216. Laryngeal warts
217. Virus infection that can be controlled by vaccination
218. Type B particles are infectious
219. Type C virus proved to be natural cause of cancer in animals

Questions 220–223

(a) IgG
(b) IgA
(c) IgM
(d) IgD
(e) IgE

220. Capable of placental transfer
221. Most important in defense mechanisms of mucous membranes
222. Binds to mast cells via Fc receptors
223. High serum levels associated with parasitic infections

Questions 224–226

(a) IgE antibody

(b) IgA antibody
(c) IgM antibody
(d) IgG antibody
(e) IgD antibody

224. Associated with the release of histamine and slow-reacting substance of anaphylaxis (SRS-A)
225. Functions primarily as an opsonin
226. Most effective in the lysis of certain gram-negative bacteria when complement is present

Questions 227–229

(a) B lymphocytes
(b) T lymphocytes
(c) Macrophages
(d) K cell (null cell)
(e) Natural killer cell (NK cell)

227. Located in the lymph node cortex around germinal centers
228. Located in the periarterial sheath of the spleen and deep cortex of the lymph nodes
229. Have integral membrane Ig on the surface of cells

Questions 230–232

(a) Humans are natural hosts
(b) Humans are accidental hosts
(c) Humans are aberrant hosts

230. Cutaneous larva migrans
231. Filariasis
232. Amebiasis (*E. histolytica*)

Questions 233–236

(a) Symbiosis
(b) Commensalism
(c) Mutualism
(d) Parsasitism

233. Two species of organism living together
234. Beneficial to both species
235. Beneficial to one species without effect on the other
236. Beneficial to one species and detrimental to the other

Questions 237–240

(a) HIV-1
(b) HTLV-I

(c) Both
(d) Neither

237. Belong to the retrovirus family
238. Virus replicates in T cells and requires IL-2
239. Causative agent of adult T-cell leukemia
240. Virus isolated from patient with "hairy cell" leukemia

Questions 241–245

(a) Molluscum contagiosum
(b) B-19
(c) Rubella
(d) HTLV-I
(e) Rotavirus

241. Fifth disease ("slapped-cheek syndrome")
242. Tropical spastic paraparesis
243. Member of the poxvirus family
244. Virus that causes intestinal diarrhea in young children
245. Virus that causes German measles

Questions 246–250

(a) Extra copies seen in relapsed breast/ovarian cancer patients
(b) Homology with NF$\kappa\beta$
(c) Allows transport of singly spliced mRNA from the nucleus
(d) Tyrosine-specific kinase; viral form causes mesenchymal neoplasias in chickens
(e) Tumor suppressor

246. Wild-type p53
247. *rev*
248. *erb*B2/HER2
249. *src*
250. *rel*

Questions 251–254

(a) Reoviruses
(b) Retroviruses
(c) Both
(d) Neither

251. mRNA has a 5' cap and 3' poly A
252. Contains intravirion transcriptaselike enzymes
253. RNA genome is in 2 or more pieces or segments
254. Maturation involves extensive proteolytic cleavages by a viral encoded protease.

Questions 255–258

(a) Viroids
(b) Prions
(c) Both
(d) Neither

255. UV-resistant single-stranded RNA circles
256. Agent that is associated with epidemics of fulminant hepatitis
257. Unconventional agent associated with several different spongiform encephalopathies
258. Virus that exhibits 5:3:2 icosahedral symmetry

Questions 259–263

(a) Polyprotein; protease
(b) gp120; CD4
(c) Primer binding site; tRNA
(d) LTR; provirus
(e) RNA polymerase; spliced mRNA

259. Adsorption of an infectious HIV particle
260. Integration of HIV DNA in the nucleus
261. Capsid assembly of HIV precursors and maturation
262. Transcription during HIV infection
263. Reverse transcription at early stages of HIV replication

Section D: Case History

Directions. This case history is followed by three numbered incomplete statements. Choose the one best answer from among the lettered items following each statement.

A mother is blood group A, CDe/CDe. Her husband, the father of their third child, is blood group O, cDE/cde. The infant is blood group O, CDe/cde. The second child had been erythroblastotic at birth but had not required exchange transfusion. The mother has had no blood transfusions. Cord blood from this new baby gave a strongly positive direct antiglobulin (Coombs) test.

264. The mother's serum probably contained:
    (a) Anti-A and anti-d
    (b) Anti-B and anti-d
    (c) Anti-B and Anti-c
    (d) Only anti-B
265. The antibody most likely to have been a threat to this last infant is:
    (a) Paternal anti-A
    (b) Maternal anti-B
    (c) Maternal anti-c

(d) Maternal anti-d

(e) None of the above

266. Administration of $Rh_o(D)$ immune globulin (RhoGAM) to this patient:

(a) Was indicated to prevent primary sensitization

(b) Would have little effect with respect to possible isosensitization in future pregnancies

(c) Would prevent the appearance of any kind of antibody potentially injurious to future products of conception

(d) Would only have potentiated the hemolytic effect on the patient's cells by sensitizing them to *in vivo* complement immune lysis

A N S W E R S

Section A

1. **d** The gametocyte is the sexual form, oocyte or spermatocyte. It develops from trophozoites, which do not undergo schizogony in the erythrocytic stage, and which, when ingested by the secondary host, such as mosquitoes, develop into male and female gametes.

2. **c** Diagnosis of cutaneous leishmaniasis due to any of a number of species of *Leishmania* is confirmed by the finding of the parasite in macrophages taken by slit-skin smears from a nonulcerated portion of the lesion, or in scrapings of a debrided ulcer. *Leishmania* amastigotes grow exclusively in macrophages.

3. **a** The plasmodial parasites are introduced as sporozoites into the host by the bite of the mosquito vector. They emerge from the liver (exoerythrocytic stage) as trophozoites, which penetrate into erythrocytes and undergo schizogony with the formation of merozoites. The latter multiply and ultimately lyse the cell, thereby freeing the progeny merozoites to continue the erythrocytic cycle.

4. **b** Filaria are metazoan (*i.e.*, multicellular), in contrast to the other genera mentioned, which are protozoan (*i.e.*, unicellular).

5. **b** In streptococci of group A, type-specific M proteins, in close association with lipoteichoic acid in the bacterial cell wall, are the chief virulence factors. Isolated M protein inhibits phagocytosis in vitro of streptococci in the absence of homologous anti-M antibody. M protein also serves as the protective antigen by evoking antibodies that protect against reinfection with the same type.

6. **b** The leukotrienes are released from allergen-challenged tissue cells and from vasoamine-stimulated polymorphonuclear leukocytes, resulting in the release of arachidonic acid. This arachidonic acid is metabolized by way of the lipooxygenase pathway to produce secondary mediators, one of which is LTB4, a chemotactically active molecule.

7. **c** Macrophages and polymorphonuclear leukocytes have receptors for C3b.

8. **b** The demonstration of specific IgM antibody to *T. gondii* in fetal (cord) blood is diagnostic of primary infection (fetal toxoplasmosis). Any IgG antibody would be of maternal origin, transmitted transplacentally to the fetus.

9. **c** *Accolé* (or *appliqué*) is the early form of *Plasmodium falciparum*, which appears as a fine, blue line with a chromatin dot that is apparently adherent to the margin of an erythrocyte.

10. **a** Flagyl (metronidazole) is an oral synthetic antiprotozoal and antibacterial (especially against nonsporing obligate anaerobes) agent, with direct trichomonacidal and amebacidal activity.

11. **c** In the final, or definitive, host the parasite passes its adult and sexual existence. In an intermediate host, the parasite is in the larval, or nonsexual, form. A reservoir host serves as a source of parasitic infection.

12. **a** Trichinosis is definitively diagnosed by examination of smears of biopsied muscle tissue and demonstration of unencysted larvae.

13. **d** Invasion of the hepatic parenchyma by trophozoites of *Entamoeba histolytica* results in focal necrosis and liquefaction of liver tissue due to the direct action of amebic cytotoxin—enterotoxin. There is little inflammatory reaction or cell damage beyond the confines of individual lesions, in which abscess cavities may contain up to 1 liter of acellular fluid.

14. **b** The diagnosis of fetal toxoplasmosis rests on the demonstration of specific IgM antibodies in cord blood.

15. **d** Yomesan (niclosamide) is a taeniacide that acts as an inhibitor of oxidative phosphorylation and is not absorbed from the gut.

16. **b** Aspergillus is an opportunistic fungal pathogen the mycelium of which may invade the tissues, particularly of immunocompromised hosts. In immunocompetent hosts, aspergillosis is characterized by simple colonization of exposed tissue, such as the external ear canal or cornea.

17. **a** *Actinomyces israelii*, the most common cause of actinomycosis, is a strictly anaerobic, nonsporulating, gram-positive rod that is sensitive to penicillin.

18. **b** Certain opportunistic fungal pathogens such as *Mucor* are identifiable in infected tissues by their characteristic nonseptate (cenocytic) hyphae.

19. **c** Conidia are the main type of asexual spores. They are born on specialized hyphae (conidiophores) in the mycelium.

20. **a** In cryptococcal meningitis, there is little or no cellular reaction. In the absence of demonstrable cryptococcal cells, the presence of capsular polysaccharide may be detected by agglutination of latex beads coated with specific antibody.

21. **c** Cell-mediated immunity (CMI) is the primary defense against fungal infection, and is manifested

by delayed-type (tuberculin-type) hypersensitivity to many fungal products, and the presence of yeast cells in histiocytes (*e.g., Histoplasma capsulatum*). Conversely, impairment of CMI enhances susceptibility to infection with opportunistic fungi (as seen in victims of AIDS).

22. **c** The genome of rhabdoviruses is single-stranded, unsegmented RNA of negative polarity, which is transcribed by the large nucleocapsid (NL) protein complex into a full-length positive RNA strand.

23. **d** Antibody to the surface antigen of hepatitis B virus (HBsAg) not only is diagnostic of past infection but also is protective against reinfection with HBV. Antibody to internal viral antigen (*e.g., core* antigen, HBcAg) is not protective, since it is unreactive with the surface of the viral particle HBsAg.

24. **c** During the development of orthomyxoviruses, M protein is laid down at sites on the inner aspect of the cell membrane at which nucleocapsid is gathered. Here viral budding and release occur after the envelopment of nucleocapsid by lipids and glycoproteins (hemagglutinin and neuraminidase) derived from the cell membrane.

25. **d** An icosahedron is a polyhedron the faces of which are equilateral triangles. Examples of icosahedral virions are adenoviruses and picornaviruses.

26. **a** Rabies virus used in vaccines for humans is grown in diploid cells of human embryonic origin (*e.g.,* WI-38, MRC-5) and inactivated with tri-n-butyl phosphate or betapropiolactone.

27. **b** RNA-dependent DNA-polymerase is reverse transcriptase, characteristic of RNA tumor viruses (*e.g.,* human leukemia viruses).

28. **b** The majority of cases of Reye's syndrome have occurred during outbreaks of influenza B, although clusters of cases have accompanied influenza A outbreaks and sporadic varicella infections, the latter particularly in patients younger than those with antecedent influenza. There is significant correlation of Reye's syndrome with salicylate consumption, although the precise role of salicylates in the pathogenesis of the disorder is still obscure.

29. **e** In order for transformation to occur, the nonpermissive cell (one in which the virus does not multiply) must remain viable so that the viral genome can be integrated into the cellular genome. In infected permissive cells, the progeny of an oncogenic DNA virus (*e.g.,* polyoma virus) is released by lysis and death of the cell.

30. **c** IgM antibody denotes primary infection with herpes simplex virus type 2 (HSV2), the usual cause of herpes genitalis. Section is advised to protect the fetus from infection during passage through the birth canal.

31. **b** The core of vaccinia virus, the prototypic poxvirus, contains a large, linear, double-stranded DNA molecule (120×10^6 daltons) with a theoretical coding capacity of approximately 150 to 200 proteins, as well as a number of core enzymes. Lateral bodies, a lipid- and glycoprotein-containing envelope, and surface tubular elements characterize the complete vaccinia virion, which is 200×250 nm in size. In contrast, the genome of human papillomaviruses is supercoiled double-stranded DNA (5×10^6 daltons), the overall size of the naked virion (capsid) being 55 nm.

32. **d** Because of their segmented genome, orthomyxoviruses undergo genetic reassortment (the biologic basis for "antigenic shift"), of which advantage is taken in developing viral strains lacking virulence but retaining desired hemagglutinin (H) and neuraminidase (N) antigens.

33. **e** Specific IgM antibody detectable by hemagglutination inhibition in cord or neonatal blood is diagnostic of fetal rubella, in which most of the fetal tissues are laden with infectious virus. By the age of 3 months, immunocompetent neonates will have developed their own IgG antibodies.

34. **e** The cytopathic effect of all types of enteroviruses is the same. The capsid antigens of poliovirus and other enteroviruses are type-specific; that is, they are neutralized only by homologous antibody.

35. **d** Viral genomes consist of double- or single-stranded DNA *or* RNA, never both. Chlamydial genomes are always DNA; the organisms also contain cytoplasmic RNA, and DNA plasmids.

36. **c** Bence Jones proteins are homogeneous L-chains (kappa or lambda) representing catabolic products of a monoclonal paraprotein characteristically elaborated by multiple myeloma (plasmacytoma) cells.

37. **a** Multimeric secretory immunoglobulin A (IgA), as distinct from monomeric serum IgA, contains the J-chain (secretory piece) that is added to the molecule during passage through the endothelium of mucous membranes. The glycoprotein secretory piece protects the antibody from the action of proteolytic enzymes normally present in secretions, but not from bacterial IgA peptidases (*e.g.,* of *Neisseria gonorrhoeae* or *Haemophilus influenzae*).

38. **b** Immune lysis of bacteria sensitized by antibody (*i.e.,* bacterial cells to which specific antibacterial antibody is attached) is analogous to immune hemolysis, in that the entire classic pathway is required, from attachment of C1 through activation of the membrane attack complex (C5b–C9).

39. **a** Patients with marked deficiency of C3 suffer from severe recurrent bacterial infections due to lowered serum chemotactic and impaired phag-

ocytic cell activities. When the C3b inactivator is defective, hypercatabolism and hence low levels of C3 result, presumably because of sustained activation of the alternative complement pathway by C3b.

40. **c** The Ir gene complex, comprising Ir-1A, Ir-1B, and Ir-1C, is included in the major histocompatibility complex (MHC) and governs the magnitude of immune responses elicited by a variety of antigens. The effect of Ir genes appears to be antigen specific and to be exerted mostly on T_H cells; the Ir genes also affect the IgM-to-IgG switch. One Ir gene in the vicinity of the D locus of the MHC governs IgE responses (augmented in atopic individuals). The MHC also includes genes controlling the expression of C2 and C4 and variants of the latter, expressed on human erythrocytes as the Chido and Rogers blood group antigens.

41. **c** In Rh-incompatible matings in which there is a basis for hemolytic disease of the newborn (*i.e.,* the mother is Rh-negative and the father is Rh-positive), concomitant ABO incompatibility (*e.g.,* the mother is group O, the father is group B) tends to be protective of the fetus, because any fetal erythrocutes (which, though heterozygous for Rh, might also be heterozygous for major group A or B antigens) entering the maternal circulation would be promptly removed by preexisting natural anti-A or anti-B in the maternal blood.

42. **d** Antihistamines block the permease activity of histamine at sites distant from the mast cell or basophil from which it is released.

43. **e** There is no risk of sensitization if the father is Rh-negative; it is paternal Rh antigen(s), when present on fetal erythrocytes, to which an Rh-negative mother might become sensitized.

44. **c** In serum sickness soluble complexes of antigen (*e.g.,* horse serum) and antibody are formed. They fix complement and are deposited in the tissues, causing depletion of serum complement components. This depletion is most readily monitored by radial immunodiffusion assays for C3 and C4.

45. **c** Antigen-activated T helper–inducer (T_H) lymphocytes are stimulated to produce interleukin-2 (IL-2), which is required for the conversion of T lymphocytes to cytotoxic (T_C) lymphocytes (CTL).

46. **c** Facultative intracellular pathogens (*i.e.,* microorganisms that are capable of survival and multiplication inside phagocytic cells) include *Mycobacterium* species, *Brucella* species, *Francisella tularensis,* and *Listeria monocytogenes.* In infection with any of these organisms, the bacteria that are engulfed by macrophages are beyond the immediate reach of circulating antibody. Monocytes/macrophages that have been activated by interaction with antigen-stimulated T cells are therefore

the main line of defense through various mechanisms of intracellular killing.

47. **d** T helper–inducer (T_H) cells react with monoclonal antisera to CD4; cytotoxic–suppressor (T_C) cells react with monoclonal antisera to CD8.

48. **e** Protein A is a major group-specific protein found only in the cell wall of *Staphylococcus aureus;* about one third of it is released into the medium during growth. Protein A is also anticomplementary, antiphagocytic, and antigenic, being capable of eliciting hypersensitivity reactions, and mitogenic, being able to potentiate NK activity of human lymphocytes. Ninety percent of protein A is linked covalently to cell wall peptidoglycan, and consists of a single polypeptide chain with a molecular weight of 42,000. Protein A, either on the intact bacterial cell or purified and attached to an inert carrier, interacts uniquely through four highly homologous domains with the Fc portion of normal IgG of almost all mammals.

49. **d** The capsule of *Haemophilus influenzae* type b, which is composed of polyribitol phosphate, confers resistance to phagocytosis on the bacterial cell and is therefore an important virulence factor; unencapsulated (*i.e.,* untypable) strains of *H. influenzae* are avirulent. The capsular material of *H. influenzae* type b constitutes an effective vaccine, which is administered to infants during their second year, the period of greatest susceptibility to *H. influenzae* b meningitis.

50. **b** The presently available pneumococcal vaccine contains purified capsular polysaccharides of the 23 types of *Streptococcus pneumoniae* responsible for 87% of recent bacteremic pneumococcal disease.

51. **b** Smooth (*i.e.,* unencapsulated) pneumococci are avirulent. In the experiment cited, only rough cells derived from type III could be transformed by type I DNA into smooth (encapsulated, virulent) type I organisms to kill the mouse.

52. **b** Pulmonary infection with *Mycoplasma pneumoniae* evokes not only specific mycoplasmal antibody measurable by complement fixation, but also cold agglutinins (CA, active only at about 4° C against human erythrocytes; group O cells are used to avoid interference by isoagglutinins). The IgM CA that appear in the serum during the course of infection with *M. pneumoniae* have specificity for the I antigen, the determinants of which are also detectable in glycoproteins solubilized from human erythrocyte membranes. The CA are therefore cross-reactive with native erythrocyte antigens that share determinants with *M. pneumoniae.*

53. **c** The M, T, and R proteins of group A streptococci are type-specific surface antigens. The M proteins determine immunity to reinfection (*i.e.,* are pro-

tective antigens). They are also the main virulence factor, as shown by the facts (1) that organisms containing M protein resist phagocytosis in serum without corresponding type-specific antibody, and (2) that isolated M protein interferes *in vitro* with phagocytosis of organisms lacking M protein.

54. **c** Acute streptococcal infection (*e.g.*, septic pharyngitis) elicits an immune response to many streptococcal group-specific antigens, most of them enzymes (*e.g.*, streptolysin-O, nucleases, hyaluronidase) detectable by serum agglutination of latex beads coated with several of these antigens (*e.g.*, the "streptozyme" test). The immune response to streptolysin-O is the most potent, and the antibody (antistreptolysin-O, ASO) in the serum can be measured semiquantitatively in tube dilution tests using a standard amount of extracted lyophilized enzyme. The ASO titer usually declines following recovery, but a continuing or rising titer usually indicates the development of a nonsupportive sequela, most importantly acute rheumatic fever.

55. **c** Gas-liquid chromatography (GLC), performed on fluid from pure cultures of microbial agents, is particularly useful in the identification of nonsporing anaerobes such as *Bacteroides* and *Fusobacterium* species. For detection of alcohols and volatile acid end-products of glucose metabolism (*e.g.*, acetic, propionic, and butyric acids), ether extracts of acidified pure cultures are chromatographed. Fumaric, pyruvic, succinic, and lactic acids are not volatile, but their methyl derivatives are. GLC is also useful in differentiating certain aerobes, including species of *Neisseria*, *Pseudomonas*, *Salmonella*, and *Mycobacterium*.

56. **a** *Bartonella bacilliformis* is the cause of Carrión's disease, in which the organism is inoculated by the bite of sandflies (*Phlebotomus* species) and initially parasitizes circulating mature erythrocytes, often causing severe hemolytic anemia (Oroya fever). Following further dissemination of the organism, the tissue phase of the infection is characterized by an eruption (verruga peruana) of highly vascularized nodules in which the organisms are found in endothelial cells and macrophages.

57. **c** On the surface of solid medium, *Mycoplasma pneumoniae* slowly forms very small, dome-shaped colonies, the central part of which grows downward into the agar to produce a denser core. Sheep erythrocytes added in saline suspension to growing cultures adhere to the surface of *M. pneumoniae* colonies (hemadsorption), thus providing a ready means of identification and differentiation from other mycoplasmal organisms. Virulent strains adhere by the same mechanism to other types of cells (HeLa cells, spermatozoa, tracheal epithelial cells) and to the surface of glass vessels. Avirulent strains of *M. pneumoniae* fail to adhere to any cell surfaces.

58. **c** In a properly prepared pour plate (*i.e.*, one in which colonies are spaced sufficiently widely to be countable), each colony is considered to represent the progeny of a single viable cell present in the inoculum, which usually is a dilution of the original broth culture. The use of replicate cultures at different dilutions increases the statistical accuracy of the viable cell count.

59. **d** The formation of glucans is a sucrose-dependent reaction involving the cleavage of sucrose by glycosyltransferase and subsequent polymerization of the glucose moiety into branched high-molecular-weight glucans. *S. mutans* also possesses lectinlike cell surface receptors that mediate binding to tooth surfaces and promote aggregation into plaque.

60. **d** The mechanism of the Gram stain appears to be generally related to the thickness of the bacterial cell wall, pore size, and permeability properties of the intact cell envelope. Gram's iodine solution is a mordant that stabilizes the complex formed between cell wall components, particularly in gram-positive bacteria, and crystal violet, and thus makes them relatively resistant to decolorization with alcohol or acetone. The counterstain, safranin, is taken up by the cell but is not evident, owing to the more intense dark blue purple of the retained primary stain. In gram-negative organisms, with comparatively much less cell wall, the primary stain is greatly diminished after decolorization, and so the red counterstain shows through. Gram-positive bacteria stain gram-negative if they lose osmotic integrity through rupture of the cell membrane.

61. **a** Pasteurization (heating to 62° C for 30 minutes followed by rapid cooling) is not sterilization but is adequate to kill most nonsporing pathogens capable of surviving, such as those in raw milk (*e.g.*, *Brucella* species, streptococci, *Mycobacterium* species).

62. **c** BCG (Bacille Calmette-Guérin) is a living attenuated strain of *Mycobacterium bovis*. Administered intradermally to tuberculin-negative subjects, the vaccine causes a localized infection that stimulates a certain degree of heightened resistance to infection with human *M. tuberculosis*, as evidenced by delayed hypersensitivity to PPD.

63. **b** Phagocytic cells constitute the primary defense against acute staphylococcal infection. Accordingly, granulocytic dysfunction. (*e.g.*, deficiency of complement component C_3, defects in intracellular killing, or degranulation of lysosomes, as in Chédiak-

Higashi syndrome) is associated with recurrent staphylococcal infection.

64. **d** When microorganisms are grown on media containing fatty acids or acetate as sole carbon sources, acetyl-CoA is formed without the intermediate synthesis of pyruvic acid. These conditions provide no mechanism for the generation of oxaloacetate from pyruvate by the phosphoenolpyruvate (PEP)–carboxylase reaction. Growth on acetate, however, induces the synthesis of isocitrate lyase and malate synthetase which, together with some of the enzymes of the tricarboxylic acid cycle, carry out the glyoxylate cycle, a modification of the TCA cycle.

65. **d** In the presence of purulent exudate and breakdown products of tissue necrosis, there is an accumulation of thymidine, purine, methionine, and serine, which together reverse the inhibitory effect of sulfonamides on bacteria by replenishing the end-products of folic acid metabolism. Sulfonamides may thus lose their therapeutic efficacy.

66. **c** Obligate anaerobes, both gram-positive and gram-negative (*e.g., Bacteroides, Fusobacterium, Clostridium,* and *Peptostreptococcus* species) constitute the major component of the normal flora of the human lower gastrointestinal tract, vastly outnumbering aerobic and facultatively anaerobic bacteria.

67. **d** Pseudomembranous enterocolitis is characterized by exudative plaques with underlying necrosis of intestinal mucosal surface. More often than not, it is associated with the prolonged administration of penicillin, clindamycin, or other antibiotics and is caused by exotoxins of *Clostridium difficile,* an obligate anaerobe that colonizes the intestinal tracts of about 3% of healthy adults and a high percentage of neonates. The mechanism of disease production, however, is not simply overgrowth by resistant strains of *C. difficile.*

68. **d** Darkfield examination of freshly obtained lymph from a suspected early syphilitic chancre will reveal spirochetes showing characteristic motility, which is the most important criterion in confirming the diagnosis. Darkfield examination may yield positive results before the appearance of Wasserman (reagin) antibody in the serum. Spirochetes may also be transiently demonstrable in secondary syphilitic lesions on mucous membranes.

69. **c** *Trichomonas vaginalis* is the third most common cause of nongonococcal urethritis (NGU) in the male, in whom the urethra, prostate, and epididymis harbor the organisms. In females, in whom the incidence of infection is higher, it causes vulvovaginitis. Coitus is the main mode of transmission, which may occur in either direction.

70. **b** T_H, peripheral blood monocytes, and mac-rophages all contain CD4 molecules on their surface, in varying amounts. $T_{c/s}$ possess CD8 but not CD4 molecules on their surface. CD4 is the receptor for HIV gp120.

71. **b** EV, which is associated with HPV-5, HPV-8, and HPV-38b, can become malignant about 60% of the time. Malignant tumors of the skin (squamous-cell carcinomas) develop at an early age in EV patients, predominantly in light-exposed areas of the skin. The time from onset of skin lesions to the onset of cancer suggests that interaction of HIV-38b with UV light and host factors are associated with development of the skin carcinoma.

72. **e** The Delta Agent, also referred to as HDV, or hepatitis D virus, represents a viroidlike RNA packaged within an HB virus surface antigen capsid. It was first described endemically in Italy in 1977 and since then has been encountered in such diverse locations as the Amazon Basin, certain areas of Africa, as well as the Middle East. Epidemics of Delta Agent–related fulminant hepatitis have been reported among drug addicts in Sweden and Worcester, Massachusetts.

73. **b** Both AZT (azidothymidine) and the recently FDA-approved ddI (2'3'-dideoxyinosine) are analogues of thymidine and inosine, respectively. The major structural modifications occur on the sugar and not the base moiety. These compounds, which can act as competitive inhibitors for deoxynucleoside-5'-triphosphates, are also chain terminators. Most patients on AZT exhibit an improvement in immune response and a decrease in virus load. However, there are some side effects, such as bone marrow suppression, myositis, and nausea. Furthermore, there has been an increased incidence of ONHL (opportunistic non-Hodgkin's lymphoma) among patients on long-term (>2 years) AZT therapy. This, as well as the appearance of drug-resistant strains, has led to the development of additional antiviral drugs, such as ddI and ddC.

Section B

74. **d** HIV (human immunodeficiency virus), the causative agent of AIDS, is specific for T-helper lymphocytes, on which the antigen receptor site is included in the site at which the virus attaches (*i.e.,* the viral receptor). HIV infects only T-helper cells, which are destroyed as a result of viral replication and release. The drastic reduction in T-helper lymphocytes removes the principal barrier to other infections, against which immune defense is largely cell-mediated.

75. **d** Bacterial sporulation (endospore formation) is a

response to nutritional deprivation, particularly limitation of C and N sources. This deprivation results in a decrease in the guanosine triphosphate (GTP) pool of growing cells, this specific deficiency being the factor actually initiating sporulation.

76. **c** Papain digestion acts at the hinge region of immunoglobulin, producing two identical Fab fragments (containing the entire light chain and the V_H and C_{H1} domains of the heavy chain) and one Fc fragment (retaining the double configuration of the intact Ig molecule).

77. **e** The first three species constitute the majority of the normal flora of the lower intestinal tract and from this site may be the cause of severe mixed anaerobic metastatic infections of body sites that are normally sterile (*e.g.*, infection of lungs, brain, and pelvic organs with septicemia). *Actinomyces israelii* is a normal inhabitant of the oral cavity and from this site may also cause local and metastatic infections.

78. **a** Endocarditis due to enterococcus (group D *Streptococcus faecalis*) is clinically relatively resistant to penicillin alone, reflecting the uniformly high penicillin resistance of the organism *in vitro*. Combined therapy with streptomycin is usually recommended. In cases of infection that may be due to initially resistant strains of *Mycobacterium tuberculosis*, four-drug therapy is usually recommended (isoniazid, rifampin, streptomycin, and pyrazinamide). When the risk of initial isoniazid resistance is small, isoniazid and rifampin are usually adequate. For disseminated cryptococcosis, amphotericin B and flucytosine are recommended, although resistance to the latter is not uncommon.

79. **a** *Mycoplasma* species have a unique requirement for cholesterol and related sterols for membrane synthesis. They also lack the enzymatic pathways for the synthesis of purines and pyrimidines. They therefore grow only on complex media, particularly those enriched with animal serum (*e.g.*, beef heart infusion with 20% horse serum), yeast extract, and nucleic acids. Colonies of L forms (L for Lister Institute, where they were first described) were first associated with certain bacilli, notably *Streptobacillus moniliformis*, but L forms of *Haemophilus influenzae* and various enteric bacteria also exist. L forms can be induced by growth of the organism in osmotically supportive medium containing sublethal amounts of penicillin, which serves to suppress cell wall synthesis.

80. **b** The alpha toxin of *Clostridium perfringens (welchi)* is a phospholipase C that splits lecithin into lysolecithin and phosphoryl choline, which is further hydrolyzed to diglycerides and choline phosphate, accounting for the areas of opalescence (Nagler reaction) surrounding colonies grown on egg yolk (lecithovitellin) agar. The same enzyme acts on lecithin in the erythrocyte membrane. Colonies of *C. perfringens* cause characteristic double zones of hemolysis on blood agar due to complete (clear) hemolysis by theta toxin and a wider zone of partial hemolysis due to alpha toxin. *C. perfringens* may invade the blood stream (*e.g.*, from injury to the lower intestinal tract, or in septic abortion) in which the sudden liberation of large amounts of alpha toxin causes massive intravascular hemolysis with lower nephron nephrosis.

81. **a** Streptococci of Lancefield group D grow in broth containing 6.5% sodium chloride and hydrolyze esculin. They are classified as *Enterococcus* or *Streptococcus faecalis*, are found among the normal intestinal flora, and are a frequent cause of urinary tract infection. Next to alpha hemolytic streptococci (*Streptococcus viridans* group, normal inhabitants of the oral cavity), enterococci are the most frequent cause of infective endocarditis, in which the organisms may have been derived from instrumentation of the genitourinary tract. Enterococci are usually highly resistant to penicillin G *in vitro*.

82. **c** Membrane-bound enzymes are involved in the synthesis of envelope polymers (*e.g.*, muramyl pentapeptide) along with a cofactor (glycosylphosphate lipid carrier) that has been identified as the phosphomonoester of C_{55}-polyisoprenoid alcohol, undecaprenol. The membrane-bound carrier forms glycosylpyrophospholipid oligosaccharide intermediates, which are then transferred to form polymers, thereby completing the synthesis of repeating units of the cell wall. Cross-linking follows. The beta-lactam structure of penicillins and cephalosporins makes them structural analogs of the D-alanyl–D-alanyl portion of the pentapeptide side chain of peptidoglycan. They inhibit the transpeptidase enzyme by binding in the catalytic site where they irreversibly acylate a serine residue because of the high reactivity of the beta-lactam structure, resulting in the formation of an inactive penicillinoyl enzyme and the inhibition of cross-linking transpeptidation.

83. **d** Respiration is a process in which molecular oxygen usually serves as the ultimate electron acceptor (aerobic respiration). In anaerobic respiration, an inorganic compound such as nitrate, sulfate, or carbonate serves as the electron acceptor.

84. **c** The Weil-Felix test is based on the titration, through serial twofold dilutions, of serum agglutinating antibody to certain nonmotile strains of *Proteus* species (OXK, OX19, OX2) that share minor antigen(s) with different species of rick-

ettsiae. If the titers are high enough, and particularly if there is a significant increase during the course of suspected rickettsiosis, the test is strongly suggestive, though not strictly diagnostic, of rickettsial infection. Antibody to *Proteus* is present in a low titer in most normal persons and may be elevated in infections due to a *Proteus* species (*e.g.,* of the urinary tract).

85. **a** Certain lysogenic strains of *Staphylococcus aureus,* usually of phage group I, elaborate an exoprotein that has been shown to be identical to pyrogenic exotoxin C (PE-C) and enterotoxin F of these same strains. Toxic shock toxin (TST) has an immunosuppressive effect, as evidenced by the depression of reticuloendothelial system clearance of microorganisms, increased sensitivity to endotoxin (*e.g.,* from indigenous gram-negative flora), and enhanced type IV acquired hypersensitivity. When these lysogenic strains of *S. aureus* colonize the vagina, particularly during menstrual flow and in the concomitant presence of tampons, the combined effect of these secreted bacterial products causes the syndrome, which is characterized by signs of acute intoxication (fever, hypotension, and scarlatiniform rash).

86. **d** Infection with *Corynebacterium diphtheriae* is limited to body surfaces (*e.g.,* mucosa of the upper respiratory tract as in tracheofaucial diphtheria) and the skin (cutaneous diphtheria). The organism is never invasive, but at the primary site of infection it elaborates a potent toxin that is disseminated hematogenously to distant sites to cause late effects such as peripheral neuritis and myocarditis. Tissue damage (*e.g.,* pseudomembrane formation) at primary sites of infection is due to the direct necrotizing action of the toxin and the consequent inflammatory reaction.

87. **a** Infection with *Corynebacterium diphtheriae* is never invasive, and the organism is never found in the blood stream. All manifestations of diphtheria are due to diphtherial exotoxin elaborated at the site(s) of infection, where it causes tissue necrosis (*e.g.,* pseudomembrane formation in the tracheobronchial tree) and is disseminated hematogenously to distant sites (*e.g.,* peripheral nerves, cardiac muscle). Toxin is elaborated only by strains of *C. diphtheriae* carrying a bacteriophage (corynephage beta) that in turn carries the structural gene (tox) for toxin. A direct correlation exists between nonlytic (*i.e.,* temperate) bacteriophage infection (lysogeny) and toxigenicity. The toxin gene can be expressed either during vegetative replication of corynephage beta or when the phage is integrated into the bacterial genome (prophage), the situation usually prevalent in nature. Infection with *C. diph-*

theriae does not confer antitoxic immunity, the quantity of unstable toxin elaborated at the primary site(s) being insufficient to evoke an antitoxic antibody response. In cases of proved diphtheritic infection, passive immunization (antitoxin in the form of "despeciated" equine serum) is used to neutralize any circulating toxin that has not already been fixed to target tissues, in combination with antibiotic therapy to eliminate the bacterial source of toxin. Prophylactic immunization with toxoid protects against diphtheria (*i.e.,* diphtherial intoxication) but not against diphtheritic infection, of which humans are the only source.

88. **b** During growth in culture, as well as during the course of infection, *Streptococcus pyogenes* elaborates a number of extracellular proteins, most of them antigenic enzymes with secondary roles in pathogenesis, including streptokinase, streptolysin O (which is oxygen sensitive), streptolysin S (which is oxygen stable), hyaluronidase, various nucleases, and erythrogenic toxin (of which there are three serotypes). Streptolysin O is the strongest antigen, so that the corresponding antibodies (antistreptolysin O, or ASO) are the most easily measured for diagnostic purposes. Antibody titers to DNase B are of great value in the serodiagnosis of skin infections in which the ASO response may be blunted.

89. **c** The elaboration of toxins (heat-labile, LT and Heat-stable, ST) by *Escherichia coli* strains is associated with two transferable plasmids. LT is similar in its action to the enterotoxin of *Vibrio cholerae* in stimulating adenyl cyclase in epithelial cells of the small intestinal mucosa, thereby increasing the permeability of the intestinal lining and causing massive fluid loss and diarrhea. ST appears to activate guanylate cyclase to produce cyclic guanosine monophosphate, thus impairing net chloride and sodium absorption; ST also decreases small bowel motility.

90. **a** Fibroblast interferon (beta or type I interferon, IFN-beta) is a glycoprotein induced in cultured fibroblasts or epithelial cells, and in macrophages by viruses, nucleic acids, or synthetic polynucleotides. The antiviral protective effect of IFN is due to the induction, in normal cells, of new protein(s) with activity that inhibits translation, and hence replication of infecting virus. IFNs are broadly species specific, but they are nonspecific with respect to viruses.

91. **a** Brucellosis is primarily a zoonosis affecting ungulates (cattle, sheep, goats, swine). Human infection is derived from contact with contaminated blood and tissues, such as decidua, and from ingestion of contaminated raw milk. Leptospirosis is con-

tracted from exposure to the urine of wild rodents and of infected domestic livestock and dogs. Spores of *Bacillus anthracis* survive indefinitely in soil and on the hides and bristles of domestic animals. Human anthrax is contracted through direct contact with contaminated animal products (cutaneous anthrax), through inhalation of spores (pulmonary anthrax), or through ingestion of contaminated meat (intestinal anthrax). All forms of anthrax are accompanied by septicemia. Brucellosis, leptospirosis, and anthrax are therefore all primary zoonoses, only sporadically affecting humans.

92. **a** An immune response to infection with group A streptococci is evidenced by the presence of antibody to extracellular bacterial products, which is most easily measured as antistreptolysin O (ASO). Included in the cumulative immune response to repeated infection with different serotypes of group A streptococci, but independent of any antienzymes, is the tissue response manifested as acute rheumatic fever, the incidence of which is fairly constant at about 5%. With each succeeding streptococcal infection, particularly if the ASO titer is significantly elevated at the outset, the risk of acute rheumatic fever becomes much greater. For the same reasons, recurrent group A streptococcal infection in a person with a previous rheumatic history is associated with a high risk recurrence.

93. **b** Lipoteichoic acid (LTA) consists of chains of polyglycerol phosphate units that may contain sugar or amino sugar substituents covalently linked to a glycolipid. The streptococcal cell membrane is attached by hydrophobic interaction with the glycolipid moiety of LTA, which extends through the width of the wall and is intertwined with M protein in surface fimbriae, held together by ionic interaction. LTA is therefore involved in the attachment and binding of streptococcal antigens to cell surfaces, and through its close association with M protein is a virulence factor. LTAs of all streptococci cross-react immunologically among themselves and with LTAs of other gram-positive bacteria. Gonococcal pili, primarily protein in nature, are found on the surface of colonies of types 1 and 2 derived from freshly isolated, and presumably fully virulent, strains. Pili recognize specific binding sites on host cell surfaces and are the chief virulence factor (*i.e.,* a protective antigen).

94. **a** So-called syphilitic reaginic antibody (Wasserman antibody, not to be confused with IgE, formerly referred to as atopic *reagin*) appears early in the course of infection but may be undetectable during the darkfield-positive stage of primary syphilis. The VDRL antigen and the rapid plasma reagin (RPR) antigen (VDRL antigen adsorbed to charcoal particles) react with IgM and IgG antibodies formed by the host in response both to lipoidal material released from damaged cells early in infection and to lipid from *Treponema pallidum* itself. In the FTA-ABS test, the serum is absorbed with antigens from nonpathogenic Reiter strains of treponemes to remove antibody to commensal spirochetes and improve the specificity of the test. Specific antitreponemal antibody, detectable with the FTA-ABS test, appears in the serum late in the primary stage of infection and in most cases is present throughout subsequent stages, unless antibiotic therapy is given early enough to abort the antibody response.

95. **b** Both *Neisseria meningitidis* and *Haemophilus influenzae* type b possess capsules that, being antiphagocytic, are determinants of virulence, and both form the basis for vaccines against infection with the respective organisms. Cholera and diphtheria are both intoxications caused by surface infection with the respective organisms, neither of which ever becomes invasive.

96. **a** *Plasmodium malariae* and hepatitis B both cause a subacute or chronic form of disease in which antigens of the corresponding pathogen are continually released into the bloodstream at a time when high levels of antibody are already present and there form immune complexes. Immune complexes with a density in the range of 19 S or larger are removed by reticuloendothelial cells, but they are also those most likely to be deposited along vessels and to damage them; in contrast, immune complexes with a lower density fix complement poorly and are only slowly cleared from the blood. The specific microbial antigens and immunoglobulin are demonstrable in immune complexes that have diffused through the normal endothelial fenestrations of glomerular capillaries and formed granular aggregates on the glomerular basement membrane.

97. **b** In transformed cells the entire viral DNA is integrated, even though it is never expressed in its entirety (*i.e.,* as infective virus). The viral genome can be "rescued," or made to express itself, by treatment with mutagens, or by fusion of transformed cells with permissive cells, only the cytoplasm of which is required for viral reactivation through excision or recombination mechanisms. Cell-to-cell fusion is accomplished by treatment with inactive (noninfectious) Sendai virus (in which the F, or fusion, envelope protein is still functional).

98. **d** Certain plant diseases are caused by infectious nucleic acid molecules lacking both lipid and protein coats. These molecules are called *viroids*. Sim-

ilar agents are associated with the hepatitis B virus in some cases of fulminant hepatititis.

99. **c** The capsid proteins of adenoviruses and papovaviruses (*e.g.*, human papilloma viruses) make primary contact with the immune system and hence contain the protective antigens of the respective viruses. In contrast, the envelope glycoproteins of herpesviruses and poxviruses serve this function, the capsid proteins being initially inaccessible to immune mechanisms.

100. **b** The hemagglutinin (H) and neuraminidase (N) of influenza virus are separate envelope glycoproteins which, being exposed at the surface of the virion, are the first antigens to encounter the immune system and hence are host-protective antigens. The H protein mediates the attachment of virions to erythrocytes as well as to susceptible cells; the N protein mediates the elution of virions from erythrocytes and the release of mature viral particles from the membrane of infected cells.

101. **a** The genomes of measles (a pseudomyxovirus) and mumps (a paramyxovirus) viruses are single-stranded, negative-polarity RNA. The genome of rubella virus (the only member of the *Rubivirus* genus in the Togaviridae family) is a single strand of positive-polarity RNA. These three classes of virus are therefore antigenically stable. The more than 40 human adenoviruses are distinguishable serologically by the monotypic specificity of their penton fiber antigens.

102. **e** Certain RNA tumor viruses are retroviruses (*e.g.*, human T-cell lymphoma/leukemia virus I, II) in which the centrally located core contains a nucleoid (C-type particles) and that acquire their envelope lipids from the cell membrane before release at the cell surface.

103. **a** Cytomegalovirus (CMV) is a herpesvirus that develops in the nucleus, from which it derives its envelope. Adenoviruses mature as aggregates of complete and incomplete particles often seen in Feulgen-positive crystalline array in the nuclei of infected cells. Human polyomavirus (*e.g.*, JC or BK virus) may be shed from the urinary tract in atypical cells, which, after Papanicolaou or H&E staining, are seen to contain intranuclear inclusions consisting of aggregates of viral particles.

104. **e** Paramyxoviruses (*e.g.*, parainfluenza and mumps viruses) are respiratory pathogens (parainfluenza virus type 2 was formerly called *croup-associated*, or *CA, virus*) that mature in the cytoplasm of infected cells, forming large eosinophilic inclusions made up of aggregated strands of nucleocapsid; some (*e.g.*, type 1, Sendai virus) fuse cells to form syncytia. The envelopes contain host-derived lipids

and a single, large glycoprotein that has both hemagglutinin and neuraminidase activates (HN protein).

105. **b** The term *heterophile* refers to "a different species" (*i.e.*, ovine or equine erythrocytes that contain the EB virus infectious mononucleosis, or IM, heterophile antigen), antibodies to which (*e.g.*, following "serum sickness" due to the therapeutic administration of horse serum) are ubiquitous in human sera and can be removed by absorption with formalinized guinea pig kidney tissue, which is rich in the corresponding Forssman antigen. Residual IM heterophile antibody is then detectable and absorbable with bovine erythrocytes, which contain IM heterophile antigen. Immune lysis of ox erythrocytes is also specific for IM.

106. **b** Hemagglutinin (H envelope protein) specific for primate erythrocytes appears in the membrane of cultured cells in which rubeola virus is developing. The envelope protein spikes of Sindbis virions (a togavirus) interact over a narrow *p*H range with receptors that on erythrocytes are phospholipid rather than glycoprotein, and with cultured cells through receptors of which histocompatibility antigens may be a part.

107. **a** In the transformation of nonpermissive cells (*i.e.*, cells in which the virus does not actively replicate), the viral genome is integrated into that of the cell, which survives without producing infective virus. Infective virus introduced into permissive cells at low multiplicity will initiate the replicative cycle, with ultimate cytolysis, which precludes transformation.

108. **b** Herpes simplex virus, most often type I, causes corneal ulcers that are frequently recurrent, and may progress to interstitial keratitis with stromal involvement. The resulting scarring is a major cause of blindness. Cytomegalovirus is the most common cause of intrauterine infection (congenital infection of the fetus), with 30% mortality and a high incidence of permanent neurological damage in survivors, even in those who are initially asymptomatic.

109. **c** The genome of poxviruses is double-stranded DNA; the segmented genome of reoviruses is double-stranded RNA.

110. **e** Arenaviruses contain four species of negative, single-stranded RNA, two of which (L and S) are virus-specific and may be shown to undergo reassortment, and the other two of which are ribosomal. The genome of reoviruses consists of ten individual segments of double-stranded RNA. The bunyaviral genome consists of three single-stranded RNA segments (L, M, and S), and that of

orthomyxoviruses consists of eight single-stranded RNA segments of negative polarity (*i.e.,* antimessage sense).

111. **d** Reverse transcriptase is found in tumor viruses with an RNA genome (*e.g.,* HTLV I and II and HIV).

112. **c** The hemagglutinin of orthomyxoviruses is one of two envelope glycoproteins (neuraminidase is the other) with affinity for sialoprotein (glycophorin) in the erythrocyte membrane and analogous receptors on host cells capable of supporting viral replication. Nonspecific sialoprotein inhibitor in serum must be inactivated to reveal any hemagglutination inhibition (HI) due to specific antibody.

113. **b** In the B cell actively producing immunoglobulin, only two genes, one for the light and one for the heavy chain, are expressed at a given time; others are suppressed. The same or similar mechanism is involved in the switch from IgM to IgG production.

114. **c** Influenza vaccine contains inactive (*i.e.,* killed) influenza virus; pneumococcal vaccine contains purified polysaccharides of various types of pneumococci. Neither vaccine is therefore infectious per se. Rubella and trivalent oral poliomyelitis vaccines comprise the respective living attenuated viruses, which have the potential for causing more serious infection in the immunocompromised host than in the immunocompetent host, in whom the induced subclinical infection is the base for subsequent immunity to natural challenge.

115. **e** Since there are no peptides in purified pneumococcal polysaccharide (S3 stands for *soluble-specific substance,* an old term for capsular polysaccharide), nitrogen in the antigen–antibody precipitates will represent antibody. At the point of maximum precipitation (*i.e.,* where only traces of antigen and no antibody are found in the supernatants), all antibody sites for cross-linking with multivalent antigen have been occupied. The equivalence zone is defined as the point at which all antibody and antigen have been completely and mutually precipitated; this does not mean that antigen and antibody are precipitated in equal amounts. If there is an excess of antigen, some S3 will remain free and some will combine with antibody to form small complexes too small to be sedimented at ordinary centrifugal speeds (*i.e.,* "soluble" complexes). In some systems, particularly protein precipitated with divalent antibody, precipitated complexes will break up (*i.e.,* dissolve) due to competition for multivalent antigen-combining sites.

116. **c** In order for the graft to survive, donor and recipient must be as closely matched as possible with respect to tissue (HLA) type. This matching can be done with the mixed lymphocyte reaction (MLR). Differences at the HLA-D or DR loci on stimulator B lymphocytes cause the blastogenesis of responder T_H cells. If the HLA-A, -B, and -C locus antigens are also different, then responder T_C lymphocytes are induced that will lyse target cells bearing the same HLA-A, -B, or -C antigens as the stimulator cells. The induction of T_C lymphocytes is greater if HLA-D locus disparity occurs and T_H cells are also produced. ABO blood group compatibility between donor and recipient is also desirable to avoid possible intravascular hemolysis due to active alloantibody formation. It has been found, however, that patients who are transfused with compatible whole blood several weeks before receiving a transplant in most instances accept the graft more freely than do untransfused recipients, perhaps because of the elimination of the most immunoreactive recipients and in part because of the triggering of an as yet unidentified mechanism of immunosuppression.

117. **d** Patients with malaria acquired in areas where chloroquine-resistant malaria is prevalent should not be given chloroquine. Pyrimethamine with trimethoprim–sulfisoxazole, or fansidar (pyrimethamine and sulfadoxine), is the drug of choice.

118. **b** The acute hemorrhage glomerulonephritis that may follow infection with certain types of group A streptococci (nephritogenic strains, e.g., types 4, 12) is caused by the intravascular formation of immune complexes and their deposition in the glomerular basement membrane, where they fix complement (accounting for the drop in serum total complement activity) and thereby trigger an inflammatory tissue response demonstrable as granular distribution of immune aggregates reactive with labeled (fluorescein, ferritin) antibody to IgG and streptococcal antigen(s).

119. **a** A large number of substances, particularly high-molecular-weight polymers of polysaccharides or proteins with repeating antigenic determinants, as well as a number of viruses, are direct B-cell mitogens and polyclonal B-cell activators not requiring the intervention of Ig receptors. Certain isolated viral proteins (not necessarily on infectious virions) may act as B-cell mitogens. Virus-specific T-helper cells may release B-cell growth and differentiation factors (*i.e.,* lymphokines that can nonspecifically activate "primed" bystander B cells).

120. **b** Monocytes/macrophages are the source of interleukin-1 (IL-1), which promotes antigen-induced activation of T cells (both helper–inducer and suppressor–cytotoxic). The latter (T_C) cells are CD8+.

121. **d** Macrophages bearing antigen are stimulated to produce IL-1, which in turn activates specific T cells to produce interleukin-2 (IL-2), formerly called T cell growth factor (TCGF), by antigen-activated T-cells. IL-2 promotes T-cell differentiation and natural killing. IL-2 has recently been produced through recombinant DNA techniques.

122. **a** Class II antigens (HLA-DP, HLA-DQ, and HLA-DR series) of the MHC are expressed mostly on B lymphocytes but are also found on T lymphocytes after activation. Class II HLA antigens are detected by the mixed lymphocyte reaction (MLR), in which peripheral blood responder leukocytes (*e.g.,* of a transplantation recipient) are mixed with irradiated peripheral blood stimulator leukocytes (*e.g.,* from a potential donor) in culture, which is then monitored for lymphocyte activation both cytologically and by measurement of radioiodine uptake from the culture fluid. Incompatible stimulator cells cause activation of responder T cells; lack of activation indicates tissue compatibility.

123. **a** Initiation of phagocytosis activates plasma membrane–associated oxidase enzymes that convert oxygen to 1- and 2-electron reduction products (superoxide anions and hydrogen peroxide). The antimicrobial activity of H_2O_2 is potentiated by myeloperoxidase.

124. **e** During sporulation, certain storage polymers (*e.g.,* poly-β-hydroxybutyrate) accumulate for later use during extensive turnover of macromolecules and synthesis of characteristic spore structures, notably two surrounding membranes of opposite polarity that, by their orientation, preclude active transport from the vegetative cell. Calcium accumulates by facilitated diffusion and chelates with dipicolinic acid, the parallel synthesis of which permits continued withdrawal of calcium from the bacterial cytoplasm. The spore-specific peptidoglycan is only 3% cross-linked (in contrast to bacterial cell peptidoglycan, which may be 60% cross-linked), and this reduced degree of cross-linking may be important in the contraction of the cortex and dehydration and hence in greater resistance to physical agents. The spore coat comprises layers of spore specific keratinlike proteins that confer most of the survival value.

125. **b** Virtually 100% of normal viable polymorphonuclear leukocytes stimulated with phorbol myristate acetate take up nitro blue tetrazolium, a yellow redox compound, the superoxide reduction product of which is a purple insoluble formazan. Subjects with only a small number of defective (*i.e.,* NBT-negative) cells can thus be differentiated from normal individuals.

126. **c** IL-2 is required for the generation of cytotoxic T (T_C) cells as well as for the induction of antigen-specific antibody responses. IL-2 also enhances natural killer (NK) cell activity. When antigen is present on the surface of activated macrophages, T cells are activated by macrophage-produced interleukin-1 (IL-1), a lymphokine formerly referred to as lymphocyte-activating factor. Once activated, T cells produce a large number of growth and differentiation factors (lymphokines) that promote their own continued proliferation as well as that of B lymphocytes. IL-2 also induces the production of tumor necrosis factors and gamma interferon. The importance of IL-2 lies in the fact that it can regulate immune functions directly as well as indirectly through the induction of other lymphokines.

127. **a** Cysts and extracystic bodies of *P. carinii* can be found in smears of needle aspirates, biopsy specimens, and sections of lung tissue stained with methenamine silver nitrate, toluidine blue, and Giemsa. The inflammatory reaction to massive infection is predominantly lymphocytic, with a high proportion of plasma cells. Although universally present as a commensal respiratory tract parasite in the normal host (up to 70% of healthy persons have antibody), in immunocompromised patients (those with leukemia, prolonged steroid therapy, AIDS) the organisms multiply rapidly, attaching to alveolar cell surfaces during a phase of the replicative cycle, and never being found intracellularly.

128. **e** *Cryptosporidium,* a species of coccidian protozoan related to *Toxoplasma,* is found in many animal species, particularly young ruminants, in which it causes diarrhea, and therefore it may be a source of human infection. In normal persons acute gastroenteritis is self-limited; in immunocompromised patients (*e.g.,* those with AIDS) cryptosporidiosis may be severe and protracted and contribute to the lethal effects of other opportunistic infections.

129. **b** *Pneumocystis carinii* is a widely distributed saprophytic protozoan that in conditions of compromised cellular immunity causes massive pulmonary infection. The diagnosis is made by direct examination of tracheal aspirates or lung biopsy material. *P. carinii* is a major cause of death in U.S. patients with AIDS.

130. **a** Infective sporozoites are injected into the susceptible human host by the mosquito and on reaching the liver multiply (exoerythrocytic forms) in hepatocytes. Trophozoites eventually reach the bloodstream and invade circulating erythrocytes, in which merozoites develop and are released, completing the erythrocytic cycle(s).

131. **a** Cell-mediated immunity is the principal element in host defense against fungal infection, involving

primarily macrophages. Asymptomatic mycosis (*e.g.*, histoplasmosis) stimulates specific delayed-type hypersensitivity, which indicates relative resistance of ths host.

132. **b** Amphotericin B is a polyene antibiotic that interacts with sterols (mainly ergosterol) in fungal cells to exert a detergentlike effect on the cell membrane with resultant alteration of permeability and leakage of cations and other cytoplasmic constituents. Interaction with cholesterol accounts for the lesser toxicity of amphotericin B for mammalian cells. A relatively unstable macrolide polyene, amphotericin B is insoluble, unstable to acid or alkali, and poorly absorbed from the gastrointestinal tract; therefore, it must be rendered colloidal with deoxycholate and stabilized with glucose for parenteral administration.

133. **a** Arthrospores (*e.g.*, *Coccidioides immitis*), chlamydospores (*e.g.*, *Candida albicans*) and blastospores (*e.g.*, *Blastomyces dermatitidis*) may be the infectious form of the fungus; ascospores are contained in a sac (ascus) representing the sexual reproductive system of certain fungi.

134. **d** The mitochondria of fungi resemble those of plant and animal cells, their number varying considerably with the levels of respiration required for different life processes, such as sporulation.

135. **d** Infection with *Coccidioides immitis*, a dimorphic fungus, is initiated by inhalation of highly infectious arthrospores. From these arthrospores, spherules (sporangia) containing endospores (sporangiospores) develop. The latter, when released by breakdown of the spherules, spread the infection through the pulmonary tissue.

136. **b** Like that of orthomyxoviruses, the genome of reoviruses is segmented; unlike that of orthomyxoviruses, the RNA of reoviruses is double stranded.

137. **b** Interferon protects only cells of the same species against any type of virus to which they may be normally susceptible.

138. **b** The bunyaviruses contain three segments of negative-polarity single-stranded RNA, and the arena-viruses contain two segments of RNA with virus-coding specificity.

139. **c** The complete "life cycle" of virulent bacteriophages spans the attachment of the infectious particle, injection of nucleic acid into the bacterial cell (*e.g.*, T-even coliphage DNA), uncoating and expression of the complete phage genome, and assembly and release through lysis of the bacterial cell. All temperate phage genes except one are completely repressed, and the phage genome either is inserted into the host genome or exists in the bacterial cell in free plasmidlike form. When integrated, the prophage (also called the lysogenic phage) is then replicated as part of the bacterial chromosome, from which it may be excised and induced to undergo its own replicative cycle as a virulent phage, ending in lysis of the cell.

140. **b** Injection of allergen in an atopic person elicits primarily IgG antibody, so-called blocking antibody, which competes for homologous IgE on mast cells and basophils and thus diminishes the hypersensitivity response to antigen challenge via the respiratory tract. IgE formation (hence type I hypersensitivity) as well as delayed-type hypersensitivity may be controlled through feedback mechanisms mediated by subsets of suppressor T lymphocytes that recognize antigen The latter exert their suppressive effects through soluble factors containing an antigen-binding site as well as other elements restricting the activity of appropriate acceptor/target cells.

141. **c** T cells are stimulated by antigen presented on accessory cells, such as macrophages, which produce IL-1. This lymphokine promotes antigen-specific T-cell blastogenesis and differentiation. Activated T_{DTH} cells then release a variety of lymphokines, including IL-2 and other mitogenic and other factors that promote the proliferation of both T and B cells. Most, but not all, of these lymphokines are nonspecific with respect to antigen.

142. **d** Pre–B cells are precommitted stem cells that differentiate in the microenvironment of the bone marrow or the fetal liver. The first identifiable post–stem cell stage contains cytoplasmic IgM. IgM, and subsequently IgD, is expressed at the membrane surface in most B cells. The cells carrying IgD are probably those representing true memory cells, a process in which the surface IgD is later lost and replaced by IgG. After repeated challenges, the antigen-specific IgM-IgG–carrying cells disappear, the memory cells remaining the only antigen-responsive B-cell population.

143. **a** C1q must be simultaneously affixed to immunoglobulins by at least two of its binding areas. Since IgG has only one such binding area (the CH2 heavy-chain region in the Fc portion), two IgG molecules bound to the same multivalent antigen molecule are required to activate the classical complement pathway. One molecule of pentavalent IgM will suffice.

144. **e** Histamine release is under the control of cAMP. Falling levels, caused by blockage of adenylcyclase (which catalyzes the production of cAMP) promotes histamine release; promotion of cAMP synthesis by increased adenylcyclase activity (stimulated by epinephrine, degranulation) reduces histamine release. Xanthines (such as theophylline) block phosphodiesterase, which is responsible for the destruc-

tion of cAMP and therefore helps effect relaxation of bronchiolar smooth muscle contraction induced by vasoactive amines released from antigen-activated IgE-sensitized basophils and mast cells.

145. **b** Secretory IgA, being in the mucous secretions, neutralizes respiratory viruses and viruses such as enteroviruses that are potentially infective via the lower intestinal tract. Secretory IgA is composed at the mucosal surface by the junction of IgA synthesized by plasma cells at local tissue sites. *Neisseria gonorrhoeae* and *N. meningitidis,* as well as *Haemophilus influenzae* (typable as well as nontypable strains), secrete neutral endopeptidases that hydrolyze the human IgA₁ heavy chain at the hinge region and are therefore thought to contribute to the pathogenicity of these microorganisms.

146. **a** Circulating antigen–antibody complexes, particularly those formed by IgM in slight antigen excess (corresponding to the point of maximum precipitation in the quantitative precipitin curve), tend to be lodged in vessel walls, where they can cause permanent tissue destruction by attracting complement, leukocytes, and phagocytes to cause a tissue-destructive inflammatory reaction. Immune complexes are also deposited in the basement membrane of the kidney, as in poststreptococcal glomerulonephritis.

147. **e** *Klebsiella* species possess O antigens and K (German *Kapsel,* capsule) antigens, the latter representing 72 antigenic types. No single serologic type of *K. pneumoniae* is more virulent than others, in which the capsular polysaccharide has antiphagocytic properties, and, hence is the virulence factor. The capsule of *Cryptococcus neoformans,* a high-molecular-weight polysaccharide, contains at least four antigenic determinants, is antiphagocytic, and evokes an immune reponse in the course of cryptococcal infection. Nine serotypes of *Neisseria meningitidis* have been identified by the antigenic specificity of capsular polysaccharides, which are antiphagocytic and, which, except for type B, constitute the protective antigens of each type. Accordingly, purified polysaccharides A and C constitute effective vaccines against infection with *N. meningitidis* types A and C, respectively. The capsule of *Bacillus anthracis* is D-glutamyl-polypeptide, which represents a single capsular antigenic type. During the early stages of infection, the capsule interferes with phagocytosis and evokes antibodies that, however, are not protective. The capsule and the soluble toxin of *B. anthracis* together account for its virulence.

148. **a** Only lysogenic strains of beta hemolytic streptococci of Lancefield group A (*i.e.,* strains infected with temperate bacteriophages) produce erythro-

genic toxin (scarlatinal toxin), three distinct serotypes of which are recognized (A, B, C). Pyrogenicity rather than dermal reactivity seems to be the primary effect of the toxins, which may in part at least be secondary to the interplay of cellular and humoral factors associated with hypersensitivity to streptococcal products.

149. **e** *Clostridium perfringens* is included among the normal vaginal flora in many women; from this source it may cause severe, life-threatening pelvic sepsis and uterine myonecrosis, especially following attempted abortion or puerperal infection. Also a normal inhabitant of the lower intestinal tract, *C. perfringens* is the cause of intra-abdominal sepsis associated with bowel disease or trauma. In both of these situations, septicemia occurs and the clostridial alpha toxin causes massive intravascular hemolysis and renal failure. In clostridial food poisoning, usually due to type A strains, and contracted through ingestion of contaminated meat, the symptoms are attributable to clostridial enterotoxin, which acts directly on the intestinal mucosa. In necrotizing jejunitis, more severe disease is due to the beta toxin of type C strains.

150. **a** Chlamydiae replicate only in viable cells, in which they undergo a complex life cycle involving two morphological forms, the elementary body and the reticulate body. Infection with *C. trachomatis* is the leading cause of sexually transmitted disease (lymphogranuloma venereum, LGV) and its complications (*e.g.,* pelvic inflammatory disease and sterility). Trachoma is one of the major causes of blindness in developing countries. *C. trachomatis* is responsible for a less severe disease, inclusion conjunctivitis (blennorrhea), as well as for neonatal pneumonia syndrome. All forms of chlamydial infection are treatable with tetracycline or erythromycin.

151. **d** Acute hemorrhagic glomerulonephritis is a sequel to infection with any of several so-called nephritogenic strains of group A streptococcus (*e.g.,* following outbreaks of acute pharyngitis due to types 1, 3, 4, 12, and 25; or following streptococcal pyoderma due to type 2 and other types). The glomerular lesions are caused by the deposition of immune complexes in which streptococcal antigens are found. Complete recovery is the rule, and recurrences are rare owing to the type-specific immunity conferred by streptococcal infection and the statistical improbability of a second encounter with a nephritogenic strain.

152. **c** R-factor–mediated resistance to antibiotics is determined by protein products of the plasmid, namely enzymes found in the periplasmic space. Chloramphenicol and aminoglycosides are inac-

tivated by the enzymatic attachment of the acetyl, phosphate, or adenyl group. In the case of penicillins and cephalosporins, beta lactamase activity destroys the antibiotic in the periplasmic space or outside of the cell wall. The single product of a plasmid in some instances reacts with a variety of compounds; for example, a given beta lactamase may destroy ampicillin, penicillin G, and cephalothin, or a given aminoglycoside-modifying enzyme may react with kanamycin, gentamicin, and tobramycin.

153. **d** Group B streptococci (four serotypes) colonize 25% of normal vaginas and from this site may cause severe and often fatal neonatal infection. "Early-onset" disease is due to any of the four serotypes and is fatal in up to 60% of cases; it occurs during the first postnatal week in association with prematurity or obstetric complications and is characterized by "respiratory distress" syndrome (pneumonia) and septicemia. "Delayed-onset" disease, with lower mortality, is caused usually by type III (either maternally acquired or nosocomial) and is characterized by meningitis, septicemia, or more localized infections.

154. **c** Even though botulism is due entirely to botulinus toxin ingested with contaminated food, the amount of the heat-labile toxin transiently entering the circulation and reaching the central nervous system is extremely small and well below the threshold necessary for an immune response. The pneumococcus does not elaborate any toxins, pathogenicity being related entirely to the antiphagocytic properties of the polysaccharide capsule of virulent strains.

155. **b** *Legionella pneumophila* is an unencapsulated, pleomorphic, motile, nonsporulating rod that stains only weakly with safranin. It is demonstrable in tissue with silver impregnation stains (*e.g.*, Dieterle) or with the Gimenez stain, which is about as sensitive. Specific immunofluorescence is the basis for typing strains. For primary isolation, charcoal yeast extract agar (CYE) at *p*H 6.8 to *p*H 7.0 is used and cultures are incubated at 36° C plus or minus 1° C in an atmosphere of 2.5 to 5.0 carbon dioxide.

156. **c** The bacillus of Calmette and Guérin (BCG) used for active immunization against tuberculosis is a strain of *Mycobacterium bovis* that has been attenuated (*i.e.*, rendered relatively avirulent) by repeated subculture on glycerol–potato–bile medium. BCG should be administered only to persons who are unreactive to tuberculin (PPD). Immunization, involving active infection with the attenuated organism, stimulates an immune response evidenced by the development of delayed-type hypersensitivity to tuberculin. BCG organisms may occasionally be isolated from abscesses formed at the site of inoculation, or from lymph nodes draining the site. Laboratory identification is therefore of great importance.

Section C

157. **C** The relatively slow elimination of antigen in segment B is due primarily to metabolic degradation; however, increasing amounts of antibody are being formed during this period, accounting for the accelerated disappearance of antigen as antigen–antibody complexes in segment C, which corresponds roughly to the equivalence zone in the precipitin curve (*i.e.*, the point at which neither antigen nor antibody is detectable in the supernatants).

158. **A** Injected antigen during this period is distributed to the tissue; hence its serum concentration falls during the hours immediately following injection.

159. **D** By day 13, most if not all antigen–antibody complexes have been eliminated either by phagocytosis or by deposition in certain highly vascular tissues (*e.g.*, kidney, pulmonary parenchyma), leaving excess antibody in the serum. In the quantitative precipitin curve, this segment corresponds to the zone of antibody excess in which only antibody is found in supernatants.

160. **C** Immune complex disease, of which the prototype is the constellation of signs and symptoms caused by therapeutic injection of horse serum (*e.g.*, type-specific horse serum therapy for pneumococcal pneumonia in presulfonamide days, equine antiserum to human lymphocytes in posttransplantation immunosuppressive therapy), also occurs with drugs (*e.g.*, penicillin) and in bacteremia (*e.g.*, infective endocarditis). Clinical recovery accompanies the appearance of antibody in the serum, signalling the elimination of circulating antigen.

161. **d** *Trypanosoma gambiense* and *T. rhodesiense* are the agents, respectively, of West African and East African sleeping sickness. The trypomastigote (or trypanosomal) forms are found in the blood in the acute stages of the disease.

162. **c** Visceral leishmaniasis (kala azar) is an infection with the viscerotropic *Leishmania* species *L. donovani*. It is usually a zoonosis transmitted sporadically to humans by *Phlebotomus* species of sandfly.

163. **b** American trypanosomiasis is caused by infection with *Trypanosoma cruzi*, which is transmitted by Hemiptera, or blood-sucking insects.

164. **a** Oriental sore, including leishmaniasis recidivans (recurrent dermal leishmaniasis), is common in the

Mediterranean basin and the Middle East. It is most often, though not exclusively, caused by *Leishmania tropica*.

165. **e** Lesions caused by *Leishmania brasiliensis* are usually large, persistent, and destructive skin ulcers, from which oronasal metastases are common (espundia).

166. **b** Killer cells and macrophages bear receptors for the Fc portion of antibody, which thus mediates the attachment of viral antigen(s) to these effector cells.

167. **c** T lymphocytes are sensitized to specific viral antigen(s) as part of the total immune response. Cells infected by viruses that develop at the surface of cells (*e.g.*, RNA tumor retroviruses) thus become specific targets of cytotoxic T-cell action, for which the presence of· at least a portion of the major histocompatibility complex on both interacting cells is required (HLA restriction).

168. **d** IgG has the lowest catabolic rate in serum, measured as percentage of loss per day. For IgG this value is about 68%; for all other Ig classes it is significantly higher.

169. **c** IgE is found in serum in only nanogram amounts, whereas the level of all. other classes is measured in milligrams per milliliter.

170. **b** Molecule for molecule, IgM, being pentavalent, attaches more efficiently to multivalent (*e.g.*, cell surface) antigens than any of the other Ig classes of smaller molecular weight.

171. **b** The IgM molecule consists of five basic four-chain polypeptide units joined by an accessory glycopolypeptide (J-chain).

172. **b** The molecular configuration of IgM as a pentamer accounts for the most part for its higher sedimentation coefficient which, however, is also influenced by molecular shape.

173. **d** At normal serum levels of up to 16 mg/ml, all four subclasses of IgG account for up to 80% of serum immunoglobulin.

174. **c** All identifiable bone marrow precursor cells and presumably also the human pluripotential stem cell, which cannot be tested *in vitro,* are unreactive with monoclonal antibodies to specific lymphocyte markers.

175. **c** The antigen receptor on B cells is membrane-bound immunoglobulin of the same class as that destined to be produced by monoclonal progeny plasmocytes. The antigen receptor on T cells is a heterodimeric structure comprising two glycosylated chains (alpha and beta), each with two extracellular Ig-like domains, an amino-terminal variable domain, and a carboxy-terminal constant domain. The general resemblance to Ig structure is obvious.

176. **a** In mature B lymphocytes programmed to pro-duce IgG, membrane-bound IgG serves as the antigen receptor. The lymphocytes programmed to synthesize any of the other three classes of immunoglobulin behave in an analogous manner.

177. **a** Immunologic memory, or recall (anamnestic response), results from the expansion of antigen-specific T- and B-cell clones without the intervention of antigen-bearing macrophages. The average affinity of the antibody molecules produced increases with time (maturation of the immune response), probably owing to the progressive selection and expansion of clones of lymphocytes with Ig receptors of relatively high affinity.

178. **c** *Chlamydia* are intermediate forms that, although they contain both RNA and DNA, are absolutely dependent on host cells for replication. All viruses are obligate intracellular parasites.

179. **a** The chlamydial genome is DNA, although the mature organism contains mitochondrial and other RNAs.

180. **d** The genome of rubella virus is single-stranded unsegmented RNA; hence the antigenic stability of the virus.

181. **a** Although chlamydiae cause disease in certain internal organs (*e.g.*, pelvic inflammatory disease), the organism is never truly invasive or found in the blood.

182. **d** Chlamydial infection is sexually transmitted, rubella presumably by contact or aerosol droplet or, in the case of congenital rubella syndrome, transplacentally.

183. **b** Rubella virus contains a hemagglutinin that is associated with one of the major proteins of the viral envelope and that agglutinates erythrocytes from a variety of species. Newly hatched chick, adult goose, and human O erythrocytes have been used most extensively for serologic (hemagglutination inhibition, HI) tests. Serum beta lipoproteins are nonspecific inhibitors, which must be removed before testing for specific HI antibody.

184. **c** *P. falciparum* may invade all erythrocytes, irrespective of age, causing "stickiness" and impaired microcirculation, particularly in liver and spleen, both of which become greatly enlarged owing to widespread capillary occlusion and deposition of malarial pigment.

185. **b** Paroxysms of fever every 72 hours are synchronized with simultaneous periodic release of merozoites of *Plasmodium malariae* from ruptured erythrocytes.

186. **c** *P. falciparum* is the cause of malignant subtertian malaria, so called because of the characteristically overwhelming parasitemia and life-threatening severity.

187. **c** In contrast to the round gametocytes of *P. vivax*

and *P. malariae,* which may fill the entire erythro-cyte, those of *P. falciparum* are distinctive and di-agnostic, having a crescent shape and causing elongation and distortion of the normal round erythrocyte shape.

188. **a** *Plasmodium vivax* (benign tertian) malaria is the most widely distributed and prevalent, although most cases seen in the United States and Europe are imported from Africa, Asia, and Latin America. *P. falciparum* fails to establish itself in areas with long, cold seasons; like *P. malariae,* it is limited to tropical and subtropical regions.

189. **c** Capillary occlusions, particularly in the brain, are most characteristic of malignant *P. falciparum* ter-tian malaria (cerebral malaria). Parasitized erythro-cytes become sticky, agglutinate (possibly owing to antigen–antibody reactions), and marginate around the lamina of vessels, which then become oc-cluded, with resulting perivascular ("ring") hemor-rhages. These lesions are seen exclusively in the subcortical and paraventricular white matter.

190. **b** In malaria due to *P. malariae,* only older erythrocytes are invaded. This accounts for the rela-tively limited hemolysis associated with *P. malariae* infection as compared with the massive erythrocyte destruction seen with *P. falciparum* infection.

191. **a** In *P. vivax* malaria, the degree of intravascular hemolysis is limited, since the parasite invades only reticulocytes, representing a maximum of 2% of the total erythrocyte count.

192. **d** Because of the predilection of *Trypanosoma cruzi* for muscle and nerve cells, particularly of the heart and gastrointestinal tract, patients with chronic American trypanosomiasis may display serious intestinal malfunction due to parasitic inva-sion and destruction of the cells of autonomic nerve ganglia, with consequent massive reten-tion of food (megaesophagus) and feces (mega-colon).

193. **c** Nodules, eye lesions, and dermatitis are constant manifestations of infection with *Onchocerca vol-vulus.* Immunologic reaction to the breakdown of microfilarial products in the tissues causes the localized formation of perivascular immune com-plexes that induce type III (Arthus) injury in the eye.

194. **b** In dracontiasis, subcutaneous and connective tis-sues are infested with adult *Dracunculus medi-nensis* (guinea worm), which alternates among hu-mans, the definitive host, and an intermediate arthropod host. The latter is a freshwater crusta-cean, *Cyclops,* which ingests the larvae and is thus the source of human infection.

195. **c** In onchocerciasis, a constant trio of man-ifestations follows the introduction of larvae of *Onchocerca volvulus* into the human skin, where they develop into adult parasites. These aggregate in superficial or deeply embedded nodules (onchocercomas), or live free in the tissues, where they cause no inflammatory reaction. Large num-bers of microfilariae are subsequently produced, which migrate to the skin and distant sites (*e.g.,* eyes, testes).

196. **d** *Trypanosoma cruzi* preferentially infects neural cells and muscle cells of the heart, causing damage initially by multiplication of the parasites and later through immunologic injury, as shown by a wide-spread inflammatory reaction in cardiac tissue in the absence of parasites, with resulting myocardial insufficiency, cardiomegaly, conduction distur-bances, and sudden death on exertion as a terminal event in chronic Chagas' disease.

197. **a** Hydrocele is probably the most common sign of longstanding infection with *Wuchereria bancrofti,* affecting up to 40% of the male population in high-ly endemic areas.

198. **a** At the onset of infection with *Wuchereria ban-crofti,* the adult worms cause lymphatic inflamma-tion and obstruction. Subsequent lymphangitis and lymphadenitis are thought to be allergic reactions to parasitic secretions or antigens liberated from dead filariae.

199. **d** Unilateral conjunctivitis is caused by an inocula-tion of chagoma in the ocular mucosa and is accom-panied by palpebral edema and satellite lympha-denitis.

200. **c** The genome of reoviruses comprises ten in-dividual segments of double-stranded RNA, each segment containing complementary positive and negative strands.

201. **d** RNA purified from concentrated infectious polio-virus will initiate infection in cultured cells, such as chick embryo fibroblasts, which are not normally susceptible to penetration by the intact virion. This process is called transfection and requires a rela-tively high input multiplicity. Alternatively, the RNA can be incorporated into liposomes and the uptake efficiency increased.

202. **e** The segmented genome of orthomyxoviruses (influenza viruses) and the attendant capacity for genetic reassortment account for their antigenic instability.

203. **b** The retroviruses include HTLV I and II and HIV. All have their RNA genomes transcribed into dsDNA, which becomes integrated into the nucleus as proviral DNA.

204. **a** For replication, paramyxoviruses transcribe the genome to an intermediate form of RNA (replica-tive intermediate) of positive polarity that acts as viral message(s).

205. **b** This is the basis for the transformation of non-permissive cells by RNA tumor viruses.

206. **b** Orthomyxoviruses have a genome consisting of segmented, single-stranded RNA.

207. **c** Cytomegalovirus (CMV) is a herpesvirus, which develops in the nucleus.

208. **d** Negri bodies are diagnostic of rabies when found in neurons infected with the virus. They are composed of aggregated nucleocapsid.

209. **a** Echoviruses are a common cause of benign meningitis with predominantly lymphocytic reaction in the cerebrospinal fluid, although the initial reaction may be predominantly polymorphonuclear. The acronym *Echo* means *E*nteric *c*ytopathic *h*uman *o*rphan virus.

210. **e** Hepatitis B virus is inactivated by heating to 60° C for 10 hours (*e.g.,* in the sterilization of human serum albumin for intravenous use), by formalin, or by chloroform.

211. **c** Both the complete hepatitis B viral particle and adenoviruses contain DNA. For adenoviruses, it is double-stranded linear DNA, while with HBV, it is an almost complete double-stranded circle.

212. **c** Hepatitis B virus, particularly in chronic hepatitis, is associated etiologically with hepatoma or hepatocellular carcinoma (HCC). Most adenoviruses can transform the cells of a nonpermissive host *in vitro*. Certain types of adenovirus (*e.g.,* types 12, 18, and 31) produce tumors when inoculated directly into newborn hamsters or rats, but are not oncogenic in humans.

213. **b** Human adenoviruses are propagable in cultures of human cells only.

214. **a** The Dane particle is the complete infectious form of hepatitis B virus (HBV).

215. **b** The penton fibers of the adenovirus particle mediate viral attachment to erythrocytes *in vitro* as well as to susceptible cultured cells.

216. **e** Laryngeal papillomas, associated with human papovirus type 11 (HPV-11), are the most common benign epithelial tumors of the larynx.

217. **c** Marek's disease (the agent is a herpesvirus) of chickens is a major problem in animal husbandry. A live attenuated vaccine made from a related herpesvirus of turkeys is effective in controlling the spread of infection.

218. **d** B-type particles of mouse mammary tumor viruses contain an eccentric, electron-dense nucleoid and bud from the infected cell membrane. A-type particles are intracellular and may in part represent immature B particles.

219. **b** Rous sarcoma of chickens was the first cancer proved unequivocally to be caused by a virus.

220. **a** Maternal IgG of all four classes can pass through the placenta to the fetus, whereas IgM, IgD, and IgE cannot.

221. **b** Secretory IgA comprises two molecules of monomeric serum IgA joined by a secretory piece that is synthesized in mucous epithelial cells and incorporated into the molecule as it passes to the external surface of the mucous membrane.

222. **e** IgE mediates type I (atopic) hypersensitivity by fixing to the surface of mast cells and basophils which, on reaction with homologous antigen(s), are triggered to produce vasoactive amines.

223. **e** Certain parasitic infections, notably helminthoses, cause marked elevation of serum IgE, which may have some protective effect by increasing the release of mediators from mast cells to affect the parasites directly or, through increasing vascular permeability and releasing eosinophil chemotactic factors, promoting accumulation of antibodies at the sites of infestation. Eosinophils can mediate IgG-dependent cytotoxic killing of schistosomula and *Trichinella* larvae, and parasite-specific IgE immune complexes can induce macrophage-mediated cytotoxicity for schistosomula.

224. **a** IgE attaches to mast cells and basophils by its Fc portion, leaving the Fab end protruding to react with homologous circulating antigen and to set in motion the release of vasoactive amines.

225. **d** Particulate antigens (*e.g.,* bacterial cells or fragments) combined with specific IgG (*i.e.,* opsonized) antibody are more readily engulfed by phagocytic cells than uncoated antigen(s) because of Fc receptors in the membrane of macrophages and neutrophils.

226. **c** Because of its multivalency, IgM is more efficient in sensitizing cells to immune lysis than are the other immunoglobulins.

227. **a** In the primary immune response to soluble antigens, the size of germinal centers in the splenic cortex increases, indicating proliferation of B lymphocytes.

228. **b** Specifically "sensitized" T lymphocytes predominate in the normal circulation.

229. **a** On B cells the receptor for antigen is specific antibody identical to that eventually produced by the plasmacyte progeny of individual activated lymphocytes.

230. **c** Creeping eruption is due to prolonged migration of canine or feline hookworm (*Ancylostoma braziliense*) larvae in the skin of infected humans, in whom the parasite is unable to complete its life cycle.

231. **a** The life cycle of *Wuchereria bancrofti* and *Brugia malayi* is limited to the human host, in whom the infectious cycle is maintained by the transfer of

infectious microfilariae through the bites of mosquitoes.

232. a The majority of cases of amebic dysentery are caused by the ingestion of cysts from sources contaminated with the feces of human carriers.

233. a The term *symbiosis* broadly connotes toleration of one another by two dissimilar organisms without detriment to either. Each is called a symbiont.

234. c This is a form of symbiosis in which both species gain from the association and are unable to survive without it. For example, lichens are thallophytic plants formed by mutualistic combination of a blue–green alga and a fungus, usually an ascomycete.

235. b Many organisms of the oral cavity (*e.g.,* the viridans group of streptococci) or the lower intestinal tract (*e.g.,* coliform bacteria, nonsporing anaerobes) are commensals that under normal circumstances are nonpathogenic. However, in certain circumstances (*e.g.,* infective endocarditis in patients with rheumatic endocardial damage), commensal organisms may cause disease.

236. d The term *parasitism* broadly includes most organisms capable of causing disease.

237. c Both HTLV-1 and HIV-1 are retroviruses. They contain the enzyme reverse transcriptase, which allows conversion of virion RNA to DNA.

238. c It was found several years ago that conditioned media from T cells contained T cell growth factors (such as interleukin-2), which allowed long-term propagation of T cells from ATL patients and the subsequent isolation of HTLV-I. Using a similar growth medium, HIV-1 was isolated from peripheral blood mononuclear cells of AIDS patients.

239. b HTLV-I has been isolated from patients with adult T-cell leukemia (ATL) and is also associated with tropical spastic paraperesis (TSP), as well as a rare form of HTLV-I-associated myelopathy (HAM).

240. d The virus HTLV-II was originally isolated from a patient with "hairy cell" leukemia. It is a virus without a disease; however, it has been found (serologically) to have infected large numbers of drug abusers in cities such as New Orleans and among Indian tribes in Panama as well as Brazil.

241. b B-19 is a recently isolated *nondefective* human parvovirus that has been linked to severe aplastic crises in children with homozygous sickle-cell anemia. B-19 preferentially infects immature red blood cell precursors in the bone marrow and kills them. In addition, fifth disease, or *erythema infectiosum,* a self-limiting febrile illness of infants and young children is associated with B-19.

242. d HTLV-I has been associated with tropical spastic paraperesis in many warmer climates, where the viral infection is prevalent. Among these are the Zairean region of Africa, Caribbean countries, and South America.

243. a Molluscum contagiosum is a poxvirus that causes benign epidermal tumors of children and young adults; these tumors usually regress and disappear in several months. Removal of the lesions is recommended so as to prevent spread to other sites.

244. e Rotaviruses are segmented double-stranded RNA viruses, whose members cause diarrhea in young animals. As with reoviruses, transcription of minus-strand RNA occurs in subviral particles, yielding plus-stranded RNA, which can be used as mRNA for translation or serve as a template in replication of double-stranded RNA. Replication occurs in a conservative mode. In contrast to reoviruses, rotaviruses appear to assemble and bud from the endoplasm reticulum.

245. c Rubella is a member of the *Togaviridae* and is classified in a separate subgenus as a *rubivirus.* Also known as German measles, if rubella is contracted during the first trimester of pregnancy, it causes severe fetal damage and results in the congenital rubella syndrome of surviving infants. This virus is to be contrasted with rubeola, or "red measles," also known as measles, which is a paramyxovirus.

246. e Wild-type p53 is a tumor-suppressor gene product. It is expressed in the nucleus of most cells and has a 20-minute turnover time. Normally, it is believed to serve a role in oncogene surveillance. As detection methods have improved, it appears that in many cancers, such as colon carcinoma or Li-Fraumeri syndrome, mutant forms of p53 predominate. In fact, a recent study has shown that p53 mutations are the most frequently observed genetic change in breast cancer. Since the mutant form of p53 can outcompete wild-type p53 and has a longer half-life (up to 24 hours), it is believed that mutant p53 overrides the activity of wild-type p53.

247. c The *rev* gene product is one of about five regulatory proteins encoded by HIV-1. It carries out its function by binding to a site on viral RNA called the RRE (*rev* responsive element). This permits it to enhance transport (from the nucleus to cytoplasm) and stabilization of large singly spliced RNA species that encodes among others, the *gag, pol,* and *env* proteins. This leads to an increased expression of these proteins in the cytoplasm, concomitant with the late stage of virion assembly.

248. a *erb*B2 (also known as HER2, or *neu*) encodes a 185kD transmembrane glycoprotein that has homology to the EGF (epidermal growth factor) receptor but is the receptor for a different growth factor. It has an intrinsic tyrosine kinase activity.

Extra copies of this gene (amplified) or its gene product (overexpressed) are seen in certain cancers. In particular, overexpression of HER2 shows a high predictability for relapse in human breast and ovarian cancer patients.

249. **d** The v-*src* gene was originally isolated from Rous sarcoma virus, which rapidly (3–4 weeks) causes sarcomas in newborn chickens. These viruses also transform chick embryo fibroblasts in culture, *e.g.*, cells become rounded, lose contact inhibition, and grow on top of one another. This is the basis of the focus assay (ffu) and contrasts with the pfu (plaque-forming unit) assay for lytic viruses. The v-*src* gene encodes a protein called pp60$^{v=src}$, which is both a tyrosine protein kinase and a phosphoprotein. When present at increased levels, certain cellular cytoskeleton proteins are modified, leading to transformation.

250. **b** The *rel* oncogene product is found in avian reticuloendotheliosis virus. Recently, it was shown to be structurally related to the NF$\kappa\beta$ family of proteins. Specifically, the v-*rel* product binds to $\kappa\beta$ cis-acting regulatory sequences in the nucleus, thereby inhibiting NF$\kappa\beta$ activated transcription.

251. **b** Reovirus, like most other virus families (except for picornaviruses), has the appropriate enzymatic machinery to cap its mRNA early in infection and thus enhance stability. However, late in reovirus infection, there is a preferential synthesis and translation of uncapped mRNA. Further, no significant poly A is added to the 3' end of reovirus mRNA, since it is predominantly found associated with polysomes or in subviral particles.

252. **c** Retroviruses contain reverse transcriptase, which is an RNA-dependent DNA polymerase and converts RNA to DNA. In reoviruses the particle transcriptase is an RNA-dependent RNA polymease and initially converts the (–) strand of genome RNA to (+) strand RNA that can serve as an mRNA or later on during the life cycle as a template for the second strand of genomic (–) RNA.

253. **c** In retroviruses there are 2 identical copies of (+) single-stranded genome RNA. For reoviruses, there are 10 double-stranded RNA segments.

254. **b** In retroviruses, at the final stage of assembly, there is an extensive cleavage of *gag* and *gag-pol* encoded polyproteins. In the former case, four polypeptides are produced, *i.e.*, MA (matrix), NC (nucleocapsid), CA (capsid), and a phosphoprotein. For the larger *gag-pol* polyprotein, the protease, reverse transcriptase, and integrase enzymes are produced after cleavage. In the case of reoviruses, one or possibly two protein cleavages occur. These are usually secondary in nature, since each of the segments predominantly encode a single uncleaved protein.

255. **a** Viroids are covalently closed single-stranded RNA circles about 300 to 400 nucleotides in length. They are not viruses or virions. Viroids do not encode proteins but are highly resistant to denaturing agents such as UV light. Their mechanism of pathogenesis may involve interference with normal transcription inside cells.

256. **a** The Delta Agent, when present in individuals already infected with hepatitis B virus, can lead to a significant increase in fulminant hepatitis. The Delta Agent or hepatitis D virus is a viroidlike RNA packaged within a capsid containing the HBsAg.

257. **b** *Prions* are small *pro*teinaceous *in*fectious particles. They do not contain nucleic acid. An example is the scrapie agent, which causes a progressive fatal neurological disease of sheep. It is considered a prototype agent to explain the unconventional, slow, viruslike infections of humans, such as Creutzfeldt-Jakob disease, kuru, and Gerstmann-Straussler syndrome (GSS). The agent is stable at 90° C for 30 min; it has an associated 27K hydrophobic protein, which seems to be needed for infectivity. This protein forms amyloidlike fibrils, which deposit in an abnormal manner around neurons in the brain, and is found both in scrapie and the above-mentioned human neurological diseases. Transgenic mice have now been created with a leucine substitution at codon 102 of the PrP gene (GSS mutant). They exhibit spontaneous neurodegenerative disease by 166 days. This is a good model for GSS. Recently in England, "Mad Cow" (bovine encephalopathy) disease was killing 2,000 cattle per month—because of being fed improperly processed bone meal from sheep (possibly contaminated with scrapie) as babies—about 8 years ago. This then stimulated amyloid fibril formation in adult cows and led to the spongiform encephalopathy.

258. **d** Neither viroids nor prions are viruses. They also do not contain capsids or nucleocapsids with icosahedral symmetry.

259. **b** During the earliest stages of HIV-1 infection, gp120 glycoprotein moieties adsorb specifically to CD4 molecules on the surface of susceptible T_H (helper), cells, macrophages, or monocytes. Current attempts at HIV-1 vaccine development involve exploitation of this interaction. Thus, hybrid molecule constructs containing the combining part of the CD4 receptor with a bacterial exotoxin protein have been successful in killing HIV-1 infected cells in tissue culture system. Similarly, recombinant

gp 120 and gp 160 (gp 120 precursor) molecules produced in bacteria or baculovirus systems are undergoing vaccine trials in several laboratories.

260. d The long terminal repeat (LTR) contains the site, whereby proviral DNA is integrated into host DNA. This recombining event involves the viral integrase protein, an enzyme that trims the HIV DNA provirus prior to covalently joining at its cut ends into a freshly nicked site on host DNA. Once integrated, the HIV proviral DNA replicates with the host nuclear DNA. All of these integration events occur in the nucleus.

261. a Capsid assembly is the final stage of HIV maturation. Assuming validity of a murine model, about 1,500 *gag* and *gag-pol* encoded polyproteins are brought to a site under the cell surface, along with the two strands of genomic RNA. A nascent budding particle forms and then after autocatalytic cleavage by the viral protease, cleavage of the polyproteins subsequently occurs (specifically noted in question 254), leading to formation of an infectious virus particle.

262. e Transcription during an HIV infection involves the host RNA polymerase and early formation of multiply spliced mRNAs. Critical to this is having the HIV-1 LTR becoming an active promoter. This occurs as a result of change in cellular transcription factors due to activation of T cells, or by synthesis of increased amounts of the HIV-1 encoded *tat* (transactivator) protein. *Tat* is a regulatory protein with several effects. It binds to TAR sequences at the 5' end of viral genomic RNA and thus can increase the frequency of mRNA initiation and also *tat* proteins interact with nascent RNA strands to increase stability of the RNA polymerase, so that full length transcripts can be made. The initial early transcripts in an HIV-1–infected cell have several splicing sites that are recognized by the cells splicing machinery and thus gives rise to several mRNAs that are translated into the early HIV-1 regulatory proteins.

263. c Reverse transcription occurs via binding of the HIV-1 reverse transcriptase (RT) [a heterodimer (66kD/51kD)] near the 5' end of genomic RNA, at the primer binding site (PBS). The PBS is where a specific tRNA has bound, so that single-stranded

DNA synthesis can be initiated. The RT has at least three enzyme activities: an RNA-dependent DNA polymerase that synthesizes the first (–) strand of DNA, an RNaseH (hybrid) activity that digests the RNA away from the newly reverse transcribed RNA/DNA hybrid, and finally a DNA-dependent DNA polymerase that completes synthesis of the second strand of proviral DNA using the (–) strand as a template. All of these events occur in the cytoplasm.

Section D

264. c Hemolytic disease of the newborn (HDN) occurs in connection with a first pregnancy only if there has been opportunity for prior maternal sensitization (*e.g.*, blood transfusion, miscarriage of an Rh-incompatible fetus). HDN in the second-term pregnancy made it probable that the third infant would be likewise affected, the mother having become sensitized during the first term pregnancy to paternal *c* antigen present on the fetal erythrocytes but not on her own. Anti-c (IgG) would therefore be found in her serum. The serum of individuals of group A (*e.g.*, the mother) normally contains naturally occurring anti-B, which in this case was no threat to the fetus.

265. e The same IgG antibody (anti-c) would have been recalled during the third pregnancy as occurred in the second term pregnancy (assuming the fetal erythrocytes had the *c* antigen). Since the group O father was homozygous only for the *c* antigen of the Rh system (cDE/cde), this was most probably the antigen involved in the maternal isoimmunization; correspondingly, anti-c would have been discovered by a direct antiglobulin test on the cord blood.

266. b RhoGAM is the commercial name for a preparation of human IgG antibody to $Rh_O(D)$, the antigen most frequently involved in HDN. It is obtained from male donors who have been hyperimmunized with $Rh_O(D)$-positive erythrocytes. It would not have been considered for use in this case, since the mother was homozygous with respect to the D antigen. Besides, RhoGAM contains little if any anti-c.

Rypins' Questions & Answers for Basic Sciences Review, Second Edition, edited by Edward D. Frohlich. J. B. Lippincott Company, Philadelphia © 1993.

C H A P T E R

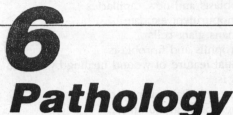

Pathology

Jack P. Strong, M.D.

Boyd Professor and Head, Department of Pathology, Louisiana State University School of Medicine

Lester J. Vial, Jr., M.D.

Associate Professor, Department of Pathology, Louisiana State University School of Medicine

QUESTIONS

Directions.   Each of the statements below is followed by five suggested answers. For each statement select the one answer that is best.

1. The first ultrastructural nuclear change in necrosis is:
   (a) Condensation of chromatin into a dense mass
   (b) Fragmentation of the nucleus
   (c) Clumping of chromatin in the nuclear membrane
   (d) Dissolution of chromatin
   (e) Rupture of the nuclear membrane

2. The location of increased microvascular permeability in the acute inflammatory reaction is best characterized as:
   (a) Arterioles
   (b) Arteriolar end of the capillary loop
   (c) Midportion of the capillary loop
   (d) Venules and venular portion of the capillary loop
   (e) Even distribution over the microvasculature

3. The emigration and accumulation of neutrophilic polymorphonuclear leukocytes in the acute inflammation reaction is primarily the result of:
   (a) Active hyperemia
   (b) Hydrostatic pressure
   (c) Increased microvascular permeability
   (d) Chemotaxis
   (e) None of the above

4. Which of the following inflammatory mediators does *not* have a chemotactic effect?
   (a) Histamine
   (b) Fragments of C5
   (c) C567
   (d) Cationic protein
   (e) Lymphokines

5. Among cells classified according to regenerative ability, an example of a permanent cell is the:
   (a) Hepatocyte
   (b) Osteocyte
   (c) Erythrocyte
   (d) Colonic mucosal cell
   (e) Acinar cell of the pancreas

6. A chemical mediator derived from neutrophils, which is responsible for increased vascular permeability, is:
   (a) Cationic protein
   (b) Acid phosphatase
   (c) Beta glucuronidase
   (d) Cholesteryl oleate
   (e) Acid mucopolysaccharide

7. The most likely cause of anemia with basophilic stippling of erythrocytes in a child is exposure to which of the following?
   (a) Arsenic
   (b) Vinyl chloride
   (c) Cyanide
   (d) Lead
   (e) Mercury

8. The most characteristic feature of granulation tissue is the presence of:

(a) Epithelial cells
(b) Fibroblasts and new capillaries
(c) Fibrinopurulent exudate
(d) Langhans giant cells
(e) Neutrophils and fibroblasts

9. An essential feature of wound healing by second intention is:
   (a) Rapid epithelial covering of the defect
   (b) Foreign body granulomata
   (c) Large amounts of granulation tissue
   (d) Need for approximation of wound edges before repair
   (e) Secondary infection

10. The characteristic fate of ischemic necrosis in the brain in a patient who survives is:
    (a) Abscess formation
    (b) Collagenous scarring
    (c) Liquefaction and cyst formation
    (d) Regeneration
    (e) Dystrophic calcification

11. The process of regeneration:
    (a) Does not restore prior function
    (b) Invariably leads to scar formation
    (c) Refers to healing by proliferation of stromal elements
    (d) Occurs in tissues composed of labile and stable cells
    (e) Is synonymous with repair

12. The most precise definition of a neoplasm is:
    (a) Cancer
    (b) Carcinoma
    (c) Tumor
    (d) Autonomous new growth
    (e) Increase in number of cells

13. Which of the following is absolute proof of malignancy of a tumor?
    (a) Invasion
    (b) Anaplasia
    (c) Metastases
    (d) Rapid growth
    (e) Mitoses

14. A substance that will not produce cancer when acting alone but that will produce cancer when acting in conjunction with another substance is best described as a(n):
    (a) Carcinogen
    (b) Cocarcinogen
    (c) Procarcinogen
    (d) Direct acting carcinogen
    (e) Ultimate carcinogen

15. Ureteral obstruction with renal failure is a frequent result of carcinoma of the:
    (a) Kidney
    (b) Urinary bladder
    (c) Cervix

(d) Prostate
(e) Endometrium

16. The least common of the following types of breast neoplasm is:
    (a) Infiltrating ductal carcinoma
    (b) Infiltrating lobular carcinoma
    (c) Cystosarcoma phyllodes
    (d) Mucinous carcinoma
    (e) Medullary carcinoma

17. Which one of the following neoplasms is most commonly associated with the acquired immune deficiency syndrome?
    (a) Sarcoma botryoides
    (b) Mycosis fungoides
    (c) Central nervous system lymphoma
    (d) Cystosarcoma phyllodes
    (e) Chronic lymphocytic leukemia

18. An autoantibody that is found in only about 30% of patients with systemic lupus erythematosus but that when present is almost pathognomonic of lupus is:
    (a) Antideoxyribonucleoprotein
    (b) Anti–single-stranded DNA
    (c) Anti-RNA
    (d) Anti-RNP
    (e) Anti–Sm antigen

19. An example of graft-versus-host disease is:
    (a) Rejection of grafted bone marrow
    (b) Hyperacute rejection of transplanted kidney
    (c) Retinitis following corneal transplant
    (d) T cells in transplanted marrow acting against the recipient
    (e) None of the above

20. Which of the following lesions is the most characteristic of an antibody-mediated transplant rejection?
    (a) Vasculitis
    (b) Interstitial mononuclear infiltrates
    (c) Interstitial granulomatous inflammation
    (d) Coagulation necrosis of proximal tubules
    (e) Vascular fibrosis

21. The fundamental difference between transudates and exudates is:
    (a) Color of edema fluid
    (b) Location of edema fluid
    (c) Cause of edema fluid
    (d) Specific gravity of edema fluid
    (e) Protein content of edema fluid

22. All of the following factors favor thrombus formation *except:*
    (a) Polycythemia
    (b) Chronic heart failure
    (c) Vitamin K deficiency
    (d) Sickle-cell disease
    (e) Atherosclerosis

23. The most common cause of meningitis in children and young adults is:
    (a) *Escherichia coli*
    (b) *Neisseria meningitidis*
    (c) *Streptococcus pneumoniae*
    (d) *Haemophilus influenzae*
    (e) *Staphylococcus aureus*

24. Primary infection with tuberculosis is most commonly characterized by:
    (a) Cavitary apical lesions
    (b) Multiple diffuse pulmonary calcifications
    (c) Peripheral lung lesions and regional lymph node involvement
    (d) Tuberculous pneumonia
    (e) Tuberculous meningitis

25. Diagnosis of a penile lesion as syphilis can best be established by:
    (a) Serologic test for syphilis
    (b) Culture of organisms
    (c) Characteristic appearance of chancre
    (d) Darkfield analysis
    (e) None of the above

26. Barr body positive cells may be found in all of the following conditions *except:*
    (a) Klinefelter's syndrome
    (b) "Super" females
    (c) Turner's syndrome
    (d) XXXXX mosaic
    (e) Females with Down's syndrome

27. A deficiency of surfactant is the fundamental defect in:
    (a) Hemolytic disease of the newborn
    (b) Primary atelectasis
    (c) Amniotic fluid aspiration
    (d) Hyaline membrane disease
    (e) Cystic fibrosis

28. The most frequent type of congenital heart disease is:
    (a) Ostium atrioventricularis communis
    (b) Tetralogy of Fallot
    (c) Coarctation of the aorta
    (d) Ventricular septal defect
    (e) Transposition of great vessels

29. The most frequent type of cyanotic congenital heart disease is:
    (a) Ostium atrioventricularis communis
    (b) Tetralogy of Fallot
    (c) Coarctation of the aorta
    (d) Ventricular septal defect
    (e) Transposition of great vessels

30. Patients who die during the first attack of rheumatic fever usually die as a result of:
    (a) Streptococcal septicemia
    (b) Myocardial failure due to myocarditis
    (c) Myocardial rupture

(d) Mitral stenosis with pulmonary edema
(e) Bacterial endocarditis

31. Thrombosis of the right coronary artery typically produces infarction of the:
    (a) Lateral left ventricle
    (b) Anterior left ventricle
    (c) Posterior interventricular septum
    (d) Apex of the left ventricle
    (e) Right atrium

32. In middle-aged men, aortic atherosclerosis is usually most extensive and severe in the:
    (a) Ascending thoracic aorta
    (b) Aortic arch
    (c) Upper portion of the descending thoracic aorta
    (d) Lower portion of the descending thoracic aorta
    (e) Abdominal aorta

33. All of the following predispose to bacterial endocarditis *except:*
    (a) Congenital heart disease
    (b) Intravenous drug addiction
    (c) Rheumatic heart disease
    (d) Coronary heart disease
    (e) Cardiac surgery

34. The most common cause of myocarditis in the population of the United States is:
    (a) Rheumatic fever
    (b) Diphtheria
    (c) Fungal infection
    (d) Viral infection
    (e) None of the above

35. A 5-year survival rate of approximately 90% is likely for patients with which of the following types of Hodgkin's disease?
    (a) Lymphocyte depletion
    (b) Nodular sclerosis
    (c) Mixed cellularity
    (d) Lymphocyte predominance
    (e) Hodgkin's disease, not otherwise classified

36. The tumor formerly known as chloroma is better designated as:
    (a) Malignant lymphoma
    (b) Monocytic leukemia
    (c) Granulocytic sarcoma
    (d) Multiple myeloma
    (e) Tumor of plant cell origin

37. The most common cause of iron deficiency in adults is:
    (a) Hemolysis
    (b) Inadequate dietary intake of meat
    (c) Inadequate intake of iron supplements
    (d) Chronic blood loss
    (e) None of the above

38. Cytochemical staining with specific and

nonspecific esterases, Sudan black B, peroxidase, and PAS is most useful in:
(a) Classifying anemia
(b) Classifying lymphomas
(c) Determining the prognosis of lymphomas
(d) Classifying types of leukemia
(e) Determining the prognosis of leukemia

39. The most common monoclonal immunoglobulin in patients with multiple myeloma is:
(a) IgM
(b) IgG
(c) IgA
(d) IgD
(e) IgE

40. Splenomegaly is characteristic of all of the following hematologic disorders *except:*
(a) Hereditary spherocytosis
(b) Idiopathic thrombocytopenic purpura
(c) Long-standing sickle-cell disease
(d) Chronic myelocytic leukemia
(e) Myelofibrosis

41. The most characteristic feature of pulmonary chronic passive congestion is the presence of:
(a) Neutrophils within alveoli
(b) Engorged alveolar capillaries
(c) Hyaline membranes
(d) Granular eosinophilic material within alveoli
(e) Hemosiderin-laden macrophages

42. The type of emphysema most closely related to cigarette smoking is:
(a) Focal
(b) Bullous
(c) Centriacinar
(d) Interstitial
(e) Panacinar

43. Which of the following is an unusual complication feature of lobar pneumonia rather than a typical classical feature or stage of the disease?
(a) Exudate containing edema fluid and numerous bacteria
(b) Organization of alveolar exudate
(c) Gray consolidation
(d) Red consolidation
(e) Resolution

44. The most characteristic microscopic feature of chronic bronchitis is:
(a) Epithelial basement membrane thickening
(b) Interstitial mononuclear inflammation
(c) Smooth muscle hypertrophy in bronchial walls
(d) Increased thickness of the submucosal mucous gland layer
(e) Decreased numbers of goblet cells in bronchial mucosa

45. Filling of the alveoli with foamy, eosinophilic material, together with interstitial mononuclear infiltration, is most characteristic of pneumonia due to:
(a) *Staphylococcus*
(b) *Mycoplasma*
(c) *Pneumococcus*
(d) Adenovirus
(e) *Pneumocystis*

46. Hyaline membranes lining alveolar walls are a characteristic feature of:
(a) Pulmonary proteinosis
(b) Goodpasture's syndrome
(c) Desquamative interstitial pneumonitis
(d) Adult respiratory distress syndrome
(e) Berylliosis

47. The most common neoplasm of major salivary glands is:
(a) Mucoepidermoid carcinoma
(b) Papillary cystadenoma
(c) Adenoid cystic carcinoma
(d) Adenolymphoma (Warthin's tumor)
(e) Pleomorphic adenoma

48. The most common malignant tumor of the esophagus is:
(a) Adenocarcinoma
(b) Lymphoma
(c) Leiomyosarcoma
(d) Mucoepidermoid carcinoma
(e) Squamous-cell carcinoma

49. All of the following are likely complications or sequelae of duodenal ulcers *except:*
(a) Hemorrhage
(b) Perforation
(c) Scarring with obstruction
(d) Complete healing
(e) Malignant degeneration

50. Most carcinomas of the colon occur in the:
(a) Transverse colon
(b) Rectosigmoid
(c) Cecum
(d) Ascending colon
(e) Hepatic flexure

51. All of the following pairings of hepatic necrosis and usual causes are related *except:*
(a) Central (centrilobular) necrosis/carbon tetrachloride
(b) Focal necrosis/mushroom poisoning
(c) Midzonal necrosis/yellow fever
(d) Massive and submassive necrosis/viral hepatitis
(e) Peripheral (periportal) necrosis/eclampsia

52. Typical microscopic features of viral hepatitis include all of the following *except:*
(a) Varying degrees of cholestasis

(b) Lymphocytic infiltration of lobules and portal tracts

(c) Focal necrosis of hepatocytes

(d) Fatty change

(e) Diffuse hepatocyte injury with lobular disarray

53. Mallory's hyaline is characteristic of:
    (a) Hemochromatosis
    (b) Aicoholic liver disease
    (c) Hepatitis B infection
    (d) Wilson's disease
    (e) Amyloidosis

54. A macronodular pattern is typically found in cirrhosis associated with:
    (a) Viral hepatitis
    (b) Prolonged biliary obstruction
    (c) Chronic alcohol abuse
    (d) Hemochromatosis
    (e) Chronic congestive heart failure

55. Hepatocellular adenomas are associated with:
    (a) Chronic exposure to vinyl chloride
    (b) Subclinical infection with non-A, non-B hepatitis
    (c) Prolonged oral contraceptive use
    (d) Ingestion of pyrollizidine alkaloids in "bush teas"
    (e) Chronic alcohol abuse

56. The most common malignant tumor involving the liver is:
    (a) Hepatoblastoma
    (b) Angiosarcoma
    (c) Hepatocellular carcinoma
    (d) Cholangiocarcinoma
    (e) Metastatic carcinoma

57. All of the following statements concerning cholelithiasis are true *except:*
    (a) Present in at least 75% of diseased gall-bladders
    (b) Obesity and pregnancy play a role in formation
    (c) Infection and stagnation of bile involved in pathogenesis
    (d) Pigment type of calculus is most common type
    (e) May be present without producing symptoms

58. An alcoholic patient presents to the emergency room with midabdominal pain, in shock, with a low serum calcium level and small mid-abdominal calcifications on x ray. The most likely diagnosis is:
    (a) Carcinoma of ampulla of Vater
    (b) Common bile duct stone
    (c) Chronic (relapsing) pancreatitis
    (d) Pancreatic pseudocyst
    (e) Pancreatic carcinoma

59. The most common primary malignant tumor of the thyroid is:
    (a) Follicular carcinoma
    (b) Medullary carcinoma with amyloid stroma
    (c) Papillary carcinoma
    (d) Large cell carcinoma
    (e) Anaplastic carcinoma

60. Dilation of the renal pelvis and calyces associated with progressive atrophy of the kidney due to obstruction of urine outflow best describes:
    (a) Chronic pyelonephritis
    (b) Acute pyelonephritis
    (c) Renal cystic disease
    (d) Hydronephrosis
    (e) Medullary papillary necrosis

61. Which of the following urinary abnormalities is the most specific for renal parenchymal disease?
    (a) Hematuria
    (b) Glucosuria
    (c) Biliribinuria
    (d) Proteinuria
    (e) Elevated specific gravity

62. The nephrotic syndrome is characterized by all of the following *except:*
    (a) Proteinuria of greater than 3.5 g/24 hours
    (b) Hypoalbuminemia
    (c) Edema
    (d) Hyperlipidemia
    (e) Azotemia

63. The most common cause of nephrotic syndrome in a 4-year-old patient is:
    (a) Minimal-change disease
    (b) Focal segmental glomerulosclerosis
    (c) Membranous glomerulonephritis
    (d) Congenital nephrotic syndrome
    (e) Membranoproliferative glomerulonephritis

64. Rapidly progressive glomerulonephritis is histologically characterized by the presence of numerous:
    (a) Intramembranous dense deposits
    (b) Atrophic proximal convoluted tubules
    (c) Hyalinized small arterioles
    (d) Epithelial cell crescents
    (e) Hyalinized, sclerotic glomeruli

65. The primary histologic lesion of benign nephrosclerosis is:
    (a) Narrowing of the lumina of arterioles by hyalinization of the walls
    (b) Focal glomerulosclerosis
    (c) Tubular atrophy
    (d) Interstitial fibrosis
    (e) Subendothelial dense deposits

66. Cerebral palsy is:
    (a) A congenital form of chronic motor neuron disease

(b) Usually the result of kernicterus

(c) Most commonly caused by congenital toxoplasmosis

(d) An early-life disability due to various causes

(e) Usually the result of physical damage to the head in forceps delivery

67. The incidence of cerebral palsy is approximately:
    (a) 2 per 100 live births
    (b) 2 per 1,000 live births
    (c) 2 per 10,000 live births
    (d) 2 per 100,000 live births
    (e) 2 per 1,000,000 live births

68. Most cases of hydrocephalus producing clinical symptoms in adults:
    (a) Are caused by overproduction of cerebrospinal fluid
    (b) Are due to obstruction of the outlets of the fourth ventricle
    (c) Cause separation of cranial sutures
    (d) Are the result of obstruction of flow of cerebrospinal fluid
    (e) Are due to postinflammatory stenosis of the cerebral aqueduct

69. The earliest pathologic change in bacterial meningitis is:
    (a) Vascular dilation
    (b) Emigration of neutrophilic granulocytes
    (c) Presence of bacteria in otherwise normal meninges
    (d) Swelling of brain tissue
    (e) Exudation of protein-rich fluid

70. Neurotuberculosis is:
    (a) Usually characterized by large tumors (tuberculomas) in brain tissue
    (b) Not associated with evidence of tuberculosis elsewhere in the body
    (c) Usually a smoldering chronic process
    (d) Characterized by fibrinous meningitis about the base of the brain
    (e) More common in adults than in children

71. Cryptococcal meningitis is:
    (a) Usually acute and rapidly fatal if untreated
    (b) Among the rarest forms of fungal meningitis
    (c) Usually characterized by intense inflammatory exudate
    (d) Rarely associated with cryptococcal infection elsewhere in the body
    (e) Usually opportunistic, occurring in patients with underlying disease

72. The intracranial vascular lesion most closely related to hypertension is:
    (a) Petechial hemorrhage in the cerebral cortex
    (b) Arteriolar sclerosis
    (c) Dissecting aneurysm

(d) Atherosclerosis

(e) Saccular arterial aneurysm

73. The most common aging change in brain tissue is:
    (a) Atrophy of neurons
    (b) Focal demyelination
    (c) Senile plaques
    (d) Multiple small infarcts
    (e) Neurofibrillary tangles in neurons

74. The most common primary malignant tumor of bone is:
    (a) Malignant giant cell tumor
    (b) Osteosarcoma
    (c) Chondrosarcoma
    (d) Osteochondroma
    (e) None of the above

Directions. For each numbered item, select the one heading most closely associated with it. Each lettered heading may be selected once, more than once, or not at all.

Questions 75–79

(a) Carcinoid of intestine

(b) Renal cell carcinoma

(c) Anaplastic carcinoma of the lung

(d) Thyroid medullary carcinoma

(e) Granulosa cell tumor of ovary

75. Erythropoietin
76. Estrogens
77. Calcitonin
78. ACTH
79. Serotonin

Questions 80–84

(a) Thrombus

(b) Clot

(c) Embolus

(d) Infarct

(e) Hyperemia

80. Can occur outside of the body
81. Dislodged mass in a blood vessel
82. Formed in flowing blood
83. Increased amount of blood in an organ or tissue
84. Localized focus of ischemic necrosis

Questions 85–89

(a) Syphilis

(b) Granuloma inguinale

(c) Chancroid.

(d) Lymphogranuloma venereum
(e) Gonorrhea

85. Acute arthritis
86. Rectal stricture formation
87. Obliterative endarteritis
88. Donovan bodies
89. Painful irregular ulcer with necrotic base

Questions 90–94

(a) Thiamine deficiency
(b) Riboflavin deficiency
(c) Deficiency of vitamin D in children
(d) Cobalamin deficiency
(e) Niacin deficiency

90. Endochondral abnormalities
91. Cheilosis
92. Megaloblastic anemia
93. Wernicke's encephalopathy
94. Dermatitis, glossitis

Questions 95–99

(a) Mercuric chloride
(b) Carbon tetrachloride
(c) Carbon monoxide
(d) Methyl alcohol
(e) Cyanide

95. No distinctive morphological findings
96. Necrosis of the efferent portion of the liver lobule
97. Degeneration of retina
98. Necrosis of proximal convoluted tubules of kidney
99. Necrosis of the globus pallidus

Questions 100–104

(a) Membranous glomerulonephritis
(b) Lipoid nephrosis (minimal-change disease)
(c) Membranoproliferative glomerulonephritis
(d) Goodpasture's syndrome
(e) Acute poststreptococcal glomerulonephritis

100. Subendothelial "humps" of immune complex deposits
101. Antibodies reacting uniformly to basement membrane
102. Double contour or "train track" glomerular basement membrane
103. Spike-and-dome appearance of glomerular basement membrane

104. Effacement of foot processes of glomerular epithelial cells

Questions 105–109

(a) Infiltrating ductal carcinoma
(b) Infiltrating lobular carcinoma
(c) Colloid carcinoma
(d) Medullary carcinoma
(e) Intraductal carcinoma

105. Small "indian file" epithelial cells
106. Solid cords of epithelial cells surrounded by dense collagen
107. Solid masses of epithelial cells with lymphoid stroma
108. Papillary or comedo pattern in center of ducts
109. Abundant mucous secretions

Questions 110–112

(a) *Clostridium tetani*
(b) *Clostridium botulinum*
(c) *Clostridium perfringens*
(d) *Clostridium difficile*
(e) *Clostridium subtilis*

110. Food poisoning
111. Pseudomembranous colitis
112. Gas gangrene

Questions 113–116

(a) XXY
(b) #5 chromosome deletion
(c) Trisomy 21
(d) Trisomy 18
(e) #22 to #9 translocation

113. Down's syndrome
114. Edwards' syndrome
115. Klinefelter's syndrome
116. Cat cry syndrome

Questions 117–119

(a) Seminoma
(b) Teratocarcinoma
(c) Choriocarcinoma
(d) Embryonal carcinoma
(e) Interstitial cell tumor

117. Most common testicular tumor
118. Frequently has lymphoid stroma
119. Androgen secretion common

Questions 120–121

(a) Hashimoto's disease
(b) Riedel's struma
(c) Graves' disease
(d) Nodular colloid goiter
(e) de Quervain's thyroiditis

120. Lymphoid follicles
121. Follicular atrophy with dense fibrosis

Questions 122–126

(a) Rheumatoid arthritis
(b) Osteoarthritis
(c) Gouty arthritis
(d) Pyogenic arthritis
(e) Osteoporosis

122. Erosion of articular cartilage
123. Nodules (Heberden's nodes) at base of terminal phalanges
124. Thinning of cortical and trabecular bone
125. Frequent with estrogen deficiency
126. Foreign body giant cell reaction

Directions. Each set of lettered headings below is followed by a list of numbered statements. For each statement answer:

A if the item is associated with *(a) only*
B if the item is associated with *(b) only*
C if the item is associated with *both (a) and (b)*
D if the item is associated with *neither (a) nor (b)*

Questions 127–128

(a) Cryptococcosis
(b) Blastomycosis
(c) Both
(d) Neither

127. Frequently seen in immunosuppressed patients
128. Causative organism not demonstrated with H&E stain

Questions 129–130

(a) Vitamin D deficiency
(b) Vitamin C deficiency
(c) Both
(d) Neither

129. Subperiosteal hematomas
130. Failure of mineralization

Questions 131–135

(a) Hepatitis A
(b) Hepatitis B
(c) Both
(d) Neither

131. Viral hepatitis
132. Incubation period of 2 to 6 weeks
133. Development of several types of chronic hepatitis
134. "Ground-glass" hepatocytes
135. Specific serologic tests not available

Questions 136–137

(a) Carcinoma of the prostate
(b) Nodular hyperplasia of the prostate
(c) Both
(d) Neither

136. Elevated serum acid phosphatase
137. Glandular elements in perineural spaces

Questions 138–144

(a) Subdural hematoma
(b) Epidural hematoma
(c) Both
(d) Neither

138. Usually arterial
139. Fracture of bone is directly involved in pathogenesis
140. Usually results from trauma
141. Tends to become encapsulated
142. Causes increased intracranial pressure
143. Directly related to systemic hypertension
144. Consists predominantly of venous blood

Directions. For each of the following answer:

(a) if only 1, 2, and 3 are correct
(b) if only 1 and 3 are correct
(c) if only 2 and 4 are correct
(d) if only 4 is correct
(e) if all are correct

145. Vasopermeability factors resulting from the cleavage of plasma substrates include:
   1. Bradykinin
   2. Histamine
   3. Anaphylatoxins
   4. Cationic protein
146. Highly radiosensitive cells include:
   1. Intestinal mucosal cells

2. Platelets
3. Lymphocytes
4. Skeletal muscle cells
147. Pigments derived from hemoglobin include:
    1. Bilirubin
    2. Hematin
    3. Hemosiderin
    4. Lipofuscin
148. Transplacental infections of the newborn may cause:
    1. Cytomegalic inclusion disease
    2. Generalized herpes simplex infection
    3. Listeriosis
    4. Toxoplasmosis
149. Serious conditions affecting the newborn infant include which of the following?
    1. Intrauterine pneumonia
    2. Hyaline membrane disease
    3. Intrauterine anoxia
    4. Caput succedaneum
150. Conditions consistently associated with eclampsia include:
    1. Peripheral zonal necrosis of the liver
    2. Disseminated intravascular coagulopathy
    3. Cortical necrosis of the kidneys
    4. Grapelike, cystic placental villi
151. Major causative factors involved in the production of cancer include:
    1. Bacteria
    2. Viruses
    3. Acute trauma
    4. Chemical substances
152. Direct-acting carcinogens include:
    1. Nitrosamines
    2. Polycyclic hydrocarbons
    3. Alkylating agents
    4. Tocopherol
153. Proven statements about tumor viruses include:
    1. Cause angiosarcoma of the liver
    2. Cause both benign and malignant tumors
    3. Strongly associated with endometrial carcinoma
    4. Include RNA and DNA viruses
154. Epidemiologic features associated with increased risk of developing breast cancer include:
    1. Nulliparous state
    2. First pregnancy occurring late in reproductive life
    3. High-fat diet
    4. Trauma
155. Tumors that are classified as malignant but that rarely metastasize include:
    1. Glioblastoma
    2. Renal-cell carcinoma
    3. Basal-cell carcinoma

4. Choriocarcinoma
156. Asbestosis leads to greatly increased risk of:
    1. Bronchial carcinoid
    2. Bronchogenic carcinoma
    3. Carcinoma of the stomach
    4. Mesothelioma
157. Cigarette smoking is associated with an increased risk of carcinoma of the:
    1. Larynx
    2. Esophagus
    3. Oral cavity
    4. Urinary bladder
158. Retinoblastoma is characterized by:
    1. Anaplasia
    2. Hereditary tendency
    3. Rosette formation
    4. Invasion of optic nerve
159. Malignant tumors with a predilection to metastasize to bone include carcinoma of the:
    1. Prostate
    2. Breast
    3. Lung
    4. Large intestine
160. Multiple myeloma is characterized by:
    1. Hypercalcemia
    2. Impairment of cellular immunity
    3. Renal involvement
    4. Polyclonal gammopathy
161. Examples of immunologic tissue injury include:
    1. Anaphylactic hypersensitivity
    2. Cytotoxic hypersensitivity
    3. Immune complex hypersensitivity
    4. Cell-mediated hypersensitivity
162. Correct statements about anaphylactic hypersensitivity include:
    1. Reaction may be local or systemic
    2. Fatal shock may occur
    3. It is mediated by IgE antibodies
    4. Local reaction may be manifested as hives
163. Mediators of anaphylaxis performed and stored in mast cell granules include:
    1. Slow-reacting substance of anaphylaxis (SRS-A)
    2. ECF-A (eosinophilic chemotactic factor of anaphylaxis)
    3. Platelet-activating factor (PAF)
    4. Histamine
164. Immune complex diseases include:
    1. Bronchial asthma
    2. Erythroblastosis
    3. Transfusion reaction
    4. Acute serum sickness
165. Autoimmune diseases include:
    1. Systemic lupus erythematosus
    2. Scleroderma

3. Dermatomyositis
4. DiGeorge's syndrome
166. Immunologic deficiency diseases in which B lymphocytes are deficient include:
 1. Bruton's disease
 2. DiGeorge's syndrome
 3. Combined Swiss-type immunodeficiency
 4. Sjögren's syndrome
167. Opportunistic infections frequently occurring in patients with acquired immunodeficiency syndrome include:
 1. *Pneumocystis carinii* infection
 2. Cryptosporidiosis
 3. Cytomegalovirus infection
 4. Streptococcal cellulitis
168. Edema is frequently associated with which of the following?
 1. Cardiac failure
 2. Sodium retention
 3. Lymphatic obstruction
 4. Hypoproteinemia
169. The most common pus-producing microorganisms are:
 1. Staphylococci
 2. Pneumococci
 3. Gonococci
 4. *Salmonella typhi*
170. Staphylococcal organisms cause:
 1. Food poisoning
 2. Erysipelas
 3. Toxic shock syndrome
 4. Scarlet fever
171. In general, rickettsial infections are characterized by:
 1. Obligate intracellular parasitism
 2. Prominence of cutaneous manifestations
 3. Transmission by arthropod vectors
 4. Formation of multiple abscesses
172. Diseases that frequently complicate intravenous drug abuse include:
 1. Viral hepatitis
 2. Thrombophlebitis
 3. Bacterial endocarditis
 4. Tetanus
173. Causes of cyanotic congenital heart disease include:
 1. Truncus arteriosus
 2. Taussig-Bing anomaly
 3. Transposition of great vessels
 4. Tricuspid atresia
174. Congenital heart diseases with increased blood flow to the lungs include:
 1. Tetralogy of Fallot
 2. Ventricular septal defect
 3. Tricuspid atresia

 4. Patent ductus arteriosus
175. Characteristic features of cardiovascular syphilis include:
 1. Narrowing of the aortic ring
 2. Dissecting aneurysm
 3. Mitral stenosis
 4. Saccular aneurysm of the thoracic aorta
176. Features of endocardial fibroelastosis include:
 1. Large globular heart
 2. Occurrence primarily in first 2 years of life
 3. Heart failure without valvular disease
 4. Thiamine deficiency as cause
177. Causes of fibrinous pericarditis include:
 1. Rheumatic fever
 2. Cardiac failure
 3. Uremia
 4. Syphilitic heart disease
178. Causes of hemolytic anemias due to intracorpuscular defects include:
 1. Glucose-6-phosphate dehydrogenase deficiency
 2. Thalassemia
 3. Pyruvate kinase deficiency
 4. Hereditary spherocytosis
179. Findings distinctive of bronchial asthma that would be found at autopsy include:
 1. Atrophy of submucosal glands
 2. Mucous plugs in bronchi
 3. Extensively collapsed lungs
 4. Thickening of basement membranes of bronchial epithelium
180. Pulmonary hypertension may occur as a result of:
 1. Mitral stenosis
 2. Chronic obstructive lung disease
 3. Multiple pulmonary emboli
 4. Right-to-left shunt in congenital heart disease
181. Pulmonary embolism may result in:
 1. Left-sided cardiac failure
 2. Pulmonary infarction
 3. Obstructive atelectasis
 4. Sudden death
182. The adult respiratory distress syndrome may occur as a complication of:
 1. Cardiac surgery
 2. Severe burns
 3. Narcotic overdose
 4. Oxygen toxicity
183. Bronchiectasis may result from:
 1. Foreign body aspiration
 2. Bronchial asthma
 3. Bronchial carcinoid
 4. Cystic fibrosis
184. Bronchopneumonia:
 1. Is a common complication of chronic debilitating diseases
 2. Is characteristically patchy in distribution

3. May be produced by virtually any pathogenic organism
4. Rarely results in abscess formation

185. Benign peptic ulcers are most commonly:
   1. Solitary
   2. Less than 3 cm in diameter
   3. Sharply punched out
   4. Located in the duodenum

186. Histologic features characteristically present in ulcerative colitis include:
   1. Crypt abscesses
   2. Fissures
   3. Inflammatory pseudopolyps
   4. Transmural inflammation

187. Histologic features characteristically present in Crohn's disease include:
   1. Noncaseating granulomas
   2. Fissures and fistulas
   3. Transmural inflammation
   4. Skip areas of uninvolved bowel

188. Hepatic fatty change is frequently associated with:
   1. Malnutrition
   2. Corticosteroid therapy
   3. Obesity
   4. Wilson's disease

189. The liver from a patient with chronic congestive heart failure characteristically shows:
   1. Marked fatty change with Mallory bodies
   2. Lymphocytic infiltration of the triads
   3. Bile duct proliferation
   4. Centrilobular congestion

190. Which of the following conditions would predispose a person to the development of urinary tract infection?
   1. Nephrolithiasis (kidney stones)
   2. Pregnancy
   3. Benign prostatic hyperplasia
   4. Neurogenic bladder

191. Which of the following conditions predispose to the development of *acute glomerulonephritis?*
   1. Streptococcal pharyngitis
   2. Tuberculosis
   3. Impetigo
   4. Rubella

192. Germ cell tumors of the testis:
   1. Are usually highly malignant
   2. Account for a large percentage of testicular tumors
   3. Occur most frequently in persons between the ages of 25 and 35
   4. Sometimes produce hormonal products

193. Hyperparathyroidism is characterized by:
   1. Osteitis fibrosa cystica
   2. Central buffalo-type obesity
   3. Formation of urinary calculi

4. Virilism in women

194. Common renal lesions in diabetes mellitus include:
   1. Nodular glomerulosclerosis
   2. Acute pyelonephritis
   3. Diffuse glomerulosclerosis
   4. Papillary necrosis

195. The pathologic process in syringomyelia is characterized by:
   1. Argyrophilic cytoplasmic inclusions in anterior horn neurons
   2. Selective atrophy of motor neurons in the spinal cord extending into brain stem
   3. Demyelination of dorsal and lateral columns of the spinal cord
   4. Cystic cavitation of the spinal cord damaging crossing sensory fibers

196. Metastatic carcinoma is the most common form of malignant brain tumor in:
   1. Children younger than 10 years of age
   2. Adults without a known primary tumor
   3. Children between 10 and 20 years old
   4. Adults with a known primary tumor

197. Glioblastoma multiforme may occur in the:
   1. Cerebrum of adult
   2. Brain stem of child
   3. Spinal cord of adult
   4. Adrenal medulla of child

198. Characteristic pathologic changes in Alzheimer's disease include:
   1. Senile plaques
   2. Loss of neurons in cerebral cortex
   3. Neurofibrillary tangles
   4. Shrinkage of caudate nuclei

199. Pathologic changes of Huntington's disease include:
   1. Argyrophilic cytoplasmic inclusions in neurons of temporal cortex
   2. Shrinkage of caudate nuclei due to nerve cell loss and gliosis
   3. Sclerosis of cerebral cortex in lobar patterns
   4. Atrophy of cerebral cortex diffusely in frontal lobes

200. In idiopathic parkinsonism, pathologic changes are characteristic in the:
   1. Temporal cortex of Ammon's horns
   2. Substantia nigra
   3. Caudate nuclei
   4. Locus ceruleus

201. Untreated glaucoma is characterized by:
   1. Opacification of the lens
   2. Progressive atrophy of the retina
   3. Impeded outflow of vitreous humor
   4. Increased intraocular pressure

1. **c** Pyknosis (a), karyorrhexis (b), karolysis (d), and rupture of the membrane (e) are late changes following the early change of clumping of chromatin in the nuclear membrane, best appreciated by electron microscopy of experimentally induced necrosis.

2. **d** Increased microvascular permeability is most pronounced in the postcapillary venules and venular portions of the capillary loop.

3. **d** Chemotaxis determines the directional motion of leukocytes.

4. **a** All of the mediators except histamine have a chemotactic effect on neutrophils and monocytes. Histamine is a vasopermeability mediator.

5. **c** The erythrocyte is an end-stage cell that is not capable of further division and regeneration. Hepatocytes, osteocytes, and acinar cells are stable cells capable of some regeneration under certain conditions. Colonic mucosal cells are labile cells that regenerate readily.

6. **a** Cationic protein, a product of neutrophils, results in increased vascular permeability, while the other choices do not.

7. **d** Lead poisoning in children produces basophilic stippling of erythrocytes. The other toxins are not especially common in children, nor do they produce stippling in erythrocytes.

8. **b**

9. **c** Large amounts of newly formed capillaries and fibroblasts (granulation tissue) are always present in healing by second intention.

10. **c** Infarcts of the brain undergo liquefactive necrosis with cyst formation rather than scarring.

11. **d**

12. **d**

13. **c** Although all of the choices listed are features of malignant tumors, metastases are the most positive proof of malignancy.

14. **b**

15. **c** Carcinoma of the cervix characteristically causes ureteral obstruction by direct extension of the primary tumor.

16. **c** Cystosarcoma phyllodes is an unusual type of breast neoplasm; the other types listed occur frequently.

17. **c** In addition to Kaposi's sarcoma, lymphoma of the central nervous system is one of the most frequent neoplasms occurring in patients with AIDS. Other neoplasms found with increased frequency in AIDS patients are Burkitt's lymphoma, immunoblastic lymphoma, and lymphoblastic lymphoma. Sarcoma botryoides is a tumor of the uterus and upper vagina in young girls. Cystosarcoma phyllodes is a breast tumor in women. Mycosis fungoides and chronic lymphocytic leukemia are not reported as being strongly associated with AIDS.

18. **e** The correct answer is anti–Sm antigen. Antibodies to anti–double-stranded DNA are almost specific for lupus. The other antibodies are not specific for lupus. Anti-RNP in high titer is distinctive for mixed connective tissue disease.

19. **a** Transplanted marrow causing disease in the recipient host is the typical GVH disease.

20. **a**

21. **c** The fundamental difference is that transudates are noninflammatory edema fluids and exudates are inflammatory edema fluids. This difference accounts for differences in the qualities of the fluids.

22. **c**

23. **b** *Neisseria meningitidis* most commonly causes meningitis in children and young adults. *E. coli* causes meningitis in newborns and sometimes in elderly debilitated adults. *H. influenzae* is the most common cause of meningitis in infants.

24. **c** The usual fate of primary or first-infection tuberculosis is the primary complex, a peripheral lung lesion, and involved draining tracheobronchial nodes, with both lesions healing and becoming calcified.

25. **d** Treponemata are abundant in material from a chancre and can best be seen by darkfield examination. Serologic tests are usually not positive at time of initial infection.

26. **c** All of these except Turner's syndrome have two or more X chromosomes and thus have Barr body–positive cells. Subjects with Turner's syndrome, although female, do not have a Barr body because they have only one X chromosome (XO).

27. **d**

28. **d** Ventricular septal defect is the most common of all congenital heart lesions. Tetralogy of Fallot is the most common cause of cyanotic congenital heart disease.

29. **b** Ventricular septal defect is the most common of all congenital heart lesions. Tetralogy of Fallot is the most common cause of cyanotic congenital heart disease.

30. **b** Patients who die during a first attack do so as a

result of myocarditis rather than of valvular disease or other conditions listed.

31. **c** Occlusion of the right coronary artery typically leads to infarction of the posterior interventricular septum and posterior portion of the left ventricle.

32. **e** In adults the abdominal aorta is usually most severely involved by atherosclerosis.

33. **d**

34. **d** Rheumatic fever and diphtheria have largely been prevented in the United States. Fungal heart infections are rare. Several viral infections, including coxsackie and echoviruses, cause myocarditis.

35. **d** The lymphocyte predominance type of Hodgkin's disease has the best prognosis. Lymphocyte depletion has the worst prognosis.

36. **c** *Granulocytic sarcoma* is now the accepted term for chloroma.

37. **d** Dietary requirements for iron are easily met in adults. The most common and significant cause of iron deficiency anemia in adults is chronic loss of blood due to a number of causes.

38. **d** These cytochemical stains are used to distinguish among myeloblastic, myelomonocytic, monocytic, and lymphoblastic leukemias.

39. **b**

40. **c** In long-standing sickle-cell disease the spleen is small and fibrotic. The other conditions typically are associated with moderate to extreme splenomegaly.

41. **e**

42. **c** Centriacinar emphysema has clearly been shown to be associated with smoking. Panacinar emphysema is the type associated with alpha-1-antitrypsin deficiency.

43. **b** Organization is a rare complication of lobar pneumonia; the other choices listed are the classical stages.

44. **d** Choices a and c are characteristic features of bronchial asthma, not chronic bronchitis. In chronic bronchitis, an increase in the number of goblet cells in the bronchial mucosa is a constant finding.

45. **e** This histologic pattern is very characteristic of *Pneumocystis carinii*.

46. **d** Pulmonary edema, alveolar lining cell hyperplasia, and hyaline membrane formation are the result of the alveolar wall injury, which occurs in the adult respiratory distress syndrome.

47. **e**

48. **e**

49. **e**

50. **b** Approximately 68% of carcinomas of the colon and rectum are located in the rectum or sigmoid and can be detected by rectal examination or sigmoidoscopy.

51. **b** Focal hepatic necrosis is seen in various infectious processes, such as typhoid fever, but is not typically seen with mushroom poisoning. Choices a, c, and e are classic associations of patterns of necrosis and usual causes. Although viral hepatitis is the most common cause of massive and submassive necrosis, when it occurs, the usual result of viral hepatitis is panlobular injury, in which all zones of the lobule are affected but not all cells are necrotic.

52. **d** Fatty change is typically absent in the usual case of viral hepatitis.

53. **b** Mallory's hyaline (Mallory bodies) is commonly found in degenerating hepatocytes in chronic alcoholic liver disease. It consists of irregular cytoplasmic clumps of hyaline material. Excessive iron deposition is present in the liver in hemochromatosis. Patients with hepatitis B sometimes have "ground-glass" hepatocytes. In Wilson's disease, excessive copper is present in the liver. In amyloidosis, the hyaline amyloid material is deposited between the hepatocytes and sinusoidal lining cells.

54. **a** Cirrhosis associated with viral hepatitis is typically macronodular. Prolonged biliary obstruction (biliary cirrhosis), chronic alcohol abuse, hemochromatosis (pigment cirrhosis), and chronic-congestive heart failure (cardiac cirrhosis) are typically associated with micronodular cirrhosis.

55. **c** Hepatocellular adenomas are benign neoplasms that have a tendency to rupture, especially during pregnancy, and cause intraperitoneal hemorrhage. These rare tumors are related to prolonged use of oral contraceptives. This tumor has not been reported to be caused by any of the other conditions listed.

56. **e** Secondary, or metastatic, carcinoma is far more frequent than any of the types of primary malignancy of the liver.

57. **d** Mixed calculi, not pigment calculi, are the most common type of gallstone.

58. **c** The features described are typical of chronic (relapsing) pancreatitis.

59. **c** Papillary carcinoma is by far the most common malignant tumor of the thyroid.

60. **d** Obstruction of urinary tract flow predisposes to acute and chronic pyelonephritis; however, the description given does not fit these conditions precisely.

61. **d** Proteinuria almost always results from changes in the kidney. Hematuria can result from changes anywhere in the urinary tract. Glucosuria indicates that the renal threshold for glucose has been exceeded. Bilirubin in the urine indicates biliary tract obstruction. Elevated specific gravity may occur from dehydration.

62. **e** The nephrotic syndrome is basically defined by choices a through d. Azotemia is not a necessary component of the nephrotic syndrome.

63. **a** Minimal-change disease or lipoid nephrosis is the major cause of nephrotic syndrome in children. The congenital nephrotic syndrome is rare. Membranous glomerulonephritis is the most common cause of the nephrotic syndrome in adults.

64. **d** Epithelial crescents are the hallmark of this form of nephritic syndrome, which leads to rapid deterioration of renal function and renal failure.

65. **a** Thickening and hyalinization of the arteriolar walls is the basic lesion of benign nephrosclerosis. All other changes of nephrosclerosis are secondary to the arteriolar changes.

66. **d** Cerebral palsy is a broad term that includes many forms of brain damage occurring in early life.

67. **b** The frequency of cerebral palsy indicates that the conditions that make up the disorder are not extremely rare but occur in less than 1% of live births.

68. **d** Hydrocephalus is usually the result of obstruction of flow of cerebrospinal fluid. In adults hydrocephalus does not cause separation of the cranial sutures because they are fused; in infants with hydrocephalus there is separation of the cranial sutures.

69. **c** Bacteria are present in the earliest stage of bacterial meningitis because they are responsible for the inflammatory changes that follow.

70. **d** This is the characteristic pathologic appearance of tuberculous meningitis. Tuberculomas in the parenchyma of the brain are rare. Patients with tuberculous meningitis usually have foci of tuberculosis elsewhere in the body. Tuberculous meningitis occurs more frequently in children than in adults.

71. **e** Cryptococcal meningitis is a fungal disease that usually occurs in immunosuppressed persons and persons with other diseases and thus is considered an opportunistic infection. It is one of the most frequent opportunistic infections in patients with AIDS.

72. **b** The characteristic vascular lesion of hypertension in the brain is arteriolar sclerosis. Severe arteriolar sclerosis with necrosis and microaneurysm formation in arterioles is the basis of hypertensive intracerebral hemorrhage. Hypertension also accelerates the development of atherosclerosis in arteries of the circle of Willis, but the basic hypertensive change is arteriolar sclerosis.

73. **a** Microscopically, the earliest and most characteristic change of aging is atrophy of nerve cells with accumulation of lipochrome pigment. Other changes may also occur, but neuronal changes are most common.

74. **b** Osteosarcoma is the most common primary malignant tumor of bone. Metastatic tumors of the bone are more common but are not primary. Malignant giant cell tumor and chondrosarcoma occur less frequently than osteosarcoma. Osteochondromas are benign.

75. **b**
76. **e**
77. **d**
78. **c**
79. **a**
80. **b**
81. **c**
82. **a**
83. **e**
84. **d**
85. **e**
86. **d**
87. **a**
88. **b**
89. **c**
90. **c**
91. **b**
92. **d**
93. **a**
94. **e**
95. **e**
96. **b**
97. **d**
98. **a**
99. **c**
100. **e**
101. **d**
102. **c**
103. **a**
104. **b**
105. **b**
106. **a**
107. **d**
108. **e**
109. **c**
110. **b** *C. botulinum* growing in improperly processed foods produces toxins that cause botulism.
111. **d** The toxin from *C. difficile* is the cause of antibiotic-associated pseudomembranous colitis.
112. **c** *C. perfringens* is the organism most commonly causing gas gangrene.
113. **c**
114. **d**
115. **a**
116. **b**
117. **a** Seminoma is by far the most common of these testicular tumors.

118. **a** Histologic features of seminoma include light-staining cytoplasm of tumor cells and lymphoid cells interspersed among the tumor cells.
119. **e** Interstitial (Leydig) cell tumors frequently produce androgens and may lead to masculinization when they occur in children.
120. **a** While foci of lymphocytes are common in Graves' disease, lymphoid follicles are characteristic of Hashimoto's disease.
121. **b** Riedel's struma is a rare form of thyroiditis characterized by a small, hard thyroid with dense fibrosis.
122. **b** Erosion of articular cartilage with overgrowth of underlying bone is characteristic of osteoarthritis.
123. **b** Heberden's nodes occur because of bone spur formation in osteoarthritis.
124. **e** Osteoporosis is characterized by generalized or localized thinning of cortical and trabecular bone with loss of bone mass.
125. **e** Osteoporosis occurs in postmenopausal women and other women with estrogen deficiency as well as in Cushing's syndrome and hyperparathyroidism.
126. **c** Deposits of urate crystals elicit foreign body giant cell reaction.
127. **A** Cryptococcosis is a common infection in immunosuppressed patients and is a frequent complication of AIDS. Blastomycosis is endemic and may occur in patients with normal immune systems.
128. **D** Both cryptococcal organisms and blastomyces are visible on H&E staining.
129. **B** Vitamin C deficiency causes scurvy, in which subperiosteal hemorrhage is common.
130. **C** The basic bone abnormality in vitamin D deficiency is decreased mineralization of bone.
131. **C** Hepatitis A and B are two of the three currently recognized types of viral hepatitis.
132. **A** Hepatitis A has an incubation period of 2 to 6 weeks; hepatitis B, 6 weeks to 6 months.
133. **B** Some patients with hepatitis B develop chronic hepatitis of variable severity; chronic hepatitis following hepatitis A is not recognized.
134. **B** Patients who develop cirrhosis or chronic hepatitis as a result of hepatitis B have "ground-glass" hepatocytes, which are morphological indicators of hepatitis B infection.
135. **D** Specific serologic tests are available for hepatitis A and B, but not for non-A non-B hepatitis.
136. **A** Elevated acid phosphatase levels in blood are increased with metastatic carcinoma of the prostate.
137. **A** Perineural involvement is a predominant feature of prostate carcinoma.
138. **B** Epidural hematoma is a result of arterial bleeding; subdural hematoma is from venous bleeding.
139. **B** Epidural hematoma is usually associated with fracture of the temporal bone overlying a branch of the middle meningeal artery; subdural hematoma is not necessarily associated with skull fracture.
140. **C** Both conditions are usually traumatic in origin.
141. **A** Subdural hematoma may develop rapidly, or the hematoma may develop slowly and become encapsulated; epidural hematoma develops rapidly.
142. **C** Both conditions lead to increased intracranial pressure.
143. **D** Neither is directly the result of hypertension. Intracerebral hemorrhage is the lesion that may result in hypertension.
144. **A** Subdural hematoma consists of venous blood from tears of venous sinuses; epidural hematoma consists of arterial blood from tears of branches of the middle meningeal artery.
145. **b** Bradykinin is formed in the kinin generation system by enzymatic cleavage of plasma substrate. Anaphylatoxins are cleavage fragments of C3 and C5 in the plasma. Histamine is preformed in basophil granules, and cationic protein is preformed in lysosomal granules of neutrophils.
146. **b** As labile cells, intestinal mucosal cells and lymphocytes are sensitive to radiation. As permanent cells, platelets and skeletal muscle cells are not highly sensitive to radiation.
147. **a** Bilirubin, hematin, and hemosiderin are breakdown products of hemoglobin. Lipofuscin is nonhemoglobin "wear-and-tear" pigment prominent in atrophic cardiac muscle cells.
148. **e** All conditions listed are important transplacental infections of the newborn.
149. **a** Caput succedaneum is a transient, non–life-threatening soft tissue injury of the infant's head.
150. **a** Grapelike placental villi are characteristic of hydatidiform mole.
151. **c** Oncogenic viruses and chemical carcinogens are two of the major types of carcinogenic agents. Bacterial infection and acute trauma have not been shown to cause cancer.
152. **b** Nitrosamines and alkylating agents are direct-acting carcinogens. Polycyclic hydrocarbons are procarcinogens. Alpha tocopherol (vitamin E) is not a recognized carcinogen.
153. **c** Vinyl chloride is a cause of angiosarcoma of the liver. Endometrial carcinoma is not reported to be caused by a tumor virus.
154. **a** Trauma is not accepted as a risk factor for breast cancer.
155. **b** Glioblastoma, a highly malignant tumor by growth characteristics and location, and basal cell carcinoma, a locally invasive and ulcerative neoplasm, rarely if ever metastasize. Renal cell carcinoma and choriocarcinoma typically metastasize.

156. c Asbestosis increases risk of both mesothelioma and bronchogenic carcinoma and also causes other pulmonary complications. Neither bronchial carcinoid nor stomach cancer is related to asbestosis.

157. e These are four of the many malignant tumors associated with tobacco usage.

158. e This malignant tumor of the eye in childhood has all of the features listed.

159. a Tumors of prostate, breast, and lung preferentially metastasize to bone compared with most other tumors. Carcinoma of the large intestine typically metastasizes to lymph nodes and liver.

160. b Hypercalcemia and renal involvement are typical features of myeloma. Cellular immunity is not impaired, since myeloma is related to B cells rather than T cells. The gammopathy in myeloma is monoclonal rather than polyclonal.

161. e The four choices listed are the four major types of immunologic injury.

162. e All are correct.

163. c Histamine and ECF-A are preformed and stored in mast cell granules, while PAF and SRS-A are generated during the anaphylaxis process. The term *SRS-A* is now better defined and includes leukotrienes C_4, D_4, and E_4.

164. d Acute serum sickness is the only condition listed resulting from immune complex disease. Bronchial asthma is an example of localized anaphylactic hypersensitivity reaction, and erythroblastosis and transfusion reactions are examples of cytotoxic reactions.

165. a The first three diseases listed are common examples of autoimmune diseases, which occur when there is loss of tolerance of self-antigens and the body reacts to these self-antigens. DiGeorge's syndrome is thymic dysplasia, a genetically determined immunodeficiency disease.

166. b B lymphocytes are deficient in Bruton's disease and combined immunodeficiency resulting in decreased or absent immunoglobulins. T cells also are deficient in combined immunodeficiency. The defect in DiGeorge's syndrome is in T cells. Sjögren's syndrome is an autoimmune disease, not an immunologic deficiency disease.

167. a The first three conditions listed are infections typical of AIDS.

168. e All the conditions listed are causes of edema.

169. a Staphylococci, pneumococci, and gonococci are examples of organisms causing pyogenic (pus-forming) infections. *Salmonella typhi* typically produces a response characterized by large numbers of monocytes and does not cause a pyogenic infection.

170. b Toxins from staphylococcal organisms are known to cause food poisoning and have been shown to be related to the development of toxic shock syndrome in women who use tampons. Erysipelas and scarlet fever are the result of streptococcal infection.

171. a The first three items listed are classical features of rickettsial infections. Abscesses are not typical lesions in any rickettsial diseases.

172. e All diseases listed occur with intravenous drug abuse as a result of contaminated needles.

173. e All of these cause cyanosis because of right-to-left shunts.

174. c Ventricular septal defect and patent ductus arteriosus lead to left-to-right shunts with increased blood flow to the lungs. The other conditions are characterized by decreased blood flow to the lungs.

175. d The aortic ring is dilated in syphilis. Dissecting aneurysm and mitral stenosis are not caused by syphilis. Thoracic saccular aneurysm is a classic lesion of cardiovascular syphilis.

176. a Thiamine deficiency is not a cause of endocardial fibroelastosis but causes beriberi heart disease.

177. b Rheumatic fever and uremia are classical causes of fibrinous pericarditis. Cardiac failure causes pericardial effusion, a transudate. Syphilis does not cause pericarditis.

178. e All the conditions listed are associated with intracorpuscular defects. Choices 1 and 3 are inherited enzyme deficiencies that cause erythrocytes to be more vulnerable to injury than normal. Thalassemia is a hemoglobinopathy with defective synthesis of a polypeptide chain. Hereditary spherocytosis is characterized by an inherited defect that causes erythrocytes to be spheroidal and fragile.

179. c Choices 2 and 4 are typical findings. Submucosal glands are enlarged; lungs are hyperinflated.

180. a The first three choices listed are common causes of pulmonary hypertension. Left-to-right shunts, not right-to-left shunts, cause pulmonary hypertension in congenital heart disease.

181. c Pulmonary embolism may lead to sudden death or pulmonary infarction. It may also have chronic effects, such as pulmonary hypertension or cor pulmonale. It may cause right-sided heart failure but not left-sided failure. It does not typically cause atelectasis, which is usually a result of bronchial obstruction.

182. e All of the conditions listed may lead to adult respiratory distress syndrome.

183. e All of the conditions listed can lead to chronic necrotizing inflammation with dilation of bronchi.

184. a Bronchopneumonia not infrequently results in abscess formation.

185. e All the listed statements about peptic ulcers are true.

186. b Crypt abscesses and inflammatory pseudopolyps

are salient features of ulcerative colitis; fissures and transmural inflammation are features of Crohn's disease.

187. **e** All of the features listed are characteristic of Crohn's disease.

188. **a** Malnutrition, corticosteroid therapy, and obesity cause fatty metamorphosis, or fatty change, of the liver. Fatty change is not typically seen in Wilson's disease, which is characterized by a marked increase in copper within hepatocytes.

189. **d** Centrilobular congestion is the characteristic liver change in congestive heart failure. Choice 1 is associated with alcoholic liver disease, choice 2 with viral hepatitis, and choice 3 with biliary cirrhosis.

190. **e** All of the conditions listed predispose to urinary tract infections because of some degree of obstruction of urinary flow.

191. **b** *Acute glomerulonephritis* almost always refers to acute poststreptococcal glomerulonephritis. The form of glomerulonephritis occurs following untreated or inadequately treated streptococcal infections, usually pharyngitis or impetigo.

192. **e** All of the listed features are true of germ cell tumors of the testis.

193. **b** Hyperparathyroidism leads to mobilization of calcium from the bones, hypercalcemia, metastatic calcification, excessive excretion of calcium in the urine, and formation of urinary calculi. Central obesity and virilism are characteristic of Cushing's syndrome, which is the result of the increased secretion of cortisol from a variety of causes.

194. **e** All of the renal lesions listed occur in patients with diabetes mellitus.

195. **d** A syrinx is a cylindrical cavity of usually unknown cause that characteristically causes dissociated sensory change by disproportionately distorting and damaging crossing fibers.

196. **c** In adults the most common form of malignant brain tumor is metastatic carcinoma, regardless of whether a primary tumor has been discovered. This is a basic principle of brain tumor pathology.

197. **a** Glioblastoma multiforme may occur at any age in any part of the central nervous system.

198. **a** In Alzheimer's disease neuronal changes are characteristically concentrated in cerebral cortex and consist of neurofibrillary tangles, nerve-cell deterioration and loss, and senile plaques. Shrunken caudate nuclei are characteristic of Huntington's disease, not Alzheimer's disease. This is important, because shrunken caudate nuclei and atrophic cerebral cortex can be demonstrated by computed scanning and magnetic resonance imaging in living patients.

199. **c** In Huntington's disease there is characteristic neuronal deterioration and loss throughout frontal cortex and exudate nuclei. Argyrophilia inclusions and lobar sclerosis are characteristic of Pick's disease (presenile dementia of lobar type).

200. **c** In idiopathic parkinsonism, the most constant changes are nerve-cell deterioration, depigmentation, and Lewy body formation in the substantia nigra and locus ceruleus, pigmented nuclei of the brain stem.

201. **c** Glaucoma is due to impeded outflow of aqueous humor (not vitreous humor), which leads to increased ocular pressure, which if untreated causes compression of blood vessels supplying the retina, atrophy of the retina, and eventual blindness. Opacification of the lens results in cataract formation.

Rypins' Questions & Answers for Basic Sciences Review, Second Edition, edited by Edward D. Frohlich. J. B. Lippincott Company, Philadelphia © 1993.

C H A P T E R

Pharmacology

Margaret A. Reilly, *Ph.D.*

Research Scientist, Nathan S. Kline Institute for Psychiatric Research

Adjunct Associate Professor, College of New Rochelle School of Nursing

Adjunct Assistant Professor, Department of Pharmacology, New York Medical College

QUESTIONS

Directions. Choose the best answer.

1. Which of the following is *not* an effect of acetylcholine?
   - (a) Constricted bronchi
   - (b) Increased heart rate
   - (c) Increased peristalsis
   - (d) Miosis

2. Use of acetylcholine in therapeutics is:
   - (a) Restricted to reversal of atropine poisoning
   - (b) Primarily related to its effects on the respiratory system
   - (c) Valuable for the management of gastric atony and urinary retention
   - (d) Minimal because of its chemical instability and lack of selectivity

3. Which is an action of atropine?
   - (a) Increased salivation
   - (b) Decreased sinoatrial depolarization
   - (c) Miosis
   - (d) Cycloplegia

4. Atropine blocks the effects of acetylcholine by:
   - (a) Blocking its release from storage sites
   - (b) Competing at receptor sites
   - (c) Enhancing the effects of acetylcholinesterase
   - (d) Inhibiting its synthesis

5. Which one of the following agents enhances cholinergic activity by forming an irreversible bond with acetylcholinesterase?
   - (a) Pralidoxime
   - (b) Neostigmine
   - (c) Diisopropylfluorophosphate
   - (d) Pilocarpine

6. The agent most useful for protection against the muscarinic manifestations of anticholinesterase poisoning is:
   - (a) Diisopropylfluorophosphate
   - (b) Muscarine
   - (c) Pralidoxime
   - (d) Atropine

7. The agent most useful for treating the nicotinic manifestations of anticholinesterase poisoning is:
   - (a) Atropine
   - (b) Diisopropylfluorophosphate
   - (c) Pralidoxime
   - (d) Muscarine

8. Which of the following agents acts by promoting reactivation of phosphorylated acetylcholinesterase?
   - (a) Atropine
   - (b) Pralidoxime
   - (c) Neostigmine
   - (d) Pilocarpine

9. Phenylephrine is similar to epinephrine in its:
   - (a) Inotropic effects
   - (b) Vasodilation
   - (c) Chronotropic effects
   - (d) Vasoconstriction

10. The drug of choice in treating severe anaphylactic shock is:
    - (a) Isoproterenol
    - (b) Epinephrine

(c) Norepinephrine
(d) Phenylephrine

11. Which drug has both cardiac stimulant and renal vasodilator properties?
    (a) Isoproterenol
    (b) Norepinephrine
    (c) Dopamine
    (d) Epinephrine

12. Which of the following can limit tissue damage caused by extravasation of an alpha adrenergic agonist?
    (a) Propranolol
    (b) Pralidoxime
    (c) Phentolamine
    (d) Physostigmine

13. Tissue sloughing following extravasation, acidosis, and renal failure are all adverse reactions associated with:
    (a) Norepinephrine
    (b) Epinephrine
    (c) Propranolol
    (d) Phenoxybenzamine

14. Which of the following reduces peripheral decarboxylation of L-dopa to enhance its therapeutic effects in Parkinson's disease?
    (a) Pyridoxal phosphate
    (b) Carbidopa
    (c) Both
    (d) Neither

15. When L-dopa is administered for the management of Parkinson's disease:
    (a) It is enzymatically converted within the central nervous system to form dopamine.
    (b) It effectively arrests the progressive nature of the disease.
    (c) It produces toxicity, which is reduced by monoamine oxidase inhibitors.
    (d) It is converted to a toxic metabolite that destroys dopamine neurons in the substantia nigra.

16. Which one of the following agents blocks neuromuscular transmission by depolarizing the muscle endplate?
    (a) Succinylcholine
    (b) d-tubocurarine
    (c) Gallamine
    (d) Pancuronium

17. Neostigmine is an effective antidote to:
    (a) Succinylcholine
    (b) d-tubocurarine
    (c) Decamethonium
    (d) All of the above

18. Hypotension caused by ganglionic blockage and by the release of histamine is most often associated with the use of:
    (a) d-tubocurarine
    (b) Succinylcholine
    (c) Pancuronium
    (d) Gallamine

19. Which of the following agents can produce tachycardia through an atropinelike effect?
    (a) Succinylcholine
    (b) d-tubocurarine
    (c) Pancuronium
    (d) Gallamine

20. Sympathomimetic agents in the presence of digitalis increase the risk of:
    (a) Ventricular arrhythmias
    (b) Atrioventricular block
    (c) Sinus bradycardia
    (d) None of the above

21. An early sign of digitalis intoxication is:
    (a) Green halos around objects
    (b) Nausea
    (c) Confusion
    (d) Any of the above

22. Digitalis-induced automaticity is enhanced by:
    (a) Hypercalcemia
    (b) Hypernatremia
    (c) Hyperkalemia
    (d) Hyperglycemia

23. The most important characteristic of chlorothiazide to consider in concomitant therapy with digitalis is its tendency to produce:
    (a) Hyperuricemia
    (b) Hyperglycemia
    (c) Hyponatremia
    (d) Hypokalemia

24. Inhibition of sodium movement out of the cardiac cell by cardiac glycosides leads to a positive inotropic response attributable to:
    (a) Enhanced potassium influx, which further inhibits the sodium pump
    (b) Stimulation of calcium influx via the sodium–calcium exchange
    (c) Synthesis of more sodium pump molecules
    (d) Phosphorylation of a protein by protein kinase

25. The use of cardiac glycosides in the treatment of congestive heart failure is based primarily on their ability to:
    (a) Slow conduction through the A-V node
    (b) Decrease heart size
    (c) Produce a positive inotropic effect
    (d) Produce diuresis

26. Amrinone is a second-line drug for the treatment of:
    (a) Essential hypertension
    (b) Congestive heart failure
    (c) Angina pectoris

(d) Cardiac arrhythmias

27. Antiarrhythmic agents such as quinidine:
    (a) Increase conduction velocity
    (b) Decrease conduction velocity
    (c) Enhance the responsiveness of Purkinje fibers
    (d) Shorten the duration of the action potential

28. Propranolol controls the ventricular rate in atrial tachyarrhythmias by:
    (a) Increasing conduction velocity
    (b) Increasing the duration of the action potential
    (c) Decreasing A-V conduction time
    (d) Increasing the degree of block at the A-V node

29. Which one of the following drugs would be the most rational choice for treating sinus tachycardia in a patient with pheochromocytoma?
    (a) Verapamil
    (b) Lidocaine
    (c) Propranolol
    (d) Quinidine

30. Which one of the following antiarrhythmic drugs directly affects sympathetic neurons?
    (a) Quinidine
    (b) Bretylium
    (c) Procainamide
    (d) Lidocaine

31. Adverse effects expected with verapamil include:
    (a) Decreased heart rate and decreased force of contraction
    (b) Increased heart rate and decreased force of contraction
    (c) Decreased heart rate and increased force of contraction
    (d) Increased heart rate and increased force of contraction

32. Which of the following is an orally active analogue of lidocaine?
    (a) Flecainide
    (b) Tocainide
    (c) Propafenone
    (d) Amiodarone

33. The beneficial effect of nitroglycerin in the treatment of angina pectoris is attributable to:
    (a) Negative inotropic action
    (b) Sinoatrial depression
    (c) Blockade of beta receptors
    (d) Relaxation of vascular smooth muscle

34. A drug may be beneficial in the treatment of angina if it will do the following:
    (a) Decrease heart work
    (b) Increase myocardial Po_2
    (c) Dilate capacitance vessels
    (d) All of the above

35. Tolerance develops to which of the antianginal drugs?
    (a) Nitroglycerin
    (b) Beta blockers
    (c) Calcium channel blockers
    (d) None of the above

36. Consumption of alcohol by persons who are using nitroglycerin can cause:
    (a) Renal failure
    (b) Hepatotoxicity
    (c) Severe hypotension
    (d) Hypertensive crisis

37. Captopril appears to produce its blood-pressure–lowering effects through:
    (a) Blockade of angiotensin II receptors
    (b) Stimulation of GABA receptors in the medulla
    (c) Inhibition of angiotension I converting enzyme
    (d) Inhibition of the synthesis of renin

38. Clonidine lowers arterial blood pressure by:
    (a) Competitive blockade of angiotensin II receptors
    (b) Blockade of alpha-1 adrenergic centers in the brain
    (c) Inhibition of angiotensin I converting enzyme
    (d) Stimulating alpha-2 adrenergic receptors in the medulla

39. Important contraindications to the use of propranolol as an antihypertensive drug may include:
    (a) Asthma
    (b) Congestive heart failure
    (c) Second-degree heart block
    (d) All of the above

40. Which is characteristic of nitroprusside?
    (a) Produces peripheral vasodilation through direct action on vascular smooth muscle
    (b) Acts centrally as an antihypertensive agent
    (c) Has no significant side effects or toxicities
    (d) Causes hallucinations

41. Which is characteristic of spironolactone?
    (a) Acts as a diuretic by inhibiting the synthesis of aldosterone
    (b) Is used in combination with other diuretics to decrease potassium loss
    (c) Enhances sodium reabsorption and potassium secretion
    (d) All of the above

42. Which diuretics can reduce hypercalciuria?
    (a) Osmotics
    (b) Thiazides
    (c) "Loop"
    (d) Potassium-sparing

43. Increase in osmolarity of tubular fluid is the principal mechanism of action of:
    (a) Chlorothiazide
    (b) Acetazolamide
    (c) Mannitol
    (d) Furosemide

44. Which one of the following diuretics would be least likely to produce potassium loss?
    (a) Furosemide
    (b) Chlorothiazide
    (c) Triamterene
    (d) Ethacrynic acid

45. Sudden hearing loss would most likely occur after the administration of which one of the following?
    (a) Mannitol
    (b) Ethacrynic acid
    (c) Chlorothiazide
    (d) Metolazone

46. Which is characteristic of thiopental?
    (a) Is one of the few drugs safe for use in patients with acute intermittent porphyria
    (b) Produces slow and incomplete analgesia
    (c) Is a primary agent of induction because of rapid onset and short duration of action
    (d) Maintains cardiovascular stability

47. Halogenated anesthetic agents gained considerable favor on their initial introduction because:
    (a) Respiratory depression was not a major complication.
    (b) They are generally nonexplosive.
    (c) They are relatively inexpensive.
    (d) They do not produce cardiovascular depression.

48. Nephrotoxicity has been reported with the use of:
    (a) Isoflurane
    (b) Ketamine
    (c) Benzodiazepines
    (d) Methoxyflurane

49. Meyer and Overton postulated that anesthetic potency is related to:
    (a) Direct effects on cellular colloids
    (b) Anesthetic alterations in cellular permeability
    (c) Lipoid solubility
    (d) Inhibition of oxidative enzyme systems

50. According to Guedel's signs and stages of anesthesia, stage II is the stage of:
    (a) Analgesia
    (b) Medullary depression
    (c) Surgical anesthesia
    (d) Excitement or delirium

51. Which of the following must be administered with nitrous oxide?
    (a) Oxygen
    (b) Succinylcholine
    (c) Atropine
    (d) Halothane

52. A prominent adverse effect of halothane is:
    (a) Ototoxicity
    (b) Hepatotoxicity
    (c) Nephrotoxicity
    (d) Neurotoxicity

53. Extrapyramidal movement disorders are most characteristic of:
    (a) Benzodiazepines
    (b) Levodopa
    (c) Phenothiazines
    (d) Phenytoin

54. Which of the following facilitates the actions of the neurotransmitter GABA?
    (a) Ethyl alcohol
    (b) Diazepam
    (c) Chlorpromazine
    (d) Amitriptyline

55. Which of the following may be useful in treating methanol poisoning?
    (a) Pralidoxime
    (b) Diazepam
    (c) Chlorpromazine
    (d) Ethyl alcohol

56. The drug of choice in the treatment of status epilepticus is:
    (a) Lithium
    (b) Amitriptyline
    (c) Chlorpromazine
    (d) Diazepam

57. Which one of the following drugs is most likely to induce hepatic enzymes?
    (a) Ethosuximide
    (b) Carbamazepine
    (c) Diazepam
    (d) Valproic acid

58. Which one of the following is a primary drug for treating absence seizures (petit mal)?
    (a) Ethosuximide
    (b) Phenytoin
    (c) Diazepam
    (d) Phenobarbital

59. Which one of the following is associated with valproic acid?
    (a) Hirsutism
    (b) Inhibition of carbonic anhydrase
    (c) Increased phenobarbital levels when the two drugs are administered concurrently
    (d) Constipation

60. Gingival hyperplasia is a common side effect associated with prolonged treatment with:
    (a) Diazepam
    (b) Trimethadione

(c) Phenobarbital

(d) Phenytoin

61. Use of which of the following may be associated with significant anticholinergic side effects?
    (a) Fluoxetine
    (b) Lithium
    (c) Trazodone
    (d) Amitriptyline

62. The clinical use of Δ^9-THC analogues has recently been approved by the FDA in the treatment of:
    (a) Pain due to cancer
    (b) Nausea due to cancer chemotherapy
    (c) Anxiety due to AIDS
    (d) All of the above

63. With regard to the action of local anesthetics, which of the following statements is true?
    (a) Sensory but not motor fibers are blocked.
    (b) Myelinated fibers are more easily blocked than nonmyelinated nerves.
    (c) Small nerve fibers are more susceptible than large fibers.
    (d) None of the above

64. Which of the following is associated with lidocaine?
    (a) Slow onset of action
    (b) Poor tissue penetration
    (c) Poor safety record
    (d) Suppression of tachyarrhythmias

65. The action of local anesthetics can be enhanced by concomitant administration of:
    (a) Acetylcholine
    (b) Epinephrine
    (c) Pseudocholinesterase
    (d) Nitroglycerin

66. The mechanism of action of H_1-receptor antihistaminic agents is:
    (a) Inhibition of histamine release from mast cells
    (b) Inhibition of histidine decarboxylase
    (c) Competition with histamine for receptor sites
    (d) Depletion of histamine from storage granules

67. H_2 blocking drugs such as cimetidine have therapeutic value for patients with:
    (a) Urticaria
    (b) Gastric hypersecretion
    (c) Seasonal rhinitis
    (d) Allergic dermatosis

68. Which one of the following may be induced by the prolonged use of glucocorticoids?
    (a) Rheumatic fever
    (b) Osteoporosis
    (c) Inflammatory skin conditions
    (d) Pulmonary fibrosis

69. Deoxycorticosterone:
    (a) Has little effect on water or electrolyte excretion
    (b) Promotes K^+ reabsorption in the distal renal tubule
    (c) Is a potent anti-inflammatory agent
    (d) Promotes Na^+ reabsorption in the distal renal tubule

70. When ACTH is administered to a subject with responsive adrenal glands, the following occurs:
    (a) A decrease in arterial blood pressure
    (b) An increase in eosinophils in the peripheral blood
    (c) An increase in plasma lymphocytes
    (d) An increase in urinary 17-hydroxycorticosteroids

71. Oral hypoglycemic agents:
    (a) Are effective in both Types I and II diabetes
    (b) Will not cause hypoglycemia
    (c) Appear to stimulate insulin release and to increase the sensitivity of cells to insulin
    (d) Are drugs of choice for management of gestational diabetes

72. Clomiphene is used as a fertility agent because it:
    (a) Prolongs the midcycle surge of LH
    (b) Mimics the action of FSH in stimulating follicular development
    (c) Inhibits ovarian secretion of estrogen during the follicular phase
    (d) Stimulates ovulation in anovulatory women who have potentially functional hypothalamic-pituitary-ovarian systems

73. Which psychotherapeutic drug is associated with weight loss?
    (a) Fluoxetine
    (b) Chlorpromazine
    (c) Imipramine
    (d) Diazepem

74. Androgens such as testosterone tend to:
    (a) Produce hypocalcemia
    (b) Increase protein synthesis
    (c) Suppress growth of prostatic carcinoma
    (d) Decrease electrolyte retention

75. Oxytocics are used principally for:
    (a) Acute treatment of migraine headache
    (b) Induction of labor at term
    (c) Controlling postpartum hemorrhage
    (d) Controlling coronary spasm

76. Which of the following is true of prophylthiouracil?
    (a) It is used in the treatment of myxedema.
    (b) It has a long half-life in the circulation.
    (c) It increases proteolysis of thyroglobulin.
    (d) It blocks thyroxine synthesis.

77. Which of the following has the greatest rapidity of action?
    (a) Thyroid extract
    (b) Sodium liothyronine
    (c) Thyroxine
    (d) Triiodothyronine

78. Which of the following is a highly effective immunosuppressant with relatively less toxicity than other agents used for this purpose?
    (a) Cyclazocine
    (b) Cycloserine
    (c) Cyclophosphamide
    (d) Cyclosporine

79. Misoprostol is approved to reduce the risk of serious toxicity of:
    (a) Colchicine
    (b) Narcotic analgesics
    (c) Acetaminophen
    (d) Nonsteroidal anti-inflammatory drugs

80. Dry cough is a characteristic adverse effect of:
    (a) Beta blockers
    (b) Nitroglycerin
    (c) Angiotensin converting enzyme (ACE) inhibitors
    (d) Alpha blockers

81. Which of the following possesses laxative action, which limits its use as an antacid?
    (a) Sodium bicarbonate
    (b) Magnesium hydroxide
    (c) Aluminum hydroxide
    (d) None of the above

82. Which one of the following antacids, if used over prolonged periods, would be most likely to produce severe toxic effects in a patient with poor renal function?
    (a) Aluminum hydroxide
    (b) Calcium carbonate
    (c) Magnesium hydroxide
    (d) Sodium bicarbonate

83. Treatment of an upper respiratory infection due to a group-A beta hemolytic streptococcus in a patient with a history of penicillin hypersensitivity is usually effectively accomplished by administration of:
    (a) Cephalothin
    (b) Chlortetracycline
    (c) Vancomycin
    (d) Erythromycin

84. Which of the following is *not* an inhibitor of microbial cell wall biosynthesis?
    (a) Piperacillin
    (b) Vancomycin
    (c) Cephamandole
    (d) Sulfisoxazole

85. Inhibition of protein synthesis at the ribosomal level is the principal mechanism of antibacterial action of:
    (a) Chloramphenicol
    (b) Amikacin
    (c) Piperacillin
    (d) Sulfisoxazole

86. A potentially fatal consequence of the administration of chloramphenicol is:
    (a) Anemia
    (b) Hepatic necrosis
    (c) Systemic lupus erythematosis
    (d) Stevens-Johnson syndrome
    (e) Parkinsonism

87. The selective toxicity of the sulfonamide class of antimicrobial agents against susceptible bacteria is based on the fact that:
    (a) Sulfonamides do not penetrate into mammalian cells.
    (b) Mammalian cells readily inactivate sulfonamides.
    (c) Mammalian cells do not utilize folate.
    (d) Mammalian cells synthesize folate.
    (e) Mammalian cells require folate from an exogenous source.

88. A bactericidal drug would be preferred over a bacteriostatic drug in a patient with:
    (a) Neutropenia
    (b) Renal insufficiency
    (c) Cirrhosis
    (d) Hemolytic anemia
    (e) Congestive heart failure

89. Use of outdated tetracycline preparations carries a risk of:
    (a) Renal proximal tubular necrosis
    (b) Hepatic centrilobular necrosis
    (c) Pseudomembranous colitis
    (d) Staphylococcal superinfection
    (e) Peripheral neuropathy

90. In the treatment of active tuberculosis, which of the following two drugs would virtually always be included in the treatment regimen?
    (a) Streptomycin and *para*-aminosalicyclic acid
    (b) Ethambutol and kanamycin
    (c) Streptomycin and capreomycin
    (d) Isoniazid and rifampin
    (e) Iproniazid and rifampin

91. The drug of choice for Lyme disease is:
    (a) A sulfonamide
    (b) An aminoglycoside
    (c) A tetracycline
    (d) Chloramphenicol

92. Anticoagulation with serious bleeding has occurred often with:
    (a) Methicillin
    (b) Minocycline

(c) Moxalactam

(d) Netilmicin

93. The principal mode of action of trimethoprim is inhibition of:

(a) Folate reductase

(b) Dihydrofolate reductase

(c) Tetrahydrofolate reductase

(d) PABA insertase

(e) Thymidylate synthetase

94. The drug of choice for treatment of an infection with *Legionella pneumophilia* is currently considered to be:

(a) Erythromycin

(b) Chloramphenicol

(c) Clindamycin

(d) Cefazolin

(e) Gentamicin

95. Misreading of the mRNA code at the ribosomal level with subsequent assembly of proteins containing inappropriate amino acids is involved in the antimicrobial action of:

(a) Ampicillin

(b) Clindamycin

(c) Griseofulvin

(d) Streptomycin

(e) Cycloserine

96. Which of the following is *not* an indication for administration of combinations of antimicrobial agents?

(a) Prevention of the emergence of resistant microorganisms

(b) Treatment of fever of unknown etiology

(c) Therapy of severe infections in which the etiologic agent has not yet been identified

(d) Treatment of mixed bacterial infections

(e) Enhancement of antibacterial activity in the treatment of specific infections

97. The incidence of microbial superinfections is typically lowest following the administration of an antimicrobial agent that:

(a) Has a narrow spectrum of antimicrobial activity

(b) Has a broad spectrum of antimicrobial activity

(c) Is well absorbed after oral administration

(d) Is poorly absorbed after oral administration

(e) Has a prolonged biological half-life

98. Treatment of antibiotic-associated colitis (AAC) caused by the overgrowth of *Clostridium difficile* is usually successfully accomplished by the administration of:

(a) Chloramphenicol

(b) Clindamycin

(c) Vancomycin

(d) Nystatin

(e) Streptomycin

99. Which of the following is active only against microorganisms that are actively replicating?

(a) Polymyxin

(b) Benzyl penicillin

(c) Methenamine mandelate

(d) Sulfamethoxazole

(e) Chloramphenicol

100. Which of the following antibacterial agents prevents the association of various amino acid-tRNA complexes with the 30-S ribosomal subunit?

(a) Streptomycin

(b) Amikacin

(c) Chloramphenicol

(d) Erythromycin

(e) Tetracycline

101. Substitution of the benzyl group of benzyl penicillin with an organic structure of different configuration can yield a compound with:

(a) Reduced antibacterial potency

(b) A different spectrum of antibacterial action than that of the parent compound

(c) Greater acid stability

(d) Greater resistance to the action of beta lactamase (penicillinase)

(e) Any of the above

102. An antibacterial agent that directly inhibits nucleic acid synthesis in some prokaryotes but not in eukaryotes is:

(a) Chloramphenicol

(b) Trimethoprim

(c) Rifampin

(d) 5-fluorocytosine

(e) 5-flurouracil

103. Treatment of tuberculosis with a combination of isoniazid and rifampin is a currently accepted practice. One disadvantage of this drug combination is that:

(a) Isoniazid retards the excretion of rifampin.

(b) Isoniazid reduces the potency of rifampin.

(c) Both are potentially nephrotoxic.

(d) Both are potentially hepatotoxic.

(e) Rifampin enhances the rate of excretion of isoniazid.

104. A patient undergoing remission-induction chemotherapy for acute lymphoblastic leukemia becomes progressively lethargic and semicomatose, and develops a rectal temperature of 105° F. A presumptive diagnosis of gram-negative septicemia is made. After the drawing of blood for bacterial culture and sensitivity tests, an appropriate antimicrobial regimen would be:

(a) Ampicillin and ticarcillin

(b) Ticarcillin and sulfamethoxazole/trimethoprim

(c) Carbenicillin and clindamycin
(d) Erythromycin and rifampin
(e) Cephalexin and amikacin

105. A useful drug for the treatment of uncomplicated gonorrhea in a patient who is sensitive to benzyl pencillin is:
    (a) Spectinomycin
    (b) Ampicillin
    (c) Nitrofurantoin
    (d) Ethionamide
    (e) Nalidixic acid

106. Which of the following antimicrobial agents would have the greatest potential for additive toxicity in a cancer patient whose antineoplastic regimen includes cisplatin?
    (a) Doxycycline
    (b) Kanamycin
    (c) Cephalexin
    (d) Erythromycin
    (e) Nalidixic acid

107. Ototoxicity is characteristic of:
    (a) Penicillins
    (b) Cephalosporins
    (c) Aminoglycosides
    (d) Tetracyclines

108. Inhibition of protein synthesis in mammalian mitochondria is thought to be associated with reversible leukopenia, which is often observed following the administration of:
    (a) Sulfamethoxazole plus trimethoprim
    (b) Chloramphenicol
    (c) Tobramycin
    (d) Amphotericin B
    (e) Griseofulvin

109. Following phosphorylation by herpes virus–infected cells, acyclovir becomes a potent inhibitor of:
    (a) Viral protein synthesis
    (b) Viral topoisomerase
    (c) Viral DNA polymerase
    (d) Viral RNA polymerase
    (e) Viral riboside reductase

110. Which of the following is most effective in eradicating strains of intracellular *Mycobacterium tuberculosis?*
    (a) Streptomycin
    (b) Capreomycin
    (c) Ethionamide
    (d) Cycloserine
    (e) Rifampin

111. Which of the following would *not* be a rational use of a cephalosporin antimicrobial agent?
    (a) Prophylaxis during and after certain types of surgery
    (b) Treatment of a staphylococcal infection in a

patient with a history of an immediate type of allergic reaction to benzyl penicillin
    (c) Treatment of septicemia caused by strains of *Klebsiella*
    (d) Treatment of meningitis caused by gram-negative enteric bacteria
    (e) Treatment of meningitis caused by *Haemophilus influenzae*

112. Clavulanic acid:
    (a) Is an irreversible inhibitor of beta lactamase
    (b) Is an excellent topical antifungal agent
    (c) Cannot pass through the bacterial cell wall
    (d) Is active against group-A beta hemolytic streptococci
    (e) Is a second-line antitubercular drug

113. If a given antineoplastic regimen effects a 3-log cell kill in a population of leukemia cells, what percentage of the original cell population would remain viable?
    (a) 3%
    (b) 10%
    (c) 1%
    (d) 0.1%
    (e) 0.3%

114. The dose-limiting toxicity of doxorubicin (Adriamycin) is:
    (a) Centrilobular necrosis
    (b) Congestive heart failure
    (c) Proximal tubular necrosis
    (d) Peripheral neuropathy
    (e) Reticulocytopenia

115. Which of the following antineoplastic agents does *not* require biotransformation to exert its cytotoxic action:
    (a) 5-fluorouracil
    (b) Cytarabine
    (c) Thioguanine
    (d) 6-mercaptopurine
    (e) Methotrexate

116. Allopurinol is often used as an adjunct in the treatment of cancer to:
    (a) Minimize emesis
    (b) Protect the bone marrow stem cells
    (c) Inhibit the metabolism of purines to uric acid
    (d) Enhance the degree of cell kill obtained with specific drug regimens
    (e) Minimize thrombocytopenia

117. Which of the following antineoplastic agents would *not* be considered cell cycle–specific?
    (a) Cytarabine
    (b) Cisplatin
    (c) Thioguanine
    (d) Methotrexate
    (e) 5-fluorouracil

118. Allopurinol can increase the plasma level of:
    (a) 6-mercaptopurine
    (b) Thioguanine
    (c) Both
    (d) Neither

119. Biotransformation of which of the following leads to the formation of an organic aldehyde that is markedly toxic to the epithelium of the urinary bladder?
    (a) Daunorubicin
    (b) Vincristine
    (c) Vinblastine
    (d) Cyclophosphamide
    (e) Procarbazine

120. Which of the following antineoplastic agents inhibits the conversion of ribonucleotides to deoxyribonucleotides?
    (a) Hydroxyanisole
    (b) Chlorambucil
    (c) BCNU
    (d) Methotrexate
    (e) Hydroxyurea

121. Following chronic cadmium (Cd) exposure, levels of metallothioneine-bound Cd in the kidneys are reduced by the administration of:
    (a) Ethylenediamine tetra acetic acid (EDTA)
    (b) Dimercaprol (BAL)
    (c) D-penicillamine
    (d) *N*-acetylcysteine
    (e) None of the above

122. Which of the following interventions should *not* be carried out in a patient who has ingested kerosene?
    (a) Gastric lavage
    (b) Induction of vomiting
    (c) Oxygen administration
    (d) Intravenous infusion of 5% dextrose
    (e) Infusion of normal saline

123. Development of hepatic centrilobular necrosis secondary to acetaminophen overdose can be prevented effectively by which of the following if given within a few hours after ingestion?
    (a) *N*-acetylcysteine
    (b) Dimercaprol
    (c) Sodium nitrite
    (d) Amyl nitrite
    (e) Phenobarbital

124. No specific antivenin is available for treatment of envenomation by which of the following?
    (a) Rattlesnake (*Crotalus* species)
    (b) Water moccasin (*Agkistrodon* species)
    (c) Brown recluse spider (*Loxosceles reclusa*)
    (d) Black widow spider (*Latrodectus mactans*)
    (e) Coral snake (*Micrurus fulvius*)

125. Treatment of chronic lead poisoning typically involved treatment with:
    (a) Ethylenediamine tetraacetic acid, calcium disodium salt
    (b) D-penicillamine
    (c) Dimercaprol
    (d) All of the above

126. Which of the following statements regarding acetylsalicyclic acid (aspirin) is *not* true?
    (a) It is not well reabsorbed from renal tubules.
    (b) It has significant anti-inflammatory properties.
    (c) It causes gastric distress in a significant number of patients.
    (d) It will inhibit platelet aggregation.

127. Which is (are) characteristic of probenecid?
    (a) Blocks renal tubular transport of carboxylic acids
    (b) Blocks renal tubular transport of uric acid
    (c) Both of the above
    (d) None of the above

128. Acetaminophen is an appropriate antipyretic to substitute for aspirin. Unlike aspirin, it:
    (a) Does not increase bleeding time
    (b) Does not possess significant anti-inflammatory properties
    (c) Can cause hepatic centrilobular necrosis if taken in high doses
    (d) Does not typically cause gastric irritation
    (e) All of the above

129. The major mode of action of ibuprofen is:
    (a) Blockade of synaptic transmission
    (b) Inhibition of prostaglandin synthetase
    (c) Stimulation of prostaglandin synthetase
    (d) Stimulation of endorphin production
    (e) Facilitation of transfer of endorphins from a central location to peripheral sites

130. A patient who is chronically receiving racemic warfarin develops a urinary tract infection. The urologist prescribes an antibacterial preparation to be taken orally. Three days later, the patient presents for a regularly scheduled measurement of bleeding time, which is found to be markedly increased. The antibacterial preparation prescribed by the urologist was most likely:
    (a) Methenamine mandelate
    (b) Ampicillin
    (c) Tobramycin
    (d) Trimethoprim-sulfamethoxazole
    (e) Nalidixic acid

131. An effective antidote for inadvertent heparin overdose is:
    (a) Vitamin K
    (b) Protamine sulfate
    (c) 4-hydroxycoumarin

(d) Heparinase
(e) Peptone

Directions. For Questions 132 through 138, select the one lettered heading from the list below that is most appropriate for each numbered statement.

(a) Riboflavin
(b) Nicotinamide
(c) Pyridoxine
(d) Ascorbic acid
(e) None of the above

132. Excessive intake ("megadoses") can cause kidney stones.
133. It is used in the treatment of pellagra.
134. Its administration corrects iron deficiency anemia.
135. Deficiency of this vitamin first presents as stomatitis and glossitis followed by seborrheic dermatitis of the face, and dermatitis over the trunk and extremities. Anemia and neuropathy follow.
136. Its coadministration with isoniazid prevents isoniazid-induced neuropathies.
137. Ingestion of moderately high doses redues the incidence of the common cold.
138. Its administration corrects the condition known as infantile beriberi.

Directions. For each of the following questions answer:

(a) if only 1 is correct
(b) if only 1 and 2 are correct
(c) if only 1 and 3 are correct
(d) if all are correct
(e) if none is correct

139. Cholestyramine:
 1. Reduces plasma cholesterol
 2. Reduces plasma low-density lipoproteins
 3. Frequently causes indigestion, constipation, and fecal impaction
140. Nicotinic acid:
 1. Reduces plasma very-low-density lipoproteins
 2. Causes marked vasoconstriction
 3. Inhibits lipolysis in adipose tissue
141. Vitamin B_{12}:
 1. Occurs intracellularly as methylcobalamine and deoxyadenosylcobalamine
 2. Requires gastric intrinsic factor for absorption
 3. Deficiency is detrimental to both the hematopoietic and nervous systems
142. Radioactive lead (Pb-210) is a useful diagnostic tool for the nuclear imaging of:
 1. Brain abscesses

2. Pulmonary infarcts
3. Osteogenic sarcoma
143. Chlorhexidine:
 1. Is one of the most important surgical antiseptics
 2. Is bacteriostatic to gram-positive and gram-negative organisms
 3. Is virucidal
144. Benzalkonium chloride:
 1. Has germicidal activity
 2. Is inactivated by soaps and other anionic agents
 3. Is highly irritating to skin
145. Radioisotopes that are useful in the nuclear imaging of various organs include:
 1. Iodine-125
 2. Cadmium-109
 3. Gallium-67
146. Cyclosporine:
 1. Blocks an early stage in the activation of cytotoxic T lymphocytes in response to alloantigens
 2. Is used for prophylaxis and treatment of organ rejection of allogeneic transplants
 3. Is usually used with adrenocortico-steroids
147. Treatment of mild to moderate intestinal infestation with *Entamoeba histolytica* would include use of:
 1. Metronidazole
 2. Iodoquinol
 3. Paromomycin
148. Diethylcarbamazine is the drug of choice for the treatment of:
 1. Filariasis
 2. Cutaneous larva migrans
 3. Pinworms
149. The treatment of acute carbon monoxide poisoning involves:
 1. Transferring the victim to fresh air
 2. Administration of oxygen with positive pressure
 3. Administration of sodium thiosulfate
150. Drug regimens for the treatment of an uncomplicated attack of malaria caused by a chloroquine-resistant strain of *Plasmodium falciparum* would include:
 1. Quinine sulfate plus pyrimethamine
 2. Quinine sulfate plus primaquine
 3. Quinine sulfate plus sulfadiazine
151. Mebendazole, pyrantel pamoate, and piperazine citrate all have a role in the treatment of:
 1. Roundworm *(Ascaris lumbricoides)*
 2. Amebic meningoencephalitis
 3. Tapeworm *(Taenia saginata or T. solium)*

152. Methyl alcohol (methanol) is sometimes inadvertently ingested as a component of illicit whiskey. Treatment of a patient with methyl alcohol poisoning would involve:
    1. Correction of acidosis
    2. Administration of disulfiram
    3. Administration of ethyl alcohol

153. The major durgs used in the treatment of leprosy include:
    1. Dapsone
    2. Clofazimine

3. Cycloserine

154. Which of the following are highly concentrated in erythrocytes following chronic occupational exposure?
    1. Methyl mercury
    2. Inorganic mercury
    3. Elemental mercury

155. Metronidazole is useful in the treatment of:
    1. Amebiasis
    2. Infection due to *Bacteroides fragilis*
    3. Trichomoniasis

1. b
2. d
3. d
4. b
5. c
6. d
7. c
8. b
9. d
10. b
11. c
12. c
13. a
14. b
15. a
16. a
17. b
18. a
19. d
20. a
21. d
22. a
23. d
24. b
25. c
26. b
27. b
28. d
29. c
30. b
31. a
32. b
33. d
34. d
35. a
36. c
37. c
38. d
39. d
40. a
41. b
42. b
43. c
44. c
45. b
46. c
47. b
48. d
49. c
50. d

51. a
52. b
53. c
54. b
55. d
56. d
57. b
58. a
59. c
60. d
61. d
62. b
63. c
64. d
65. b
66. c
67. b
68. b
69. d
70. d
71. c
72. d
73. a
74. b
75. c
76. d
77. b
78. d
79. d
80. c
81. b
82. c
83. d Oral administration of 250 mg to 500 mg every 6 hours of the estolate, or 30 mg/kg/day of the other forms of erythromycin, is usually curative.
84. d
85. b Amikacin, an aminoglycoside antibiotic that binds to the bacterial 30-s ribosomal subunit, blocks protein chain formation at the N-formyl-methionine stage on the bacterial 50-s subunit.
86. a The incidence of pancytopenia following administration of chloramphenicol is estimated to be about 1 in 30,000.
87. e Mammalian cells are incapable of synthesizing folate and thus require it from an exogenous source. It is reduced in a two-step reaction to tetrahydrofolate, which acts as a coenzyme with several apoenzymes to carry out essential one-carbon transfers in both mammalian and bacterial cells.

88. **a** The neutropenic patient is immunosuppressed and thus cannot fully evoke the defenses to assist in controlling infections when given a bacteriostatic drug.

89. **a** Nausea, vomiting, polyuria, polydipsia, proteinuria, acidosis, glycosuria, and gross aminoaciduria (a form of the Fanconi syndrome) have been observed in patients ingesting outdated tetracycline. Patients should always be instructed to discard any capsules not taken.

90. **d** Both isoniazid and rifampin are mycobactericidal, and rifampin is effective against intracellular mycobacteria.

91. **c** A tetracycline is preferred except for children or during pregnancy and lactation, when penicillin can be used if allergy does not contraindicate these drugs. Erythromycin and ceftriaxone are also effective.

92. **c**

93. **b** Trimethoprim is a potent inhibitor of bacterial dihydrofolate reductase. Sensitivity of the corresponding mammalian enzyme is several orders of magnitude lower. See Question 87.

94. **a** Clinical evidence as well as studies in experimental animals have shown that erythromycin is the most active antimicrobial agent available. In particularly severe cases, it is sometimes given in combination with rifampin, or rifampin alone is sometimes used for a patient who does not respond to erythromycin.

95. **d** This is thought to be a secondary effect of streptomycin, and possibly of other antibiotics of the aminoglycoside class. Uridine is read as adenine by the 30-s ribosomal subunit, with consequent assembly of inappropriate peptides and proteins.

96. **b** Fever of unknown cause is not an indication for the administration of antimicrobial agents. Most instances of pyrexia of brief duration, in the absence of specific signs to the contrary, are viral in origin. Prolonged pyrexia may be secondary to tuberculosis, occult intra-abdominal abscess, endocarditis, as well as various neoplasms and collagen disorders. Several other disorders may be characterized by fever, including metabolic aberrations, hepatitis, and certain forms of rheumatoid arthritis.

97. **a** Superinfections are more common following administration of broad-spectrum antimicrobial agents. These may be bacterial or fungal in nature and represent the emergence of a resistant strain of an originally sensitive organism, or overgrowth of an organisms that is inherently resistant, such as *Candida albicans.*

98. **c** Oral administration of nonabsorbable vancomycin is highly effective in controlling the growth of *C. difficile,* an anaerobic rod that produces the toxic substance responsible for the colitis.

99. **b** The bactericidal action of any penicillin or cephalosporin can be expressed only when the bacteria are dividing. They are thus typically ineffective against populations of bacteria that are in their plateau stage, as in abscesses.

100. **e** Tetracycline and its analogues block access of the amino acid–transfer RNA complex to the 30-s ribosomal subunit. The result is inhibition of protein synthesis by sensitive bacteria.

101. **e** All semisynthetic penicillins are substituted on the primary amine nitrogen atom of 6-aminopenicillanic acid. Depending on the chemical nature of the aryl substituent, congeners may possess any of the characteristics listed.

102. **c** Rifampin binds to the beta subunit of bacterial RNA polymerase and prevents interaction of the enzyme with the DNA template; ribonucleic acid synthesis is thus directly inhibited.

103. **d** Isoniazid is partially acetylated; the acetylated adduct breaks down with the formation of isonicotinic acid and acetylhydrazine. The latter undergoes further biotransformation by the hepatic cytochrome P_{450} mixed-function oxidase system to form hydrazine and an alkylating moiety that can covalently bind to hepatic macromolecules. Rifampin can also cause hepatitis, especially in alcoholics and in patients with previous liver disease. Its mechanism of hepatotoxicity has not been well defined; however, certain of its other toxic actions (*e.g.,* a flulike syndrome) may have an immunologic basis.

104. **e** In a patient such as this, two bactericidal agents that have broad spectra of action as well as different modes of action would be the treatment of choice. Cephalexin (a cephalosporin) and amikacin (an aminoglycoside) best meet these criteria.

105. **a** Spectinomycin may be administered intramuscularly, 2 g/dose twice a day for 3 days. It is also effective against penicillinase-producing strains of *N. gonorrhoeae.* It is not useful in the treatment of gonococcal pharyngitis or syphilis.

106. **b** The dose-limiting toxicity of cisplatin is often proximal renal tubular necrosis. Kanamycin, an aminoglycoside, is also toxic to the proximal renal tubules.

107. **c**

108. **b** Chloramphenicol inhibits protein synthesis in ribosomal preparations from mammalian mitochondria. This has been implicated as the basis of the reversible leukopenia associated with its use. In contrast, the aplastic anemia that occasionally ensues following chloramphenicol administration is through a different (unknown) mechanism.

109. **c** Acyclovir triphosphate is a potent inhibitor of DNA polymerase of viral origin; it has virtually no effect on mammalian DNA polymerase.

110. **e** Rifampin readily passes into mammalian cells and inhibits the replication of sensitive strains of *M. tuberculosis*. See Question 90.

111. **b** As a general rule, a cephalosporin should not be administered to a patient with a history of an immediate (anaphylactic) reaction to any penicillin derivative.

112. **a** Clavulanic acid is combined with amoxicillin for oral use and with ticarcillin as a parenteral preparation. It inhibits beta lactamase (penicillinase) and allows the action of the corresponding penicillin to be expressed.

113. **d** A 1-log cell kill is the same as a 90% kill of the existing tumor cell population, with 10% remaining viable. Since the action of antitumor agents is first order in nature (*i.e.*, a specific proportion rather than a specific number of cells will be killed), a 3-log cell kill would leave 0.1% of the cell population viable.

114. **b** At a cumulative dose of about 550 mg/meter^2, doxorubicin produces a cardiomyopathy with accompanying congestive heart failure that is refractory to digitalis glycosides.

115. **e** Methotrexate (amethopterin) is a potent inhibitor of mammalian dihydrofolate reductase. All of the other drugs listed must undergo some type of metabolic biotransformation before becoming pharmacologically active. After methotrexate is actively transported into cells, it may become polyglutamylated. This may serve to retard its egress from the cell but is not involved in its action on dihydrofolate reductase.

116. **c** Upon initiation of cancer chemotherapy, there is usually a large cell kill. Intracellular purines are released that would normally be converted to hypoxanthine, xanthine, and uric acid. The latter is a weak acid, is quite insoluble in acid urine, and tends to crystallize with the formation of crystalluria and frank renal calculi. Allopurinol inhibits the conversion of hypoxanthine to xanthine and the subsequent conversion of xanthine to uric acid. As the two uric acid precursors are more soluble in urine, the likelihood of crystalluria is diminished.

117. **b** Cisplatin forms both inter- and intrastrand bonds with DNA; this can occur at any phase of the cell cycle, even though its action may not be fully expressed until the cell enters the S (synthetic) phase of the cell cycle. The other drugs listed are antimetabolites and are considered to be cell cycle-specific for the S phase, during which DNA is synthesized.

118. **a**

119. **d** Acrolein, an organic aldehyde, is one of the several biotransformation products of cyclophosphamide. Unless the drug is given with large volumes of fluid, with or without sodium lactate, hemorrhagic cystitis may ensue. This condition can be fatal if it is not treated surgically in an aggressive fashion.

120. **e** Hydroxyurea is a highly specific inhibitor of ribonucleotide reductase. Without the deoxyriboside precursors, DNA synthesis cannot occur.

121. **e** There is no clinically acceptable antidote for cadmium poisoning. Although EDTA can promote some degree of Cd excretion, the EDTA-Cd complex is nephrotoxic.

122. **b** Kerosene is thought to produce pulmonary inflammation following transport to the lungs. Aspiration brought about by emesis can aggravate this condition.

123. **a** *N*-acetylcysteine has recently been approved by the FDA for treatment of acetaminophen overdose. It is rapidly deacetylated to cysteine and elevates hepatic glutathione levels more readily than L-cysteine. The elevated glutathione levels ameliorate the hepatic toxicity of the arylating acetaminophen metabolite.

124. **c** A polyvalent antivenin is available that is effective against the venoms of rattlesnakes, water moccasins, and copperheads. Another antivenin is specific against the neurotoxic venom of the coral snake. There is also a specific antivenin for the black widow spider.

125. **d** Chelation therapy should be initiated with all three drugs in patients who have a blood lead level in excess of 50 μg/dl.

126. **a**

127. **c** The ability of probenecid to block the renal tubular secretion of carboxylic acids is used to advantage in maintaining elevated blood levels of penicillin in treatment of gonorrhea. Conversely probenecid enhances the rate of elimination of uric acid in patients with chronic gout.

128. **e**

129. **b** Inhibition of prostaglandin synthetase is considered to be the major mode of action of ibuprofen as well as many other nonsteroidal anti-inflammatory agents, including aspirin, phenylbutazone, indomethacin, fenoprofen, sulindac, naproxen, and tolmetin.

130. **d** About 99% of ingested warfarin is bound to plasma albumin during chronic administration. Trimethoprim-sulfamethoxazole, as well as metronidazole and sulfinpyrazone, selectively prolong the half-life of levo-warfarin and thus enhance the efficacy of the racemic drug mixture. Acetylsalicylic

acid ingestion by a person who is also on oral anticoagulants will also cause prolonged bleeding times via reduction of release of ADP by platelets, which impairs their aggregation.

131. **b** *In vivo,* protamine antagonizes the anticoagulant effect of heparin; however, the action of heparin on platelet aggregation may persist. The recommended dose of protamine is estimated as 1 mg for every 100 units of heparin remaining in the patient. The mechanism of antagonism is an ionic interaction between the strongly acidic heparin with the strongly basic protamine. Protamine itself has anticoagulant action.

132. **d** Ascorbic acid in high doses can cause urinary excretion of oxalate, which precipitates in the kidneys.

133. **b** Pellagra occurs usually secondary to chronic alcoholism, coupled with protein–caloric malnutrition. Erythematous eruptions appear first on the hands and later on other areas exposed to light. Cutaneous manifestations are characterized by their symmetry. The tongue may be red and swollen. Pellagra should be considered as a possible diagnosis in any malnourished chronic alcoholic.

134. **c**

135. **a** Symptoms of riboflavin deficiency are usually accompanied by other vitamin deficiencies. It most frequently occurs in urban alcoholics of low economic status.

136. **c** Coadministration of pyridoxine with isoniazid prevents the neuropathies often associated with isoniazid administration without ameliorating the antitubercular action of isoniazid.

137. **e** No vitamin or combination of vitamins has been documented to reduce the incidence of colds.

138. **e** Infantile beriberi is an acute disease in infants that can run a rapid and fatal course. Its onset is characterized by a loss of appetite, vomiting, and green-colored stools. Muscular rigidity follows. Aphonia is diagnostic. Cardiac involvement is prominent. Death may occur in 12 to 24 hours. The condition is corrected by oral or intravenous administration of *thiamine.*

139. **d**

140. **c** Nicotinic acid is a vasodilator and causes an intense cutaneous flush, which appears to be mediated by a prostaglandin.

141. **d**

142. **e** Pb-210 is a weak gamma-emitting isotope. However, it decays to bismuth-210 and then to polonium-210. The latter is an alpha emitter that can cause severe damage to several organs.

143. **a** Chlorhexidine is bactericidal but is not virucidal.

144. **b** Quaternary ammonium compounds are relatively nonirritating to skin. They penetrate tissue surfaces and possess detergent, keratolytic, and emulsifying actions.

145. **c** The radioisotopic half-life of cadmium-109 (453 days) coupled with its extensive biological half-life (>10 years) and severe hepatic, renal, and testicular toxicity make it totally unacceptable as a radiodiagnostic imaging nuclide.

146. **d**

147. **d** Metronidazole and iodoquinol together are considered the drugs of choice; paromomycin is a suitable alternative.

148. **a** Cutaneous larva migrans is usually treated with thiabendazole, while pinworms are treated with pyrantel pamoate or mebendazole.

149. **b** The affinity of carbon monoxide for hemoglobin is about 220 times that of oxygen. Only oxygen can displace it from hemoglobin. Thiosulfate is used in treatment of cyanide poisoning because it converts the cyanide ion to the relatively nontoxic thiocyanate ion under the influence of the mitochondrial enzyme rhodanese (transsulfurase).

150. **c** Primaquine is the drug of choice for the prevention of relapses of malaria due to *P. vivax* or *P. ovale.*

151. **a** Amebic meningoencephalitis has been treated successfully with amphotericin B, but this drug is currently considered investigational for the condition by the U.S. Food and Drug Administration. Tapeworm due to *T. solium* or *T. saginata* is typically treated with niclosamide or praziquantel; paromomycin is considered a useful alternative.

152. **c** Correction of acidosis is of utmost importance. Ethyl alcohol administration may also be lifesaving, since ethyl alcohol competes with methanol for metabolic conversion. Disulfiram has no role in the treatment of methanol or acute ethanol poisoning.

153. **b** Cycloserine is a second- or third-line drug for the treatment of tuberculosis.

154. **a** Inorganic mercury tends to be concentrated in the kidneys and brain; elemental mercury is primarily a CNS toxicant. In a patient who presents with a vague history of working with "mercury," a high RBC/plasma ratio of mercury is diagnostic of methyl mercury intoxication.

155. **d**

Rypins' Questions & Answers for Basic Sciences
Review, Second Edition, edited by Edward D.
Frohlich. J. B. Lippincott Company, Philadelphia
© 1993.

C H A P T E R

8 Public Health and Community Medicine

Richard H. Grimm, Jr., M.D., M.P.H., Ph.D.*

*Associate Professor, Division of Cardiovascular Diseases,
Department of Internal Medicine, and Division of
Epidemiology, School of Public Health,
University of Minnesota School of Medicine*

1. Figure 8-1 shows recent trends in crude and age-adjusted death rates for the United States. How can we best explain the widening gap between these rates?

2. At most ages and for most causes, death rates are higher for men than for women in the United States. This sex contrast is less marked for:
   (a) Cardiovascular disease
   (b) Respiratory disease
   (c) Lung cancer
   (d) Motor vehicle accidents
   (e) Diabetes mellitus

3. When we compare the crude death rate of a developing country with that of the United States, we expect the rate:
   (a) To be lower for the United States
   (b) Not to be available for the developing country
   (c) To exclude infant deaths in both countries
   (d) To be based on the total population of each country
   (e) To rise in successive years in each country

4. To summarize the contrast in mortality between two countries, it is wise to use:
   (a) Infant mortality
   (b) Crude death rates
   (c) Age-specific death rates
   (d) Age-adjusted death rates

   (e) Sex-specific death rates

5. Trends in population size differ between developed and Third World countries in that:
   (a) Low death rates in developed countries cause the population to expand rapidly.
   (b) Death rates in Third World countries respond poorly to recent socioeconomic and health advances.
   (c) Immigration to Third World countries expands the size of their populations.
   (d) Populations are growing rapidly in developed countries and are contracting in the Third World.
   (e) Birth rates in most Third World countries have dropped too slowly to compensate for the falling death rates.

6. Total populations are important in setting government policy and planning health services. However, the group of most interest in describing the frequency of disease is the:
   (a) Population at risk
   (b) Young population
   (c) Population that recovers from disease
   (d) Economically productive population
   (e) High-income population

7. For all causes combined, and for most specific disease groups, death rates are lower in the married than in the single, widowed, divorced, and separated populations. One likely explanation for this is that:
   (a) Persons who marry and remain married are already more healthy than those who do not.

*The author would like to credit the original author, Charles M. Wylie, M.D., Dr.P.H., for his contributions to this chapter.

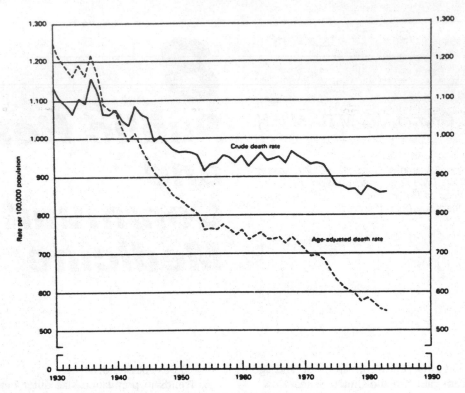

Figure 8-1. Crude and age-adjusted death rates per 100,000 U.S. population, 1930–1983. The crude rate hides part of the fall in deaths, since it does not adjust for the expanding elderly population.

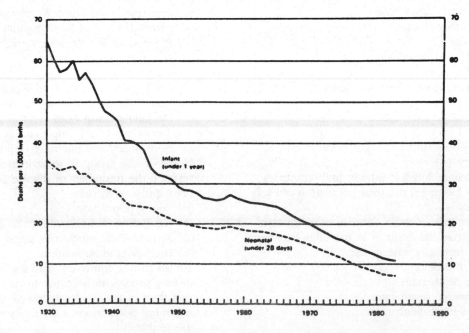

Figure 8-2. Infant and neonatal death rates per 1,000 live births in the United States, 1930–1983.

(b) Married persons take fewer risks than unmarried persons.

(c) The social stress of being married is greater than that of being single.

(d) The married population includes more women than men.

(e) The married population includes proportionately more blacks than whites.

8. When studied in the Seattle-Tacoma area in the 1970s, the frequency of prior hysterectomy was found to be much higher in married than in unmarried women. How might this finding by reasonably explained?

9. Figure 8-2 shows a falling infant mortality in the United States with passing years. A probable explanation for this fall is:

(a) Improved prenatal and infant care

(b) Advances in nutritional status

(c) Improvements in socioeconomic status

(d) Advances in infectious disease control

(e) All of the above

10. The leading causes of death in the United States have changed markedly since 1900. These changes involve:

(a) A reduction in deaths from infectious diseases

(b) A fall in deaths from noninfectious diseases

(c) A rise in the frequency of industrial accidents

(d) The less accurate reporting of causes of death

(e) The younger age of dying in recent years

11. Figure 8-3 shows time trends in the average life expectancy of newborns in the United States. This "positive" measure of health:

(a) Is determined from the death rates of the population

(b) Rises equally for males and females

(c) Falls when the population ages

(d) Is more readily calculated than death rates

(e) Reflects the frequency of both nonfatal and fatal disease

12. Name and briefly discuss two indices often used to describe the frequency of disease in a population.

13. How do the figures for incidence and prevalence relate to each other?

14. Under what circumstances is it preferable to use the prevalence ratio over the incidence rate?

15. The population at risk, the focus of many epidemiologic studies, is the population that creates the new cases of the condition being studied. If we review the phenomenon of patients leaving the hospital against medical advice (AMA), the appropriate population at risk would be:

(a) All patients discharged alive

(b) Total discharges from hospital

(c) Newborn infants

(d) All elderly patients

(e) All hospital admissions

16. A confounding variable may relate closely in time to the onset of disease but:

(a) Is not necessary for its occurrence

(b) Is one of several causal agents

(c) Is more difficult to measure than other variables

(d) Exacerbates rather than causes the disease

(e) Cannot be alleviated through disease prevention programs

17. For many diseases there is a continuum of severity. At one end of the spectrum is a mild, initial biological change; at the other is disease so advanced that it is about to cause death. Describe an important group of exceptions to this generalization.

18. What characteristic of test performance is assessed when a diagnostic test is found to be positive in only a proportion of all cases at which it aims?

19. In infectious disease epidemiology, the concept of herd immunity reflects the finding that populations:

(a) Stop spreading an infection well before 100% of individuals are immune

(b) Can be immunized by vaccines developed in animals

(c) Continue to be infectious when crowded together

(d) Receive some infectious agents from other animals

(e) Tend to panic when threatened by serious infections

20. We must often introduce disease control measures before we have complete knowledge of the cause of a disease. Give two historical examples of such situations.

21. Physical-social closeness is important in determining the frequency of:

(a) Much infectious disease

(b) Hepatitis B infection

(c) Hypertensive heart disease

(d) Cancer of the cervix

(e) Atherosclerotic heart disease

22. Keeping the frequency of illness within acceptable limits is best described as disease:

(a) Control

(b) Prevention

(c) Eradication

(d) Surveillance

(e) Treatment

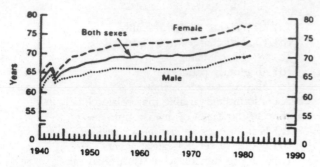

Figure 8-3. Average life expectancy in years of male and female newborns in the United States, 1940–1981. The gap between the sexes has widened with passing time.

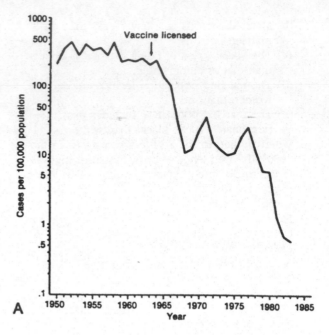

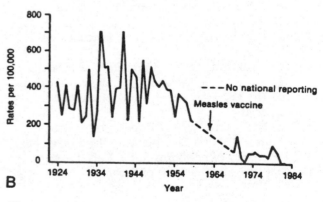

Figure 8-4. Reported new cases of measles per 100,000 population, 1950–1983 in the United States and 1924–1982 in Canada. In both countries, rates fell more steeply when immunization began in 1963.

23. Give three examples of data used in the surveillance of infectious disease in the United States.
24. Figure 8-4 shows the incidence rates of reported measles in Canada during the last six decades. From the 1920s through the 1950s, a new epidemic produced a peak about every third year. What is the best explanation of this pattern?
25. The time trends in reported measles cases showed a marked fall when the measles vaccine became available in the early 1960s (Fig. 8-4). However, lower peaks of measles outbreaks in the United States in the 1970s are best explained by what possibility?
26. How many cases of a disease are needed to produce an epidemic?
27. Infectious diseases rarely cause death in the United States but are:
    (a) A common cause of visits to physicians' offices
    (b) A frequent cause of absence from work
    (c) Acquired fairly often in patient care institutions
    (d) Often well controlled when less than 100% of the population is immunized
    (e) All of the above
28. A group of infectious diseases is transmitted through sexual contact. In the United States in the mid-1980s, the most common sexually transmitted diseases were:
    (a) Nonspecific genital infection and gonorrhea
    (b) Trichomoniasis and syphilis
    (c) Genital warts and herpes genitalis
    (d) Pelvic inflammatory disease
    (e) Acquired immunodeficiency syndrome (AIDS)
29. In an analysis of factors that seem to relate to the frequency of disease in populations, it is common to group variables under three headings. List these headings.
30. The frequency of certain disease groups relates inversely to the amounts of certain variables in the environment. Give three examples.
31. Many epidemiologic studies show a direct relationship between an outside factor and the frequency of disease. Give three such examples.
32. Prevention and treatment cannot be mutually exclusive activities. In the 1980s the priority given to prevention is:

(a) Rising partly in an effort to control costs of care
(b) Falling because consumers do not demand preventive measures
(c) Greater among men than women
(d) Rising because it increasingly appeals to practicing physicians
(e) Falling because of the high cost of most preventive measures

33. The effectiveness of maternal and child health care is partly reflected in maternal and infant mortality. The greatest single problem associated with a high risk of dying in infancy is low birth weight. List five groups of mothers who have a high risk of producing low-birth-weight infants.

34. Screening is a systematic process that separates those who probably have abnormalities from those who probably do not. In such early detection efforts, the ideal tests used should:
(a) Aim at treating disease before damage has occurred
(b) Include tests that have been useful in diagnosis
(c) Ignore screening for genetic abnormalities
(d) Focus on diseases that are rarely seen by physicians
(e) Give priority to disease that rapidly becomes symptomatic

35. Persistently elevated blood pressure is a risk factor for:
(a) Coronary heart disease
(b) Cerebrovascular disease
(c) Renal failure
(d) Congestive heart failure
(e) All of the above

36. Family planning is based on the voluntary decision and actions of persons who wish to control family size or correct infertility. In the United States:
(a) Government policy debates in the 1980s have focused strongly on family size.
(b) The public has tended to advocate one child per couple.
(c) Most wanted pregnancies are in teenagers.
(d) Fewer unintended pregnancies than average occur in low-income women.
(e) Social debates have focused more on the ethics of abortion.

37. In the late 1980s, a number of parts of the U.S. Federal Government participated in public health and environmental health services. Such agencies included:
(a) Public Health Service (PHS)
(b) Occupational Safety and Health Administration (OSHA)
(c) Environmental Protection Agency (EPA)
(d) Health Care Financing Administration (HCFA)
(e) All of the above

38. The state government is the sovereign power in the United States. In what ways, then, do federal health agencies affect the activities and decisions of state governors and state departments of health?

39. Although the United States has no reliable statistics on the incidence of occupational disease, the group that is most frequently reported is:
(a) Industrial injuries
(b) Spontaneous abortions and stillbirths
(c) Conditions caused by repeated motion
(d) Lung disease
(e) Dermatitis and other skin conditions

40. Within the U.S. Federal Government, the agencies concerned with health and industry include:
(a) Department of Labor
(b) National Institute of Occupational Safety and Health (NIOSH)
(c) Environmental Protection Agency (EPA)
(d) Occupational Safety and Health Administration (OSHA)
(e) All of the above

41. Accidents rank fourth as a cause of death in the United States in the mid-1980s. However, they could be held to be more important than that ranking because:
(a) They are the leading cause of death in persons between 1 and 43 years of age.
(b) Many accidents do not result in death but impair function.
(c) The label of accidents has included many cases of child and spouse abuse.
(d) They produce a serious socioeconomic loss, compared with disease in advanced age.
(e) All of the above

42. Some organized efforts in health are not part of government health activities. These non-governmental organizations are best described as:
(a) Voluntary health agencies
(b) Local health departments
(c) Health maintenance organizations
(d) State and local medical societies
(e) Blue Cross–Blue Shield agencies

43. Fluoridated water supplies serve about 60% of the U.S. population. Extending fluoridated water to the remaining population faces the following barriers:
(a) Community inaction
(b) Financial inability—fluoridation requires local funds

(c) Closer supervision to maintain the optimal level

(d) All of the above factors

44. Cigarette smoking has been positively associated with:

(a) Chronic bronchitis and emphysema

(b) Peripheral artery disease

(c) Retarded fetal growth

(d) Lowered resistance to infection

(e) All of the above

45. The use of tobacco, alcohol, and other drugs have pervasive effects, including:

(a) Biological consequences for the user

(b) Psychological and social effects on family members

(c) Increased risk of injury and death to both user and family

(d) Psychological and social consequences for the user

(e) All of the above

46. A large part of a person's eating habits is determined by culture. The best example of the truth of this statement in the United States is:

(a) The high prevalence of obesity

(b) The reluctance to use horse meat as food

(c) Calcium loss with osteoporosis

(d) Iron-deficiency anemia in reproductive women

(e) Elevated blood pressures in older age groups

47. Increased physical activity has been widely publicized as a preventive factor in coronary heart disease. Less well publicized has been its beneficial effect in treating:

(a) Changes associated with advancing age

(b) Higher mortality in males

(c) Depression and anxiety

(d) Diabetes insipidus

(e) Osteomalacia

48. Comprehensive programs to help persons manage stress are held to improve health. Advocates of this effort face the problem that:

(a) The scientific base for stress management is limited.

(b) Stress in large amounts may be beneficial to health.

(c) Past claims about stress management have been pessimistic.

(d) Well-controlled trials of stress management have produced conflicting results.

(e) A person's perception of stress is constant over time.

49. The social-psychological approach to health behavior suggests that a number of conditions are important in seeking and following professional advice. These factors include:

(a) The belief that the person is truly ill

(b) The belief that the illness can benefit from treatment

(c) Social approval of the patient's use of health care

(d) Willingness to overcome obstacles to health care

(e) All of the above

50. List three economic aspects in which health care differs from other goods and services.

51. A number of factors have been involved in the steep rise in the cost of health care since the 1960s in the United States. List four important factors.

52. When health insurance, Medicaid, and Medicare pay for patient care, the phenomenon is usually described as:

(a) Third-party payments

(b) Government subsidies

(c) The Robin Hood technique

(d) A national health service

(e) Social Security payments

53. The organization of health care should meet a number of desirable objectives. List four good purposes.

54. Patients using health services can be classified in different ways. For the purpose of controlling costs, the classification system used in the mid-1980s is described as:

(a) The International Classification of Diseases (ICD)

(b) Activities of daily living

(c) Diagnosis-Related Groups (DRG)

(d) The health care index

(e) All of the above

55. When steps to reduce the future cost of care are discussed, alternatives to institutional care are often mentioned. These lower cost alternatives usually include:

(a) Day hospital care

(b) Community hospice care

(c) Home-care programs

(d) Ambulatory care centers

(e) All of the above

56. The strength of the medical profession is based primarily on:

(a) The legally supported monopoly of medical practice

(b) The high prestige and incomes of physicians

(c) The ability of physicians to reach unanimous views

(d) Supporting the right political party at the right time

(e) The evident benefits from their care

57. Physicians are permitted to control their own

performance in delivering ambulatory care to private patients. In the competitive marketplace of the 1980s, however, physicians formed groups primarily to minimize charges to consumer groups. The usual term for these cost-control groups is:
(a) Group practices
(b) Local medical groups
(c) Peer review organizations
(d) Preferred-provider organizations
(e) Medical staff organizations

58. In the United States in the mid-1980s, physicians tended to monitor the quality of care given by colleagues through:
(a) Utilization review committees
(b) Health maintenance organizations
(c) Group practices
(d) Informal "colleagueal networks"
(e) All of the above mechanisms

59. Physicians behave in ways that reflect their views of the medical role. This role may change with the severity and urgency of the patient's condition. Give three examples of these changes.

60. Although physicians are classified as in abundant supply in the mid-1980s in the United States, considerable debate has been given to training a mixed group of "physician extenders." At least in theory, their shorter training results in:
(a) A lack of theory covered in their training programs
(b) A low capacity to decide about changes in treatment
(c) A continued need for supervision
(d) A focus on practice in their training programs
(e) All of the above

61. The group of "physician extenders" recently trained in the United States have included such personnel as:
(a) Licensed practical nurses
(b) Occupational therapists
(c) Physical therapy assistants
(d) Respiratory therapists
(e) Physician assistants

62. A Type I error, or alpha (α) error, is:
(a) A false-positive
(b) A false-negative
(c) Both A and B
(d) Neither A or B

63. The characteristic that is unique to randomization is:
(a) Equal chance
(b) Unpredictability
(c) Haphazardness
(d) Blocking

64. Usually the most important factor in the success of funding and carrying out a large multicenter clinical trial is:
(a) Complexity
(b) Population to be studied
(c) Type I error probabilities
(d) Significance of the question

65. The WHO definition of health is:
(a) The absence of disease
(b) The ability to function free of pain
(c) A state of complete physical, mental, and social well-being
(d) Living to one estimated life expectancy

66. What estimated percentage of deaths in the United States are autopsied?
(a) 80%
(b) 10%
(c) 25%
(d) 33%

67. Which statement best describes what an incidence rate is:
(a) The number of new cases of disease that occur during a prespecified interval of time
(b) The number of numerator of cases in the population
(c) The case occurrence at one point in time
(d) The amount of disease that occurs in the population in a "snapshot" survey

68. What is the most appropriate parameter for examining secular changes in death rates in a population?
(a) Crude death rate
(b) Prevalence ratio
(c) Incidence rate
(d) Age-adjusted death rates

69. Which statement is valid concerning life-expectancy at birth in the United States since 1970?
(a) Life expectancy has gone down primarily because of increased AIDS and cancer incidence.
(b) Life expectancy has slowly risen since the 1970s in both whites and blacks.
(c) The prospective study of populations shows a decrease in neonatal care in the United States.
(d) Life expectancy has increased in recent years because of progress in treating and preventing infectious diseases.

70. Epidemiology as a science is defined as the:
(a) Study of dermatologic diseases
(b) Study of cases versus matched controls in defined groups
(c) Prospective study of populations
(d) Study of disease as it manifests itself in the population

71. The "gold standard" for evaluating the effectiveness of new treatments is:
    (a) The clinical trial
    (b) Prospective observational studies
    (c) Treatments using historical controls
    (d) Case-control studies

72. The type of study that gains statistical power by pooling the results of several different similar studies is called:
    (a) Multivariate analysis
    (b) Multicenter clinical trial
    (c) Meta-analysis
    (d) Analysis of variance

73. *Independence,* one of the epidemiologic criteria inferring causation:
    (a) Means that the suspected causal factor always precedes the onset of the disease
    (b) Means that the suspected factor is working directly to influence the disease
    (c) Means other fields of scientific investigation
    (d) Means that there is a biologically plausible explanation about how the factor might cause the disease

74. The predictive value of a new diagnostic test is defined as:
    (a) The number of positive tests in the population
    (b) The number of true-positives in the population
    (c) The ratio of true-negatives to true positives
    (d) The percentage of true-positives of all positives (true-positives and false-positives)

75. Specificity is best defined as follows:
    (a) The ratio of true negatives to true-negatives and false-positives
    (b) The predictive value of the test
    (c) The reciprocal of the sensitivity
    (d) All of the above

76. Which of the following best describes the term *null hypothesis?*
    (a) It is the same as a Type I error.
    (b) The hypothesis that a new treatment is better than a placebo or established treatment
    (c) The chance of not making a Type II error
    (d) The hypothesis that a new treatment and placebo or established treatment are no different

77. Which of the following are important in establishing the power of a study?
    (a) Sample size
    (b) Treatment effect
    (c) Accuracy and precision of study measurements
    (d) All of the above

78. How can one minimize or eliminate regression to the mean in carrying out studies?
    (a) Use a cutpoint to select patients that is considerably below the mean to the population
    (b) Carrying out multiple measures over time and averaging those measures
    (c) Careful training of observers taking the measurements
    (d) Entering only those patients into a study with high values

79. Which of the following measures of blood pressure is most closely related to disease outcomes such as coronary heart disease and stroke?
    (a) Diastolic pressure
    (b) Mean blood pressure
    (c) Systolic blood pressure
    (d) Postural hypotension

80. Which of the following best describes the recent results of meta-analysis concerning whether lowering blood pressure with drugs prevents coronary heart disease and stroke?
    (a) Lowering blood pressure with active drugs in the major trials clearly reduced stroke and CHD at the levels predicted according to the observational study data.
    (b) Active drug therapy reduced diastolic pressure by 5–6 mmHg compared to controls, and reduced CHD but not stroke.
    (c) Active drug therapy did not reduce blood pressure to significant levels.
    (d) Active drug treatment prevented stroke (~ 40% reduction) but only prevented CHD at approximately two thirds of the levels predicted.

A N S W E R S

1. The crude death rate is falling in a population that is becoming older. When the death rate is adjusted for the increasing age, the fall in death rate steepens to cause a progressively wider gap. In Figure 8-1, the age-adjusted rate has been calculated by application of the most recent age-specific death rates to the population of the United States as it was in 1940, when the observed crude and calculated age-adjusted rates were identical.

2. **e** In the mid-1980s, age-adjusted death rates for diabetes mellitus were about the same for men as for women. In previous decades, diabetes mellitus caused higher death rates for women than for men, partly because of the biological stress of pregnancy.

3. **d** The crude death rate for the United States is relatively high because of this country's large elderly population; most developing countries have a younger average age. However, most developing countries also have counts of total deaths each year and of population size. These counts allow calculation of the crude death rate, which includes all infant deaths, which has tended to fall in successive years because of improvements in environmental control, nutrition, and preventive health services.

4. **d** Age-adjusted death rates are calculated so that they correct for the different age distributions of the populations. Thus, the large elderly population of a developed country would not adversely affect a comparison with the younger population of a Third World country. Crude death rates are not comparable because of such age differences. Infant immortality rates would show differences in death rates only in the first year of life. Age-specific death rates also show the mortality of limited age groups. Sex-specific death rates need further adjustment for the different age distributions of each sex.

5. **e** Third World countries do have falling death rates, reflecting recent socioeconomic and health advances. However, family planning activities have not been sufficient to produce a corresponding fall in birth rates. Thus, the populations of most Third World countries continue to grow, while those of most developed countries are stationary or grow slowly.

6. **a** The *population at risk* is the population with a reasonable chance of developing a disease. Thus, females would be excluded from the denominator of a rate that describes the frequency of cancer of the prostate.

7. **a** It is thought that married persons are more healthy than unmarried persons, although it must still be proved definitively. Also needing more study is the possibility that being married promotes health. Current values and perhaps even wishful thinking affect the debate on this explanation.

8. Some married women may request hysterectomy to prevent future pregnancy. Furthermore, conditions provoked by pregnancy may be treated by hysterectomy. Married women in the United States visit physicians more often than unmarried women of the same age, raising their risk of being advised to have a hysterectomy. Most unlikely is the possibility that women with hysterectomies are more liable to get married than women without hysterectomies.

9. **e** Many factors contribute to the falling infant mortality, which cannot be attributed only to improved health care.

10. **a** Tuberculosis, influenza and pneumonia, and childhood infections are all more effectively prevented and treated now than in the past. An increasing number of deaths, therefore, have been attributed to long-term noninfectious diseases. Meanwhile, deaths from industrial accidents have much diminished, and death occurs at an older average age. The reporting of causes of death has also changed; most changes have probably resulted in greater accuracy in recent decades.

11. **a** Average life expectancy at birth is inversely related to the populations's death rate—the lower the death rate, the longer the survival. The death rate has fallen more for women than men, so life expectancy has also risen more for women than for men. These trends slowly broaden the gap between the sexes in Figure 8-3.

12. The *incidence rate* is usually calculated as the number of new cases of a disease occurring annually per 100,000 population at risk. The *prevalence ratio* is usually calculated as the number of cases of disease present at one moment in time per 100,000 population at risk.

13. The longer the average duration of illness, the greater the number of cases to be found at any one moment. The relationship can be summarized as follows:

Prevalence ratio = Annual incidence rate
× Average duration in years

Thus, if the average duration of an illness is 5 weeks (one tenth of a year), we would find an incidence rate ten times that of the prevalence ratio. A high prevalence ratio may reflect a high incidence rate, a long duration of illness, or both. Moreover, when you know two of these variables, you can calculate the third.

14. When an illness is rare but lasts a long time, the prevalence ratio is the larger and more easily understood number. For example, most studies of multiple sclerosis use prevalence ratios rather than incidence rates, since the frequency of new cases is small. In contrast, incidence rates are more useful in studying short-term illness, which lasts only days or weeks. Particularly in a study of the effects of preventive measures, incidence rates change more swiftly than prevalence ratios. Thus, the effect of the polio vaccines in the 1950s was best reflected by the rapid fall in new cases of poliomyelitis, and only slowly lowered the prevalence of paralytic poliomyelitis in the population. Most polio cases paralyzed in 1949 were still paralyzed and counted for the prevalence ratio in 1956; prevalence was still high in 1956, even though the polio vaccine had much reduced new cases and lowered incidence.

15. a Patients who die in the hospital cannot decide to leave AMA, nor can newborns. Elderly patients include a higher-than-average proportion who die. Decisions about leaving AMA are made close to discharge, not at the time of admission. Thus, live discharges form the population that is at risk of leaving AMA.

16. a For example, many lung cancer patients may consume alcohol, but alcohol is a confounding variable, not necessary for lung cancer to occur.

17. Genetic disease with high penetrance, such as achondroplasia, is described as either present or absent and cannot be placed along a continuum of severity.

18. *Validity* is the term given to the characteristic described. In the test for diabetes mellitus, for example, the postprandial blood sugar level has high validity, while the urine sugar level has low validity, being negative in many newly developing diabetics.

19. a The phenomenon of herd immunity makes it unnecessary to have 100% participation in some immunization programs. The proportion needed to produce herd immunity varies with the infectivity of the agent, and with the size and social behavior of the community.

20. In 1798 Jenner introduced vaccination against cowpox to reduce the incidence of smallpox, without knowing that these conditions were caused by separate but related viruses. In the 1840s Snow re-

moved the handle of a pump that gave contaminated water in Broad Street, London, long before the organism causing water-borne cholera had been isolated. In 1861 Semmelweis required medical students to wash their hands in chlorinated water before visiting women in labor, without knowing that puerperal fever was caused by organisms that the students gathered from infected patients.

21. a Physical-social closeness is important in direct person-to-person spread of disease. When one case of an infection such as tuberculosis occurs, the search for new cases should focus first on household contacts.

22. a Prevention, eradication, surveillance, and treatment are all part of disease control. Prevention involves avoiding the occurrence of disease. Eradication ensures that the disease will no longer occur, now or in the future. Surveillance involves collecting, analyzing, and distributing data about the disease, followed by the stimulation of appropriate control activities. Through appropriate treatment, we speed recovery from curable disease and reduce the spread of infectious disease.

23. Morbidity data arise from the reports of cases seen by practicing physicians; these data are usually seriously underreported. Field data come from the investigation of epidemics, such as outbreaks of food poisoning. Laboratory data, showing an unusual frequency of positive tests such as cultures, may give the first indication of an abnormal outbreak. Special survey data, such as the results of tuberculin testing of hospital workers, may also indicate unexpected cases before they become symptomatic.

24. It took about 3 years to develop a new population of susceptible individuals. This population consisted of newborns and immigrants from other countries.

25. The measles vaccination was not sufficiently intense to reach the level of herd immunity.

26. *Epidemic* is a relative term, depending on what is expected as the usual number. We use past data to determine the approximate expected numbers. When the observed, real-life number is markedly higher than expected, the word *epidemic* is often used. These criteria change over time. Thus, an epidemic of tuberculosis in 1986 is a much smaller outbreak than in 1886.

27. e Short-term infections still cause many physician visits and absences from work. The low resistance of many inpatients in hospitals results in nosocomial infections. When an immunizing agent is available, spread is stopped before 100% of the population is immunized.

28. **a** Pelvic inflammatory disease is usually a complication of the more common gonorrhea. AIDS is widely publicized but is less frequent than the other conditions.

29. Either Host, Agent, Environment, or Time, Place, Person is correct. The latter triad is used when multiple factors play a part in causation, so no single agent is present. This is primarily the case with major noninfectious diseases, such as coronary artery disease and hypertension.

30. Within limits the following are inversely related: fluoride in the water and dental caries; physical activity and coronary artery disease; ascorbic acid and scurvy; insecticide use and malaria; dietary iron and iron deficiency anemia; number of pregnancies and breast cancer. Whenever these inverse relationships are found, their possible use in disease prevention is worth considering.

31. Well-known examples include cigarette smoking and lung cancer, sunlight and skin cancer, psychosocial stress and blood pressure levels, and sexual intercourse and cancer of the cervix. Particularly when studies show this direct dose-response relationship, we become certain that control or eradication of the causal agent is needed for health promotion and disease control.

32. **a** The high cost of treatment services in the 1980s has stimulated politicians and consumers to support more preventive measures. However, in the United States women tend to use more preventive services than men. Although most preventive techniques are inexpensive, the practicing physician gets less feedback from recipients of preventive care than when symptoms are relieved or disease is cured.

33. High-risk groups include mothers who are unusually young or elderly, of minority status, of high parity, of low socioeconomic status, or of nutritional status; who are cigarette smokers, alcohol abusers, or drug abusers; or who are late in seeking prenatal care. These groups need special help and advice during prenatal care.

34. **a** Screening implies early detection. It is most valuable when it leads to rapid diagnosis and prompt treatment while disease is still symptomatic. Many tests used in diagnosis are too uncomfortable or expensive to be used to screen large populations that are free of symptoms. Fetal screening and prenatal diagnosis now help reduce the frequency of genetic disease; however, the controversial step of abortion is the sole method of preventing the birth of the genetically impaired infant. Screening should focus on diseases that are fairly common and that have a long asymptomatic period during which patients would not seek physician care.

35. **e** When elevated blood pressures are detected early and treated well, death rates fall for all of the conditions listed. Thus, when death rates are adjusted for the advancing age of the population, they are seen to have been falling in the United States since the 1970s.

36. **e** The federal government and public discussions do not press strongly for an optimum family size. Teenagers and low-income women have the highest proportion of unwanted pregnancies; they need high priority in receiving prompt obstetric care and family planning advice.

37. **e** The PHS is the principal federal agency concerned with public health. In contrast, HCFA has the largest budget, since it is responsible for the high-cost personal health services delivered through Medicare and through the federal portion of Medicaid. The federal government's main focus on the general and industrial environments is through OSHA and the EPA. Many health activities remain in other departments of the national government, whose organization has changed often in recent years.

38. This is done primarily through the financial strength of the federal government, which subsidizes and gives grant-in-aid to support state health activities that are approved at the federal level. Thus, through the federal income tax, some state priorities have been shaped by federal funding. Federal grants also permit low-income states to have stronger health services than they could support on their own, helping equalize access to personal and environmental health services.

39. **e** Conditions caused by the effect of industrial agents on the skin form the most commonly reported group of occupational diseases.

40. **e** The different agencies focus on different aspects of health and industry. Thus, NIOSH performs research and recommends standards for toxic substances used in industry, OSHA promulgates the standards and inspects industries to ensure compliance, and EPA focuses on the effect of industry on the surrounding environment.

41. **e** Accident prevention and injury control have received greater attention since the 1960s than in previous decades.

42. **a** Voluntary health agencies are formed by members who want to pursue a common interest in health. Membership is voluntary (not compulsory) and the agency's policy is basically independent of government. To expand activities, however, some voluntary health agencies apply for and accept government funds as long as the funding purpose is compatible with the goals of the agency.

43. **d**

44. **e**
45. **e**
46. **b**
47. **c** There is evidence that exercise helps treat depression and anxiety. Exercise has little or no effect on changes with age, male mortality, diabetes insipidus, or osteomalacia. However, exercise plays a part in treating diabetes mellitus, osteoporosis, and obesity.
48. **a** Limited amounts of stress may benefit health, but the amount varies from person to person and for the same individual at different times. Claims about the value of stress management have erred on the side of optimism, and there is no well-controlled trial of stress management in humans.
49. **e** In addition, the patient must be willing to follow professional advice. It becomes clear that conveying information about health and disease is not sufficient to ensure appropriate use of health services, including use of preventive services.
50. Some health services produce "external benefits," helping society as well as the individual who receives the service. Improved health can be regarded as an "investment good," in which resources used now are returned with interest through raised future productivity. Certain health services are of a "collective nature"; when used by one person, such as drinking fluoridated water, an abundance remains for all other consumers. However, other health services form a "consumption commodity"; a sudden rise in the use of institutional care makes hospital beds less available to others.
51. Hospitals have changed from low-wage institutions before World War II to competitive-wage institutions. Each scientific advance tends to raise the complexity and cost of care. Moreover, considering the rapidly expanded number of physicians and other providers, health services have not raised their productivity as fast as has the economy at large. Finally, educational and training programs for providers have increasingly been financed by additions to patient-care charges.
52. **a** The first and second parties are regarded as the client and provider, with a third party paying for the service. Medicare and Medicaid are sometimes viewed as government subsidies, but many health insurance programs are not. Health insurance does not steal from the rich to pay the poor, as implied by the term *Robin Hood*. A national health service involves government administration of the health services, not only payment for them. Finally, Social Security forms the background for the Medicare program, but not for Medicaid or health insurance.
53. Health services should be readily accessible, adequate in quantity, and comprehensive enough to cover the range of needed care. They should be effective in reaching their stated goal, efficient in reaching goals with reasonable economy, and of good quality, satisfying consumers as well as providers.
54. **c** DRGs are based partly on the principal diagnosis, complications, patient age, and treatment procedures used. This system is used primarily to control costs in Medicare and Medicaid programs in the United States. In contrast, the ICD (or its adaptations) is used worldwide to classify patients and those who die by their most important diagnosis. Some measures of performance of activities of daily living are used to assess response to treatment and rehabilitative care.
55. **e** For patients who are appropriately selected, each activity is a possible alternative to institutional care.
56. **a** In every area of the United States, state laws give physicians a monopoly in delivering medical care. However, if physician care did not produce good results in general, consumers would elect politicians who could change these laws and cancel the monopoly.
57. **d** Preferred-provider organizations are formed to negotiate agreed low charges to consumer groups. In the mid-1980s, however, there was no clear knowledge of the effect of such economy measures on the quality of care.
58. **e** All of the efforts listed permit physicians to observe one another's performance. Probably the oldest and least formal is the "colleagueal network," in which physicians refer patients to colleagues whom they most respect. Consumer and government dissatisfaction with this intangible effort have speeded the formation of more organized efforts.
59. In treating a critically ill patient, the physician can rely on biological and technical skills and may ignore that the patient is passive. In less desperate situations, the physician guides while the patient cooperates; the latter knows what goes on and exercises some judgment. A third relationship is that of mutual participation, whereby the physician helps the patient help himself or herself; this is particularly useful in cases of chronic disease and disability. Finally, some patients undertake self-care for less serious conditions and use the physician as an occasional consultant; patients guide themselves while the physician cooperates.
60. **e** Most groups who undergo shorter training programs cover the practical aspects of care and have weak education in the theoretical knowledge that helps with diagnosis and treatment changes. Nevertheless, they do gain further knowledge through

delivering patient care. In some studies of long-term care, the shorter trained personnel have been viewed by patients as giving care of high quality, difficult to differentiate from the care given by physicians.

61. **e** Choices a through d cover areas that differ from medical care as supplied by physicians.

62. **a** Two types of errors are possible when carrying out an experiment. A Type I error, or alpha error, refers to a false-positive result. In other words, the study indicates statistical benefit for the treatment ($p < .05$) even though truly the treatment has no effect. A Type II error, or beta error, refers to a false negative result.

63. **b** The characteristic that is unique to randomization is unpredictability. Although with randomization allocation of subjects is usually done equally to study groups, a larger number may be randomized to one group versus the others. Blocking is a method to ensure that the appropriate numbers are distributed across study groups.

64. **d** Because large multicenter clinical trials are very expensive, usually only questions of high medical and social significance are studied. Example: Drug treatment of isolated systolic hypertension (ISH) affects more than 3 million older Americans and benefit of drug treatment was highly controversial. A trial Systolic Hypertension in the Elderly Program (SHEP) was carried out, comparing active drug treatment to placebo to prevent total stroke. This study had great significance, its objective being to establish solidly the benefit of active drug therapy.

65. **c** The WHO defined *healthy* in 1948 as a state of complete physical, mental, and social well being.

66. **b** In the 1990s only about 10% of deaths are autopsied and this percentage has been steadily decreasing in recent years.

67. **a** The incidence rate is the occurrence of disease during a prespecified interval of time in a population. The prevalence ratio is the number of cases of disease that occur in the population at one point or cross section in time, also referred to as a "snapshot." Both incidence rates and prevalence are expressed as the number of cases per 100,000 population.

68. **d** The most appropriate parameter for examining secular change in death rates over time in a population is age-adjusted death rates. Crude death rates are greatly influenced by the proportion of elderly in the population and by other factors such as gender, race, and socioeconomic factors.

69. **b** Life expectancy at birth has slowly risen since 1970 in the United States in all races and in men and women, but the increases has been greatest in women and whites.

70. **d** Epidemiology as a science can be defined as the study of disease as it manifests itself in a population. Epidemiology involves study of disease (cases) in relation to normals, without disease (the former making up the numerator, the latter the denominator, in mathematical comparisons).

71. **a** The clinical trial is considered the "gold standard" for evaluation of the effectiveness of new treatments. Observational studies and in establishing factors or exposures that place individuals at higher risk of disease. Case-control studies are helpful in generating causal hypotheses. Studies using historical control are frequently biased and are almost always overly optimistic about the value of new treatments.

72. **c** Meta-analysis examines specific scientific questions by pooling the results of several studies. The posted data set is much larger and more powerful. Meta-analysis will often allow a more confident estimate of the benefit (or lack of benefit) of a treatment.

73. **b** Independence means that the factor is directly related to the disease and is not confounded by some other factor that is more directly related.

74. **d** The predictive value of a test is the number of true-positives of all positives.

$$\frac{\text{True-positives}}{\text{True-positives and False-positives}}$$

The higher the proportion of true-positives, the greater the predictive value of the test.

75. **a** Specificity is defined as the ratio of true-negatives to true-negatives plus false-positives. Sensitivity is the ratio of true-positives to true-positives plus false-negatives. Generally, as the specificity of a test increases, the sensitivity will decrease, and vice versa.

76. **d** The null hypothesis is the statement that a new treatment is no different from placebo or established therapy. The alternative hypothesis states that the treatments are different.

77. **d** The answer is all of the above—larger sample size, larger treatment effect, and low variability of measurements will all increase the study's power.

78. **b** *Regression to the mean* is the tendency for measures or values that were initially selected in persons above or below the mean of the group to become more like the mean of the group on subsequent measures. A means to minimize regression to the mean includes doing multiple measures over time and averaging the measure.

79. **c** Epidemiologic data indicates that although diastolic pressure is independently associated with risk of CHD and stroke, systolic pressure is more strongly associated with these diseases.

80. **d** On pooling results of 14 unconfounded randomized trials, meta-analysis indicated that a reduction in 5 to 6 mmHg in diastolic pressure resulted in an estimated 42% reduction in stroke and a 14% reduction in CHD. The predicted reduction in stroke was 35% to 40% and in CHD, 20% to 25%. Therefore, CHD reduction was only about one half to two thirds of that predicted by observational studies.

Rypins' Questions & Answers for Basic Sciences Review, Second Edition, edited by Edward D. Frohlich. J. B. Lippincott Company, Philadelphia © 1993.

C H A P T E R

9
Behavioral Sciences

Ronald S. Krug, Ph.D.

David Ross Boyd Professor and Interim Chairman, Department of Psychiatry and Behavioral Sciences, University of Oklahoma Health Sciences Center

QUESTIONS

Directions. Choose the best answer.

1. Which of the following statements concerning mental abilities and aging is correct?
   (a) Both verbal and performance abilities remain intact.
   (b) Memory for recent events is less susceptible to interference than is memory for remote events.
   (c) Reaction time is slower with aging.
   (d) New learning is easier than old learning.
   (e) Both verbal and performance abilities decline.

2. Of the U.S. population 65 years of age or older:
   (a) 15% to 25% are in total care residential institutions.
   (b) 50% to 60% live alone.
   (c) 70% of males are sexually active.
   (d) 30% to 40% need significant assistance in their homes.
   (e) 90% to 95% have at least one chronic medical condition.

3. In the control of aggression, which of the following is not indicated?
   (a) Specifically teach stress coping skills
   (b) Positively reinforce nonaggresive behavior
   (c) Teach people to avoid frustrating situations
   (d) Decrease alcohol consumption
   (e) Aversive reinforcement of aggressive behavior

4. Which of the following is the best indicator of high suicide risk?
   (a) Female
   (b) Married
   (c) Non-Caucasian
   (d) 31 years old
   (e) Live alone

5. Regarding the human sexual response, which of the following statements is *incorrect*?
   (a) Thrusting preferences at orgasm are different in the majority of males and females.
   (b) The sympathetic-center firing rate is 0.8 per second for both males and females.
   (c) Ejaculation in males is equivalent to orgasm in females.
   (d) Vaginal lubrication in the female is the equivalent of erection in the male.
   (e) The refractory phase prevents males from being multiply orgasmic.

Questions 6–10

Mr. Ralph Smithers, age 37, and his wife Joan, age 33, have lived together for 18 years. They have two children: Gary, age 13, and June, age 12. They moved to the city in which you are practicing 1 year ago and you have been treating the family for 6 months.

Joan Smithers called Monday morning for an appointment that afternoon, but you could not see her until Wednesday. She refused to tell your receptionist her reason for the appointment, but your receptionist indicates she sounded "upset."

Mrs. Smithers gives both subjective and objective evidence for anxiety and anger, and there is congruence established. She tells you she walked into her son's room Sunday evening and found him "playing with himself."

6. Your initial response should be:
   (a) Explain that this is normal 13-year-old behavior.
   (b) Ask what she means by "playing with himself."
   (c) Encourage her to talk about her feelings regarding this.
   (d) Indicate your willingness to talk with her son about his behavior.
   (e) Arrange an appointment between her and her husband to plan alternate strategies.

7. Because you handled the above situation appropriately, Mrs. Smithers sets an appointment with you for her "annual pelvic." After you talk with her in your office, she accompanies your nurse to the examination room and changes her clothes to a drape, and you assist her into the stirrups. Upon attempting to insert your finger into the vaginal canal, you find the opening is too constricted to allow entrance. Your symptom diagnosis of this condition is:
   (a) Dyspareunia
   (b) Vaginismus
   (c) Frigidity
   (d) Penis phobia
   (e) Turner's syndrome

8. The problem is resolved. Two years later, the son, Gary, appears for a school physical. You have not seen Gary before. In the interview your impression is that he is intellectually "dull." His attention span is short, and he laughs and angers very easily and somewhat extremely. Physical examination reveals pubescent breasts and testicles that are underdeveloped. Your diagnostic impression is:
   (a) XYY syndrome
   (b) Down's syndrome
   (c) Klinefelter's syndrome
   (d) Testicular feminization syndrome
   (e) Turner's syndrome

9. Mrs. Smithers and June (the daughter), now 14, have been in the waiting room while you examined Gary. As you and Gary enter the waiting room, June asks to speak with you for a minute. You agree and in your office she asks when she will begin her "period." Your response should be:
   (a) "Any day now."
   (b) "Are you sexually active?"

   (c) "You seem to be concerned about something."
   (d) "Hasn't your mother talked to you about this?"
   (e) "Why are you asking?"

10. You set up an appointment for June, and with completion of the workup, among other things, you know she has no ovarian tubes or uterus. Your best diagnostic syndrome impression is:
    (a) Turner's syndrome
    (b) Down's syndrome
    (c) XYY syndrome
    (d) Klinefelter's syndrome
    (e) Testicular feminization syndrome

Questions 11–22

11. Countertransference is defined as:
    (a) Feeling responses by the physician in response to patient behaviors
    (b) Feeling responses on the part of the patient in response to physician behavior
    (c) Feelings within either the patient or the physician that mimic the feelings displayed by the other
    (d) Feelings displaced by the patient from important people in the past onto the physician
    (e) Feelings displaced from important people in the past by the physician onto his patients

12. The longitudinal research approach is characterized by:
    (a) The same group of children being studied over extended periods of time
    (b) Different groups of individuals being studied over extended periods of time
    (c) Children being studied at different intervals throughout their life cycle
    (d) Groups of children of overlapping ages being tested periodically on similar dimensions
    (e) Different dimensions of behavior being examined at different stages of development to determine short-range effects of longitudinal analysis

13. Which of the following is *not* a warning sign of child abuse in parents?
    (a) Appearance of abusing drugs and alcohol
    (b) A fear of losing control in discipline
    (c) Feeling that the child is purposely frustrating the parent
    (d) Low developmental expectations for the child
    (e) Few social contacts and activities

14. In a normal developmental picture within the Freudian-Eriksonian framework, a 5-year-old child would most likely be focused on which of the following areas?

(a) Trust and oral themes

(b) Autonomy and anal themes

(c) Mastery and anal themes

(d) Phallic and initiative themes

(e) Generativity and phallic themes

15. Gender identity is best defined as:

(a) The appearance of the genitalia as a man or woman

(b) The orientation toward homosexuality or heterosexuality

(c) The individual's preference for aggressive, active behaviors or passive, dependent behaviors

(d) The individual's belief and feeling that he or she is male or female

(e) Masculinization or feminization resulting from hormonal determinants

16. By repeated exposures to a physician in a white coat followed by an inoculation or injection, a child learns to cry and withdraw in response to the physician alone. This example is likely an illustration of:

(a) Reflexive behavior

(b) Classical conditioning

(c) Imprinting

(d) Shaping

(e) Instrumental conditioning

17. A parent spanks a child when the child runs amok in the house. The frequency of the behavior increases despite the spankings. Spankings are likely functioning as:

(a) Punishing stimuli

(b) Aversive stimuli

(c) Unconditional stimuli

(d) A positive reinforcer

(e) A primary reinforcer

18. Approximately what proportion of IQ scores fall between +1 standard deviation and –1 standard deviation on the normal curve?

(a) 62%

(b) 65%

(c) 68%

(d) 71%

(e) 74%

19. Mild mental retardation is associated with which of the following IQ scores?

(a) Below 20

(b) 20 to 34

(c) 35 to 49

(d) 50 to 70

(e) 71 to 86

20. A person who is mentally retarded is considered educable if he or she has an IQ of:

(a) 38

(b) 41

(c) 44

(d) 47

(e) 50

21. You pick up a 9-month-old infant and carry it to your operating room. It begins to cry as you carry it. This is an example of:

(a) Stranger anxiety

(b) Separation anxiety

(c) Both

(d) Neither

22. Which of the following disorders of consciousness is *least likely* to be identified even by a trained observer?

(a) Fugue

(b) Stupor

(c) Somnambulism

(d) Delirium

(e) Twilight state

Directions. Each group of questions consists of several lettered headings followed by a list of numbered statements. Select the one lettered heading that is most closely associated with each statement.

Questions 23–25

(a) Pharmacological and biochemical cellular effect, demonstrable on abrupt withdrawal

(b) Psychological compulsive use

(c) Same dose produces decreased effect

(d) Probably a function of impaired metabolism in the liver

23. Habituation

24. Dependence

25. Tolerance

Questions 26–29

The normal grief and bereavement process is expressed differently by different age groups. Match the age group with the expected reaction:

(a) Antisocial behavior

(b) Marasmus

(c) Hypochondriasis

(d) Social withdrawal

(e) Laughing/hypomania

26. Children

27. Infants

28. Elderly

29. Adults

Questions 30–32

A patient, Sam, has lost his wife, Mary. Match the stage of normal grief and bereavement with the statement most characteristic of that stage.

(a) "I'm drinking six or seven highballs a night."
(b) "Yes, doctor, but don't you think a sleeping pill will help Mary get more rest?"
(c) "Doctor, I have these headaches that simply won't go away."
(d) "I've been sad now for a year and a half."
(e) "I take flowers to Mary's grave each Memorial Day."

30. Stage I
31. Stage II
32. Stage III

Questions 33–36

Assume you have told a patient he has a terminal carcinoma from which there is minimal hope of survival. Match the patient's statement (verbal or nonverbal) with the stage:

(a) "Why couldn't it have been my alcoholic brother?"
(b) "But I'm still a medical student."
(c) Upon your entering the room, the patient is sitting in a chair with hands folded comfortably across the stomach.
(d) "Just keep me alive long enough to make a will."
(e) "Okay, I'll do whatever you want me to do."

33. Stage I
34. Stage III
35. Stage IV
36. Stage V

Questions 37–39

(a) Transsexuality
(b) Tranvestism
(c) Homosexuality
(d) Heterosexuality
(e) Klinefelter's syndrome

37. Mr. B, a 33-year-old white male, requests transsexual surgery. He relates a history of having been involved in a relationship with another man for seven years. He cross-dresses and wants to legally marry his lover.
38. Ms. C, a 37-year-old white female, requests sex

change surgery. She has worn pantsuits since late adolescence, preferring jeans and denim shirts. She has had sexual intercourse but usually relates to men as "buddies." She states that she has always felt like a man rather than a woman.
39. Mr. D, a "limp-wristed," effeminate, 24-year-old male, requests sex change surgery. While in the Navy he was on a nuclear submarine and became involved as a passive partner in anal intercourse for 9 months. He reached orgasm and ejaculation during these experiences. He had no homosexual experiences before the Navy but has been exclusively heterosexual since.

Questions 40–44

Consider the usual stages of awareness and response in a dying patient and match the following. The statements are made sequentially over several days by a 45-year-old man who has lung cancer with widespread metastases.

(a) "Doc, there's gotta be some way that you can keep me going long enough to see my youngest graduate from high school."
(b) "I'm so depressed I can hardly stand it. Sometimes I even find myself wondering if I'm being punished for something."
(c) "I think the docs have it all wrong. There really isn't that much wrong with me."
(d) "Well, I'm grateful to my family and my friends for all the good times we've had."
(e) "Damn it, I don't know why this kind of thing couldn't be prevented or at least found sooner when something could be done about it."

40. Statement from first phase
41. Statement from second phase
42. Statement from third phase
43. Statement from fourth phase
44. Statement from fifth phase

Questions 45–47

(a) Anxiety–fear
(b) Anger–disgust
(c) Sadness–sorrow
(d) All of the above
(e) None of the above

45. Usually linked to the affect grief
46. An emotion directed at an object with the aim of its destruction, perhaps by incorporation
47. Usually triggered by the psychological stress of threat of injury, real or imagined

Questions 48–49

A health professional asks each of his adult patients the opening question. "What brings you to see me?" The patient's immediate verbal and nonverbal responses are noted.

(a) Subjective evidence for anxiety
(b) Subjective evidence for anger
(c) Subjective evidence for sadness
(d) Objective evidence for anxiety
(e) Objective evidence for anger

48. The patient shifts in her chair, arches her eyebrows slightly, licks her lips, and says, "Well, actually, there is nothing in particular bothering me. I just believe in having a medical checkup every 6 months or so." She smiles.
49. The patient sits quietly in the chair and replies in an even-toned voice, "I'm surprised you asked that. I always think it's so obvious. I am trembly and shaky. I think everyone notices."

Questions 50–52

A health professional asks each of his adult patients the opening question, "What brings you to see me?" The patient's immediate verbal and nonverbal responses are noted.

(a) Objective evidence for sadness
(b) Subjective and objective evidence for anxiety
(c) Subjective and objective evidence for anger
(d) Subjective and objective evidence for sadness
(e) No convincing evidence, subject or objective, for any of the above emotions.

50. The patient listens intently to the question, with head cocked slightly to the side. He nods and replies, "I've just moved into town. I've had diabetes since I was a young child. You've been recommended to me. I'm hoping you will accept me as your patient." He hands a folder of medical records to the physician.
51. The patient frowns, his masseters tense, and he says almost explosively, "Well, I'll tell you if you give me a chance." His voice softens, "Doc, I'm sorry. Actually I guess that's why I'm here. I blow up at the least little thing lately and that is really unlike me."
52. At the end of a deep sigh, the patient says, "I just have to talk to someone. I've just received this disappointing letter from my son. He's in college. Well, it's actually more than that. When I read it, I cried and cried. He says he's never coming home again and I just don't know what to do." Tears swell in the patient's eyes. Her fist tightly clenches a handkerchief.

Questions 53–57

(a) Approach–approach conflict
(b) Avoidance–avoidance conflict
(c) Approach–avoidance conflict
(d) Insight
(e) None of the above

53. A second-year medical student says to his personal physician, "I began coughing up blood three months ago, and it's gotten worse every day."
54. In a conversation between a faculty member and his living partner, the faculty member says, "Sunday let's go to your parents' home for dinner." The partner replies, "That's great!"
55. A first-year medical student says to her living partner, "Stop treating me like your mother."
56. A third-year medical student talking to her living partner on Monday morning says, "I have to take those damned National Board Exams today."
57. A fourth-year medical student talking to his advisor says, "Pediatrics is a very attractive specialty, but I really like the hours that radiologists have."

Questions 58–61

(a) Generalization
(b) Discrimination
(c) Extinction
(d) Primary reinforcement
(e) Satiation

58. An adolescent male is very aggressive at school, although at home no aggressive behavior is reported.
59. Food is used to increase cooperative play between children.
60. A person has an automobile accident and now refuses to enter a bus, train, or plane.
61. A person has an accident while horseback riding and begins to avoid horses. The physician recommends that the person ride as much as possible so that what will occur?

Questions 62–66

(a) Fixed ratio
(b) Fixed interval
(c) Variable ratio

(d) Variable interval
(e) None of the above

62. A patient with low back pain is given analgesics sometimes after he complains three times; sometimes after he complains seven times; and sometimes after he complains five times.

63. An 11-year-old child can "get his way" by asking permission from the father within 5 minutes after his father comes home from work.

64. A 10-year-old child can "get her way" by asking permission from her father even though her mother has already denied permission.

65. A patient is directed to come of your office every Friday at 1:00 P.M.

66. You return a colleague's call sometimes when she has waited 1 hour, sometimes after 3 hours, and sometimes after 4 hours.

Questions 67–70

(a) Imprinting
(b) Classical conditioning
(c) Operant conditioning
(d) Cognitive learning
(e) Social learning

67. A 23-year-old single male from Istanbul moves to America. He does not know how to interact with American females. His instructor recommends that he go each night to a different night club to "see how it's done."

68. A psychotherapist requires that a patient recognize his responsibility for an argument that developed between the patient and his boss.

69. A prisoner in jail for stealing is given money credits for picking up refuse in city streets. The money credits can be cashed in for real money to pay restitution to the prisoner's victim. When restitution is completed, the jail sentence ends.

70. A patient with a fear of elevators is required to ride on elevators 12 hours a day for 2 weeks.

Questions 71–72

(a) Standard deviation of a test
(b) Validity of a test
(c) Reliability of a test
(d) Test norms
(e) Correlation coefficient

71. The degree to which a test measures what it purports to measure

72. The degree to which a test consistently produces the same result each time it is used

Questions 73–75

Match the corresponding stages of Freud with those of Erikson:

(a) Anal
(b) Genital
(c) Oral
(d) Phallic
(e) Latency

73. Autonomy vs. shame and doubt
74. Industry vs. inferiority
75. Intimacy vs. isolation

Questions 76–77

Match the appropriate stages of Erikson with those most accurately corresponding to Piagetian structures:

(a) Initiative vs. guilt
(b) Industry vs. inferiority
(c) Trust vs. mistrust
(d) Generativity vs. stagnation
(e) Philanthropy vs. stinginess

76. Sensory motor stage
77. Formal operations stage

Questions 78–80

(a) Value
(b) Opinion
(c) Belief
(d) Attitude
(e) Prejudice

78. "People who sexually molest little children should be put in prison."

79. "People who smoke (including cigarettes) should have segregated areas where their habit doesn't affect nonsmokers."

80. "When I was 17 I decided that I would only use my sexual behavior with another person to express real love."

Questions 81–84

(a) Stimulants
(b) Narcotics
(c) Both
(d) Neither

81. Chemical blockade is available
82. Has euphoric effects
83. Toxicity is characterized by perceptual dis-

tortions, poor concentration, disorientation, and ultimately, hallucinations and delusions
84. Can be effectively treated by substitute chemotherapy

Questions 85–88

(a) MMPI
(b) Halstead-Reitan Battery
(c) Meyers-Briggs
(d) Rorschach
(e) Strong

85. Objective personality test
86. Used to assess effects of brain dysfunction
87. Vocational interest test
88. Subjective personality test

Questions 89–91

(a) Associated with affective depression
(b) Has a central role in pain modulation
(c) Central role is programming CNS sex differences
(d) Clinically implicated in Klinefelter's syndrome
(e) Correlated with schizophrenia

89. Dopamine
90. Norepinephrine
91. Endorphins

Questions 92–95

With regard to moral development, match the following.

(a) Punishment
(b) Satisfaction of one's own needs
(c) "Good boy/girl"
(d) General rights and standards
(e) Decisions of conscience

92. "I'll treat anyone who comes to see me regardless of sex, age, race, sexual orientation, or religious belief, as long as it's within my level of skills and ability."
93. "I will do the restorations in your mouth for a total of $1,500.00."
94. "Even though I'm a dentist, I think it's okay if I write the prescriptions for pain medication for my next door neighbor's chronic low back pain as long as I don't get caught."
95. "It's okay if I cheat on this test, because I'll get a higher grade."

Questions 96–100

Match the following stages of death and dying with the appropriate sentence.

(a) Stage I
(b) Stage II
(c) Stage III
(d) Stage IV
(e) Stage V

96. "Please help me stay alive until my daughter graduates from medical school."
97. "Damn you! At my last checkup you said everything was all right."
98. "I want a second opinion."
99. "I'd like to discuss my funeral arrangements with you. Is it appropriate for me to be buried with my dentures in, or can someone else use them?"
100. "I just give up. There's nothing I can do anymore. I've lost everything."

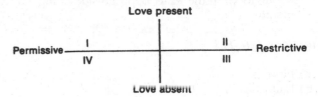

Disciplinary techniques

Questions 101–104

(a) Quadrant I
(b) Quadrant II
(c) Quadrant III
(d) Quadrant IV

101. Is correlated with a dependent, non–free-thinking child
102. Is correlated with a creative, spontaneous, independent child
103. Is correlated with an obedient, other-centered, self-controlled child
104. Is correlated with a belligerent, rebellious, selfish child

Questions 105–107

A dentist has just administered nitrous oxide to a 35-year-old patient. Match the type of disorientation with the statement the patient makes.

(a) Disorientation to person
(b) Disorientation to place

(c) Both
(d) Neither

105. "Boy, it seems like I've done this exact thing before."
106. "God, I'm floating out of my body to the corner of the room."
107. "A dentist's office in full daylight is a funny place to interview for a movie role."

Questions 108–109

(a) Retrograde amnesia
(b) Anterograde amnesia
(c) Both
(d) Neither

108. Following a bout of infection of the brain, a patient doesn't recall the work you did before the infection.
109. A third-year dental student always works on the wrong tooth in the exact opposite side of the mouth.

Questions 110–113

(a) Illusion
(b) Hallucination
(c) Both
(d) Neither

110. While talking with you, a patient in your operating chair turns her head away from you and says, "What did you say?" (There is no one in the room except you and her.)
111. As you proceed, you start to examine her mouth with a probe and she says, "Don't stick me with that needle yet."
112. You reassure her that it's a probe and she says, "Well, I saw a needle and I heard your assistant tell me you were going to inject me!"
113. The patient's next statement is, "I've done this before. I've been in this same situation before."

Questions 114–117

(a) Instincts
(b) Imprinting
(c) Classical conditioning
(d) Operant conditioning
(e) Social learning

114. A child receives a painful dental procedure on her first visit to the dentist. Thereafter, the child displays a fear reaction when she sees any dentist.
115. A child who is uncooperative with the dentist is administered the "hand over the mouth" (HOM) technique, and the child responds with fear.
116. The dentist demonstrates appropriate brushing and flossing techniques to a patient who subsequently performs these acts correctly.
117. After a particularly painful procedure the dentist smiles at the patient, pats the patient on the shoulder, and says, "You really were great. I know it was painful, but you really handled it very well. Thank you for your cooperation."

Questions 118–119

Match the following defense mechanism with the appropriate description.

(a) Repression
(b) Denial
(c) Projection
(d) Displacement
(e) Regression

118. A physician "forgets" his 6:30 A.M. apppointment with a patient who always complains about treatment.
119. While working with his assistant on a difficult patient, the dentist's hand slips and he lacerates the gingiva severely. The dentist says to the technician. "Don't bump my arm like that."

Directions. Choose the best answer.

120. Which of the following is *not* considered to be the basic psychogenic cause of "normal sexual dysfunctions"?
    (a) Going into the past or anticipated future experiences
    (b) Asking oneself about adequacy of performance
    (c) Expression of other interpersonal problems in the sexual relationship
    (d) Inadequate basic education
    (e) Being involved in the pleasure of the here and now
121. An attitude:
    (a) Has an affective component
    (b) Forces you to interpret new data in a given way
    (c) Implies an evaluative dimension
    (d) Has a cognitive or belief component
    (e) Rarely has a behavior component

122. Correct statements regarding sexuality and aging include all of the following *except:*
     (a) There is delayed vaginal lubrication.
     (b) There is increased time to erect in males.
     (c) Prostatic contractions are frequently absent.
     (d) The resolution phase is slowed for both.
     (e) Loss of erection for up to 1 hour is common.

123. Suicide is *less* likely in:
     (a) People who live alone
     (b) Patients who have made previous attempts as opposed to those who have not
     (c) The fifth and sixth decades of life as opposed to the third and fourth
     (d) Men than women
     (e) Blacks than whites

124. Unconditioned responses to unconditioned stimuli are not:
     (a) Innate to the organism
     (b) Present from an early age
     (c) Difficult to extinguish
     (d) Learned
     (e) Physiologically based

125. Negativism of a 2½-year-old child is most prominent during:
     (a) Piaget's sensory motor phase
     (b) Erikson's initiative vs. guilt period
     (c) The early stage of the attachment process
     (d) Freud's anal period
     (e) Piaget's concrete operations stage

126. The following statements are true about the APGAR *except:*
     (a) It has five basic indicators—heart rate, respiratory effort, reflex irritability, color tone, and muscle tone.
     (b) A perfect score is 10.
     (c) A score of 0 to 3 is an indicator of likely death.
     (d) The test is administered at 5- and 15-minute periods following birth.
     (e) The most valid indicator is birth weight and the 5-minute score.

127. Correct statements about adolescence include:
     (a) Intellectual changes in adolescence include the potential for a more hypothetic, speculative, and divergent form of thought.
     (b) The word *adolescence* means "a time of turmoil."
     (c) Egocentrism in adolescence is reinforced by the physiological changes that take place during this period.
     (d) Preadolescence or early adolescence is most definable by the egosyntonic nature of anxiety over sexuality.

     (e) Adolescents are in Erikson's stage of identity versus role confusion.

128. During the preschool years:
     (a) The child's thought is concrete.
     (b) There is rapid growth in muscle and skeletal tissue, reducing the top-heavy appearance of the toddler.
     (c) Speech is most often viewed as sociocentric.
     (d) Emotions become increasingly complex, and the emotions of jealousy, rivalry, and aggression surface.
     (e) The child is in Freud's phallic-urethral stage.

129. During the elementary school years (ages 6–12) all of the following are true *except:*
     (a) The growth rate slows down considerably.
     (b) Exhibiting control in the social, psychological, cognitive, and motoric dimensions becomes a major developmental theme.
     (c) Cognitive advances are characterized by the child's developing capacity for concrete operations.
     (d) Boys get fewer learning experiences and more admonitions when their school experience is compared with that of girls.
     (e) The child is forming his or her gender identity.

130. In cases of child abuse it is common:
     (a) For parents to take meticulous care of their child's appearance
     (b) For parents to have remembered themselves as favored in the family
     (c) For parents to have good social contacts in the community
     (d) For the parents to fear death at appearance of mild diarrhea or cold in the child
     (e) For the pregnancy to have been wanted

131. A 5-year-old boy should be capable (in the Piagetian sense) of:
     (a) Sensory motor information processing
     (b) Concrete thinking
     (c) Symbols and thought imagery
     (d) Conservation
     (e) Egocentric thought

132. If a group of people is prejudicially scapegoated, they would most likely be:
     (a) Unusual in appearance
     (b) Strong enough to keep a fight going
     (c) Readily available
     (d) Prejudiced against before
     (e) Resistant to taking on the prejudicial attributes

133. Unsupervised, abrupt withdrawal is potentially lethal in the person addicted to which of the following drugs?

(a) Stimulants
(b) Narcotics
(c) Sedative-hypnotics
(d) Psychedelics (including marijuana)
(e) Volatiles

134. Death from overdose is a strong possibility with all of the following drugs *except:*
    (a) Alcohol
    (b) Narcotics
    (c) Sedative-hypnotics
    (d) Psychedelics (including marijuana)
    (e) Phencyclidine

135. Poor muscular coordination is a sign of toxicity with all of the following *except:*
    (a) Alcohol
    (b) Narcotics
    (c) Sedative-hypnotics
    (d) Marijuana
    (e) Stimulants

136. Which of the following regarding grief work is *not* correct?
    (a) It should be completed within 3 months.
    (b) "Perpetual mourning" is an abnormal grief pattern.
    (c) Anniversary reactions are considered a normal grief reaction.
    (d) Long-term antianxiety medication is not appropriate.
    (e) Problems with sleep occur in early stages.

137. The committed mentally ill adult is entitled to all of the following rights *except:*
    (a) To refuse treatment
    (b) A jury trial to determine sanity
    (c) To vote
    (d) To come and go at will
    (e) The right to marry or divorce

138. The major correlates of sensory deprivation include all of the following *except:*
    (a) Profound calmness
    (b) Depressed level of consciousness
    (c) Stimulus hunger
    (d) Visual hallucinations
    (e) Auditory hallucinations

139. A 5-year-old female patient comes into your office with her mother and her 11-year-old brother. You observe the following. The girl sits on the floor and plays beside another child who is 4 years old. The girl looks at her mother anxiously when the other child begins to cry. The girl is very dependent on her mother and never shows curiosity. The girl's movements and behaviors are very "tomboy" in nature. Correct assumptions regarding this child include:
    (a) Her gender identity is appropriate.

(b) She is displaying parallel play.
(c) She has been raised in a restrictive home.
(d) She may be a victim of child abuse.
(e) She has been raised in a "love absent" home.

140. The girl in the above question enters your operatory without her mother and is hugging her "teddy bear," but becomes frightened of your x-ray machine, saying it will bite her. She tells you her tooth (baby tooth) fell out because she did something wrong. When you place your hand on her shoulder to comfort her, she cringes into the corner of her chair and asks "What's next?" From these data, further correct statements regarding this child include:
    (a) She is too old to be using transitional objects.
    (b) She is in the correct stage of cognitive development (Piaget).
    (c) She is demonstrating stranger anxiety.
    (d) Her animistic thoughts are not appropriate for her age.
    (e) You have no further legal responsibilities with this child.

141. Adherence by patients can be enhanced by:
    (a) Making telephone referrals for patients
    (b) Keeping the frequency of a treatment regimen to less than four times per day
    (c) Having the patient arrive a considerable time earlier than his or her appointment
    (d) Keeping interaction with the patient directed to the medical point of the visit
    (e) Giving the most important instructions at the end of the office visit

142. You might suspect child abuse in a child who exhibits all of the following behavior *except:*
    (a) Breaks all the toys in your waiting room
    (b) Shies away whenever you touch him or her
    (c) Looks overly mature for age
    (d) Steals toys and food
    (e) Has poor hygiene

143. Narcolepsy is associated with which of the following?
    (a) Sudden awakening from REM sleep
    (b) Heightened muscle tone in emotional situations
    (c) Vivid visual violent nightmares
    (d) Sudden onset of REM sleep
    (e) Apnea during REM sleep

144. The dying child's concern is with:
    (a) Life after death ("going to heaven or hell")
    (b) Parents' going away forever
    (c) Death as an end to playing and having fun
    (d) Who will take care of his or her pets
    (e) How soon he or she can come back and see everyone

145. The correct statement about phencyclidine is:
    (a) An antagonist is available.
    (b) Chemical blockade is available.
    (c) Abrupt withdrawal can be fatal.
    (d) It can be fatal in overdose.
    (e) Its actions are short-lived.

146. Mr. Smith presents at the Emergency Room after being involved in a traffic accident. He has sustained a severe head injury. Which of the following states of consciousness would *not* be expected as a normal sequela of his concussion?
    (a) Clouding of consciousness
    (b) Coma
    (c) Confusion state
    (d) Fugue
    (e) Stupor

147. A student did poorly on an examination that was given in a specific room. The student is afraid to fail the course. On the next occasion the student walks into the room and experiences fear. This is an example of:
    (a) Classical conditioning learning
    (b) Cognitive learning
    (c) Fixed-schedule learning
    (d) Inhibition learning
    (e) Social learning

148. The IQ is most characteristically expressed by which of the following formulas?

    (a) $\dfrac{\text{Mental age (MA)}}{\text{Chronological age (CA)}} \times 100 = \text{IQ}$

    (b) $\dfrac{\text{CA}}{\text{MA}} \times 100 = \text{IQ}$

    (c) $\dfrac{\text{Social age (SA)}}{\text{CA}} \times 100 = \text{IQ}$

    (d) $\dfrac{\text{CA}}{\text{SA}} \times 100 = \text{IQ}$

    (e) $\dfrac{\text{SA}}{\text{MA}} \times 100 = \text{IQ}$

149. Which of the following is *not* a symptom of the Kluver-Bucy syndrome?
    (a) Hypersexuality
    (b) Increased REM sleep
    (c) Oral exploration
    (d) Submissiveness
    (e) Visual agnosia

150. A patient presents to the Emergency Room with the complaints that 6 months earlier he took LSD and had not ingested any since that time. His presenting complaints at this time revolve around walls not maintaining their perpendicular and assuming a waving shape, and objects in the environment that he knows to be stationary appearing to move. This man is experiencing:
    (a) Autisms
    (b) Concretisms
    (c) Confabulations
    (d) Delusions
    (e) Illusions

1. **c** The major compromise to mental abilities from aging is that reaction time is slower and recent memory is impaired. Also, new learning is difficult.

2. **c** A large number of males 65 years of age and older are sexually active.

3. **e** The major concept in the control of aggression is to teach nonaggressive mechanisms of handling frustrating situations.

4. **e** High suicide risk indicants are being male, single, Caucasian, and either in the 15- to 24-year-old age group or in the over-65-year-old age group. Living alone is an extremely high suicide risk indicator.

5. **b** The sympathetic firing rate for males is 0.8 per second; however, for females, it is at 0.75-second intervals. All other statements in this question are correct.

6. **c** The important issue with Mrs. Smithers is to allow her to talk about her feelings. Her son's behavior is not inappropriate. The major issue is her being able to discharge her feelings to allow her to accept further counseling on this issue.

7. **b** Mrs. Smithers is demonstrating vaginismus, which is strong involuntary contractions of the muscles of the vaginal barrel. This condition occurs when any object (finger, penis, catheter) approaches the vaginal opening.

8. **c** This clinical presentation of subaverage intelligence, short attention span, emotional lability, and cross-sex characteritics is diagnostic of Klinefelter's syndrome.

9. **c** When a patient approaches the physician with a concern, it is important to determine what the underlying feeling is and the underlying stimulus for the concern. The only other possible choice would have been e but this choice is invalidated by the word "why," which is judgmental and punitive and has no place in the doctor–patient interaction.

10. **e** The absence of ovarian tubes or uterus, particularly in combination with the presenting complaints, is diagnostic of testicular feminization syndrome.

11. **e** Countertransference is the inappropriate placement of feelings from the past by the physician onto the patient. Transference is when the patient inappropriately displaces feelings from the past onto the physician.

12. **a** Longitudinal research entails the tracking of same subjects over a long period of time. The advantage of this procedure is to control for environmental events; the disadvantage is the tremendous expense and tracking problem.

13. **d** Child abuse tends to appear with drug and alcohol consumption, the fear of losing control in discipline, perception of the child as purposely doing something bad to the parent, social isolation, and extremely high developmental expectations for the child.

14. **d** Phallic and initiative stages in child development occur in the 4- to 6-year-old age range.

15. **d** Gender identity is the individual's private feeling of being male or female. Gender identification, on the other hand, is the learned behavioral public expression of gender.

16. **b** Classical conditioning is the association of two events that are not normally linked in nature. Classical conditioning is also sometimes called stimulus substitution.

17. **d** Positive reinforcers tend to increase a given behavior. In the instance described in the question, the child probably receives attention only in the form of spankings; therefore, the attention is misinterpreted by the child as affection and is sought by the child.

18. **c** The area under +1 and –1 standard deviations on a normal curve is approximately 68%.

19. **d** Mild mental retardation is defined as an IQ score falling between 50 and 70.

20. **e** An educable mentally retarded person has an IQ of at least 50. Persons with IQs below this level are not considered to be educable.

21. **a** Both separation and stranger anxiety appear at about 6 months and last until about 12 months of age. The stranger anxiety indicates the child can recognize "not mother," and when the child is separated from its mothering person, anxiety develops.

22. **a** In a fugue state, the person operates normally. This is the classic case of a person going out at 5:00 in the evening to buy a pack of cigarettes and never coming back. The person sets up a new life, with his previous identity unavailable to him. All the other choices listed imply a decreased level of consciousness, which would be easily observable.

23. **b** Habituation refers to the psychological reinforcing properties of a drug or taking the drug out of habit (*e.g.,* every night at 5:00 after work).

24. **a** Dependence means that the body has become physiologically dependent on a drug to function normally. When the drug is not in the body, the

individual experiences distressing psychophysiological symptoms called *withdrawal.*

25. **c** Tolerance means that the body becomes tolerant to the effects of a given dose of a drug. Once this happens, the dose must be increased for the desired effect to be obtained.

26. **e** Children normally react to the death of a significant other by joking and hyperactive behavior.

27. **b** Infants commonly respond to the loss of a significant other by withdrawal and sometimes death; this response is called marasmus.

28. **d** Elderly persons who lose a loved one tend to withdraw socially, if there is no care given to keep them involved in the world, they frequently die within a year after the loss of the significant other.

29. **c** Adults tend to have a reoccurrence of previous physical difficulties or a preoccupation with misinterpretation of normal physical signs for a pathological process.

30. **b** Stage I of the grief and bereavement process is shock and disbelief. Statement b implies that Sam is in such a state of shock that he does not realize that Mary is dead.

31. **c** Stage II is the working through of the relationship with the dead person and is often accompanied by psychophysiological symptomatology such as headaches.

32. **e** Stage III is the resolution of the relationship in which the surviving person has formuated a new relationship with the dead person so that the surviving person can get on with forming other intimate relationships. An acceptable ritualized interaction with the dead person is established, such as taking flowers to the dead person's grave each Memorial Day.

33. **b** Stage I of the death and dying process is denial. Statement b implies that the results must be wrong because of the person's medical student standing. This is clearly denial.

34. **d** Stage III is bargaining, in which the patient hopes to say alive long enough to experience some particular event.

35. **e** Stage IV is sadness, which is a "giving up" type of response acknowledging the loss of life in the near future.

36. **c** The last stage is acceptance, in which the person is resigned to the impending death and comfortable with the reality.

37. **c** Mr. B is clearly homosexual from his emotional involvement of some long standing with another man. The request for surgery to change his gender is not to make internal feelings compatible with external feelings, but rather for legal purposes.

38. **a** Ms. C is clearly a transsexual. Her request is to make external characteristics compatible with internal feelings.

39. **d** Mr. D is basically heterosexual. Although he had a short period of homosexual behavior in the Navy, he has had only heterosexual experiences since. His effeminate behavior simply reflects a gender identification with females, but that does not mean that he is transsexual, a transvestite, or a homosexual or that he has Klinefelters's.

40. **c** The first phase of death and dying is denial, which is reflected by statement c.

41. **e** The second phase is anger, most clearly reflected by statement e.

42. **a** The third stage is bargaining, as shown in statement a by the patient's asking the doctor to keep him alive until a given event occurs.

43. **b** The fourth phase is sadness.

44. **d** The fifth stage is acceptance. Statement d reflects the patient's ability to accept the fact that his life is rapidly drawing to a close and his level of comfort with having had a good life.

45. **c** The emotional expression of the underlying affect grief is sadness–sorrow.

46. **b** Anger and disgust are the emotions that are directed at the removal of an object that is frustrating a person.

47. **a** Anxiety or fear is usually triggered by an individual's feeling threatened with injury, whether that threat is real or imagined.

48. **d** This patient is showing objective signs of anxiety with the shifting in her chair, arching of her eyebrows, and licking of her lips; however, nothing she says indicates that she is aware of the anxiety.

49. **a** The patient is describing the anxiety in the subjective statement of being trembly and shaky; however, the external objective behavior does not indicate any anxiety.

50. **e** The patient described in this vignette gives no objective or subjective evidence for any primary emotions like anxiety, anger, or sadness. This is a clear demonstration of an adult interaction that is to the point of medical management.

51. **c** The patient is showing both subjective and objective evidence of anger. The frowning and tense masseters are objective evidence, and the verbal or subjective statements indicate that the patient is aware of the anger response.

52. **d** This patient is giving both subjective and objective evidence for sadness. The objective data are the deep sigh and the tears; the subjective data include the statement of disappointment and the statement that the patient has cried considerably.

53. **c** This is a demonstration of an approach–avoidance conflict, since the person has been coughing up blood for months but has not gotten

to his personal physician until the condition has reached the point that he can no longer ignore it.

54. **e** There is no conflict noted in this conversation.

55. **d** This statement indicates that the first-year medical student has suddenly understood that her living partner has been treating her as he used to treat his mother. This is an insight into or understanding of a relationship.

56. **b** This is an avoidance–avoidance conflict, in that the person must take the National Board exams or another negative event will occur.

57. **a** This is an example of an approach–approach conflict in which there are two equally attractive choices.

58. **b** Discrimination is the concept underlying this question. The adolescent male in the question has learned where it is permissible to be aggressive and where it is not.

59. **d** Food is a primary reinforcer, since it works on a primary drive.

60. **a** This is an example of generalization, where an event that has been associated with one particular stimulus generalizes to other related types of stimuli.

61. **c** This recommendation by the physician is an example of extinction, in which the person is placed in a situation that is frightening and is forced to stay in that situation until the anxiety is "burned out," or extinguished.

62. **c** This vignette describes a variable ratio schedule; that is, the reinforcement is given on a variable proportion of the time that the patient complains.

63. **b** This is an example of a fixed interval. The interval is within 5 minutes, and the reward comes every time the child operates within that fixed interval of time.

64. **e** This is not reflective of a partial reinforcement schedule but is indicative of conflict between the mother and father.

65. **b** This is a fixed interval format, the interval being exactly 1 week.

66. **d** This is a variable interval schedule, the interval being in terms of hours and the time being variable.

67. **e** This is an example of social learning whereby modeling is the major mode of acquisition of behaviors.

68. **d** This is cognitive learning, whereby attention must be fully directed at the interaction, and understanding is the major goal.

69. **c** This is operant conditioning, whereby a reward is given for a particular behavior.

70. **b** This is an example of classical conditioning, whereby extinction is taking place and acquisition of a nonanxious response to the elevator is substituted for the anxiety.

71. **b** This is the definition of validity of a test. Validity means the ability of a test to perform as it was designed.

72. **c** The reliability of a test is how repeatable are the results of the test. Reliability may be high and validity may be low, but it is very difficult to get validity without reliability.

73. **a** The autonomy vs. shame and doubt stage in Eriksonian theory occurs at the same time as the anal stage of Freud.

74. **e** The industry vs. inferiority stage of Eriksonian theory occurs at the same age as the latency theory of Freudian theory.

75. **b** The intimacy vs. isolation stage in Eriksonian theory occurs at the same age as the Freudian genital stage.

76. **c** Piaget's sensory motor stage occurs in the same period as Eriksonian theory's trust vs. mistrust period.

77. **d** The formal operations stage in Piaget's theory occurs at the Eriksonian stage of generativity vs. stagnation.

78. **e** This is a prejudicial statement, since it does not recognize any attenuating circumstances in a person who might become sexually active with a child. It is destructive to the person who receives the prejudice.

79. **d** This is an attitude that contains both information and emotion but allows people who are the recipients of the attitude their own personal freedom without affecting others.

80. **a** This is a value, because it is personal behavior that is decided from full cognitive awareness at an age when it is possible to think through personal decisions.

81. **b** Chemical blockade is only available for narcotic drugs.

82. **c** Both stimulants and narcotics have euphoric effects.

83. **a** This description of perceptual distortion, poor concentration, disorientation, and (if the dose is high enough) hallucinations and delusions is consistent with stimulant toxicity but not narcotic toxicity.

84. **b** Methadone maintenance is an effective treatment for narcotic addiction. There is no similar treatment at this time for stimulant addiction.

85. **a** The Minnesota Multiphasic Personality Inventory is the only objective personality test listed. It was not developed from a theoretic base, but rather by statistical analysis of what types of patients answer what questions yes or no.

86. **b** The Halstead-Reitan battery is the set of psychological tests that have been designed to reflect brain dysfunction.

87. **e** The Strong is a vocational interest test.

88. **d** The Rorschach is a subjective personality test, in that it comes from theory and requires a considerable amount of skill from the examiner for appropriate interpretation of the results. There are no statistical norms on this test.

89. **e** Dopamine is the central nervous system neurotransmitter that is most strongly implicated in schizophrenia.

90. **a** Norepinephrine has been associated with affective depressions.

91. **b** The endorphin neurotransmitter system has the most implication for pain modulation.

92. **e** This is clearly a decision of conscience and speaks to the equality of all persons.

93. **d** This is a moral decision based on general rights and standards of contracts between people.

94. **a** This is a very low level of moral development, because it operates on the simple issue of getting punished or not.

95. **b** This is again a rather low level of moral development, because it reflects the satisfaction of one's own needs regardless of the consequences.

96. **c** This is the bargaining stage of the death and dying sequence.

97. **b** This is clearly an anger stage, or stage II.

98. **a** This is the stage of denial in which the person requests a second opinion, implying that the first opinion from you is incorrect.

99. **e** This is the acceptance stage.

100. **d** This is the sadness, or "giving up," stage in which the person recognizes that loss of life is imminent.

101. **c** Dependent, non–free-thinking children are associated with restrictive parents who do not have an emotional investment in them.

102. **a** Disciplinary techniques in which there is affection and a permissiveness for exploration tend to be correlated with creative, spontaneous, independent children.

103. **b** Obedient, other-centered, and self-controlled children are associated with disciplinary techniques in which love is present but there is restrictiveness of the child's behavior.

104. **d** Children who are belligerent, rebellious, and selfish tend to be correlated with disciplinary techniques in which there is permissiveness for their behavior but with no love present.

105. **b** This statement is an example of *déjà vu*, which is reflective of a disorientation to place.

106. **a** The statement is reflecting a depersonalization episode, which is associated with disorientation to person.

107. **d** In this statement, the person is oriented for person, place, and time but disoriented for situation, which is not one of the options available.

108. **a** Retrograde amnesia is the forgetting of events before a specific trauma.

109. **d** The situation described is a portion of a dyslexia and has nothing to do with amnesia.

110. **b** A hallucination is lacks a perception that a sensory event in the environment.

111. **a** An illusion is defined as a sensory event that is misinterpreted.

112. **c** This is both an hallucination and an illusion by the patient's report.

113. **d** *Déjà vu* does not represent either an illusion or hallucination. It is a disorientation to place.

114. **c** This is an example of classical conditioning, or stimulus substitution.

115. **a** The situation described is an example of an instinctive response to occlusion of the airway.

116. **e** This is social modeling of appropriate behaviors to the patient by a dentist.

117. **d** Operant conditioning is described here, in which a secondary reinforcer, the praise from the dentist, is used as a reinforcer to elicit cooperative behavior.

118. **a** Repression is defined as automatic forgetting.

119. **c** This is an example of projection defense mechanism, whereby the dentist assigns the responsibility to the assistant and not to himself.

120. **e** Staying in the here-and-now pleasure of sexual activity prevents "normal sexual dysfunctions."

121. **e** An attitude has both an affective and a belief component. Attitudes force individuals to interpret data in a given way and have an evaluative dimension as well. Attitudes are one of the determinants of behavior.

122. **d** With aging and sexuality, there is delayed vaginal lubrication, frequently requiring assistance; often males need increased time to erect; and, at orgasm for males, prostatic contractions frequently are absent. There is a slowed resolution phase for males, but not necessarily for females. Loss of erections for up to 1 hour during the plateau phase can occur.

123. **e** More whites than blacks commit suicide per capita, although the rate in black males is increasing.

124. **d** Unconditioned responses to unconditioned stimuli are not learned. They are responses that occur if triggered by the stimuli.

125. **d** The negativism of a 2½-year-old child is most prominent during Freud's anal period, which extends from 18 months to 3 years.

126. **d** With the APGAR, there are five basic indicators that are each rated on a scale of 0, 1, or 2 at 1 and 5 minutes after birth. An extremely low score on the

APGAR indicates that the child will probably die. The best indicator is the birth weight and the 5-minute score.

127. **d** The only characteristic of adolescence that is incorrectly stated in this question is that in pre-adolescence and early adolescence, there is an egodystonic situation with sexuality in that there is a great deal of anxiety that the adolescent or early adolescent would like to avoid.

128. **c** In the preschool years, there is rapid growth in muscle and skeletal tissue, and the emotions become increasingly complex. Speech is most likely to be egocentric, and the child is tied to concrete thought processes. The child is in the latency stage of Freudian theory.

129. **e** Gender identity is formed by age 2 to 3 years old. The child at this age is forming gender identification.

130. **d** Child abuse is to be suspected when one sees the parents being overanxious at the appearance of mild physical disruptions. The other statements are the opposite of what is correct.

131. **d** A 5-year-old child does have sensory motor information processing as well as symbols of language and thought imagery; however, children of this age cannot yet do abstract reversible thinking because they are concrete in their thought processes and, as a general rule, are ruled by their perceptions without the ability to conserve the basic identity of a substance. For instance, if a sponge looks like a rock, it is reacted to as a rock, not as a sponge that looks like a rock. They have very egocentric thought processes.

132. **e** Persons who are scapegoated must be easily identified and easily located. They must be strong enough to put up a fight, and to keep the fight going but not to win; and they usually have been prejudiced against before. Over time, people prejudiced against take on the attributes of the prejudice.

133. **c** Abrupt withdrawal from sedative-hypnotics can precipitate convulsions and potentially death. No lethality is, for all practical purposes, attendant to narcotic, psychedelic, stimulant, or volatile withdrawal.

134. **d** Overdose is certainly possible on alcohol, narcotics, and sedative-hypnotics and phencyclidine, but there are no reported instances of human death from overdose of psychedelics. The major cause of death in psychedelic use is response to delusions; for example, a delusional belief that one is made of metal might cause a man to try to stop a semitruck with his body.

135. **e** Coordination is not affected by stimulants.

136. **a** Grief work should be completed within a year; therefore, perpetual mourning of more than a year is an abnormal grief pattern. Anniversary reactions are normal. The long-term use of antianxiety medication generally postpones grief work and is not indicated. Sleep problems in the first 2 or 3 weeks are to be anticipated.

137. **d** The committed mentally ill can refuse treatment, can demand a jury trial to determine their sanity, and can still vote. They lose only the ability to come and go at will. They can marry or divorce.

138. **c** The major correlates of sensory deprivation include depressed levels of consciousness and visual and auditory hallucinations. Sensory-deprived persons feel anxious, not calm, and they are stimulus hungry.

139. **d** This is a complex question that involves many different pieces of data. Her gender identity does appear to be intact, since she does not protest being a girl. She is not displaying cooperative play, but rather parallel play. Her dependent behavior reflects love-absent and restrictive disciplinary techniques, but her looking at her mother anxiously when the other child cries suggests she may be a victim of child abuse.

140. **c** This vignette describes a child ~~ho is in the correct stage of cognitive developme~~ Piaget (concrete operations), and her behavior ~~~~ interact with her—withdrawing from your physi~~ approaches—suggests that she may be a victim of child abuse. She is not demonstrating stranger anxiety, and she is not too old to be using transitional objects. You do have legal responsibilities to pursue the issue of your suspicion of child abuse.

141. **b** Adherence in patients can be enhanced by a treatment regimen that does not require activity more than four times a day and by the patient's knowing the name of the activity and how to perform it (this includes the names of medications). However, letter referrals instead of telephone referrals tend to enhance adherence, and having the patient come at a particular time and having that patient seen at that time also improves adherence. The more the patient likes the physician, the better the adherence. Patients tend to remember what is told early in the session, not at the end.

142. **c** Children who are victims of child abuse tend to be destructive of toys, shy away from physical contact, are overly mature for their age, and tend to steal toys and food from other persons. A child's personal needs such as clean clothing and good hygiene tend to be ignored by parents who are child abusers.

143. **d** Narcolepsy is associated with the loss of muscle tone in emotional situations, also called cataplexy, and is defined by the sudden onset of REM sleep.

The other responses in this question are irrelevant for narcolepsy.

144. **b** The dying child's concern is with parents' abandoning him or her. The child is not preoccupied with life after death, does not consider death an entity, and therefore does not consider it an end to playing and having fun. Most children think of death as simply going to sleep, believing that they will wake up from that sleep. They are not concerned about pets since they do not see death as a permanent situation.

145. **d** Phencyclidine can be fatal in overdose. However, there is no antagonist available, chemical blockade as a treatment mechanism is not available, and there is no indication that abrupt withdrawal is lethal. It is lipophilic; therefore its actions are very long-lasting.

146. **d** Fugue is a psychological condition, not a physiologically induced state.

147. **a** This is an example of autonomic classical conditioning.

148. **a** This is the correct formula.

149. **a** A change in REM sleep is not a part of this syndrome.

150. **e** These are misperceptions of real sensory events; therefore, they are called *illusions*.